T0132903

EXPELLING
THE PLAGUE

McGill-Queen's/Associated Medical Services Studies in the History of Medicine, Health, and Society

Series Editors: S.O. Freedman and J.T.H. Connor

Volumes in this series have financial support from Associated Medical Services, Inc. (AMS). Associated Medical Services Inc. was established in 1936 by Dr Jason Hannah as a pioneer prepaid not-for-profit health care organization in Ontario. With the advent of medicare, AMS became a charitable organization supporting innovations in academic medicine and health services, specifically the history of medicine and health care, as well as innovations in health professional education and bioethics.

Contents

Figures and Tables

FIGURES

TABLES

A Note on Names

Personal and place names in Dubrovnik have several variants – Latin, Italian, and Croatian. For example, Lopud Island or Isola de Mezo. Dubrovnik was also known as Ragusa in the past. *Ragusan* was used as an adjective pertaining to Dubrovnik, and the inhabitants of Dubrovnik were called Ragusans. The patrician families of Dubrovnik also had Latin, Italian, and Croatian versions of their last names – for example, Zamagna, Giamagno, or Džamanjić. All these options are equally valid. The Croatian form is used throughout this volume because the patricians were commonly known under those names. However, since the archival sources use the Latin or Italian form, these variations have been added in brackets – for example, Gundulić (Gondola).

The most common Latin/Italian/Croatian alternatives of Ragusan names are:

Babalio or Bobali = Bobaljević
Basilio = Basiljević
Benessa = Benešić
Binzola = Binčulić
Bocignolo or Bucignolo = Bučinčić
Bodaca or Bodaça = Budačić
Bona = Bunić
Bonda = Bundić
Caboga = Kabužić
Cerva or Zrieva = Crijević
Crosio or Croze = Krušić
Dersa = Držić
Georgio or Giorgi = Đurđević
Gondola = Gundulić

Goz(z)e or Goçe = Gučetić
Grade or Gradi = Gradić
Luccari or Luchari = Lukarević
Menze or Mençe = Menčetić
Palmota = Palmotić
Poz(z)a or Poça = Pucić
Proculo = Prokulović
Ragnina = Ranjina
Resti = Rastić
Saracha = Saraka
Sorgo = Sorkočević
Stay = Stojković
Tudisio = Tudišić
Zamagna or Giamagno = Džamanjić

A Note on the Pronunciation
of Croatian Names

C is pronounced as *ts* in "its," e.g., Cavtat

Č is prununced as *ch* in "chatter," e.g., Čibača

Ć is pronounced similarly, but more like *ty* as in "future," e.g., Orebić

Đ is pronounced *j*, but harder as in "joke," e.g., Đurđević

G is always pronounced hard as in "gig," e.g., Gundulić

H is pronounced *ch* as in "loch," e.g., Hercegnovi

J is pronounced *y* as in "yet," e.g., Janjina

Lj is pronounced *ly* as in "lewd," e.g., Ljubinje

Nj is pronounced *ny* as in "new," e.g., Senj

R is sometimes pronounced as a semi-vowel, e.g., Brsečine

S is pronounced *s* as in "since," never like *s* in "nose," e.g., Ston

Š is pronounced *sh* as in "shape," e.g., Šipan

U is pronounced *oo* as in "boot," e.g., Ulcinj

Ž is pronounced *s* as in "pleasure," e.g., Žuljana

A Note on Money, Weights, Measures, and Prices

MONEY

Dubrovnik used a variety of coins and units of account but those referred to in this book are:

1 Venetian ducat = 2–3 *hyperperi* = 30–40 *grossi*
1 *grossus* = 30 *follari*
1 *hyperperus* (perper) = 12 *grossi*
1 *scudo* (škuda) = 3 *hyperperi* = 36 *grossi*
1 *soldo* (solad) = 1/6 *grossus*

DRY WEIGHTS

1 *libra ad pondus subtile* = the "thin" pound used for gold, silver, and pearls
  Estimated at 328 grams
1 *libra ad pondus grossum* = the "fat" pound used for other goods
  Estimated at 358 grams
1 *starium* (star) = 6 *cupelli* (used for grain)
  Estimates of the equivalent metric weight of a *starium* vary from 64.5 kg to 71.5 kg

MEASURES OF LENGTH

1 Ragusan ell (*lakat*) = 0.55 metres
1 small piece of fabric = 36 ells
1 big piece of fabric = 60 ells

FOURTEENTH-CENTURY RETAIL PRICES IN DUBROVNIK*

Wheat:

In 1320 = 18 *grossi* per *starium*

In 1381 = 5 *hyperperi* per *starium*

In 1383 = 3 *hyperperi* per *starium*

Wine:

1 *quinquo* (about 18 litres) = 0.25 to 0.5 *hyperperi*

Olive Oil:

In 1390s = 20–25 *follari* for 1 *quartoço* (about 0.4 litres)

Cheese:

358 grams = 10–15 *follari*

Honey:

1 *centenarium* (about 35.8 kg) = 3 *hyperperi*

Meat:

Mutton = 8–10 *follari* for 358 grams

In 1380, pork with bones = 15 *follari*

In 1380, boneless pork = 20 *follari*

Salt:

In 1380 = 8 *grossi* per 1 *modium* (about 32.5–35.75 kg)

Tallow candles:

16–26 *follari* per 358 grams

---

* Mahnken, *Dubrovački patricijat*, 107–9.

Acknowledgments

At the end of this long road, it is a pleasure to thank those who helped us so generously along the way.

First of all, we are deeply indebted to Zdravko Šundrica, the expert archivist at the State Archives of Dubrovnik who transcribed the *Libro deli Signori Chazamorbi* and was always a source of support for our research in Dubrovnik. He introduced Zlata Blažina Tomić to the mysteries of mediaeval Latin and with his invaluable guidance she was later able to transcribe Latin texts on her own. Zdravko Šundrica, a scholar to whom Ragusan studies owe so much, did not live to see this book but his spirit and learning have been present during the entire endeavour. We dedicate this book to him.

We remember with gratitude the assistance we received over the years from the staff of the State Archives in Dubrovnik. At the Institute for the Historical Sciences of the Croatian Academy of Arts and Sciences in Dubrovnik we were offered advice and cooperation by the director Nenad Vekarić and Zdenka Janeković-Rőmer who were instrumental in preparing the Croatian edition of this work for publication. We are also grateful to their colleagues Nella Lonza and Vesna Miović. Our stay in Dubrovnik was made infinitely more agreeable by the generous hospitality and kindness of Ana and Nikša Kurtela.

We are especially indebted to Magdalene Peters Georgiades who devoted countless hours of her precious time to reading and rereading every single version of this work. Thank you dear friend, we could not have done it without you!

We owe our warmest thanks to the external reviewers who offered many helpful suggestions for organizing the material in this work. Alan Bartulović, who made the maps for this volume, deserves our heartfelt gratitude for his fine contribution. We also owe a great deal to those most immediately concerned with the preparation and production of this complicated book – the editorial staff at McGill-Queen's University Press: Kyla Madden, senior editor, for her unwavering support for this work; Helen Hajnoczky, editorial assistant; Ryan Van Huijstee and Jessica Howarth, managing editors; Elena Goranescu, production manager; Jacqui Davis, marketing; Joanne Muzak, copyeditor, for her painstaking and ingenious effort.

During the research phase of this project, Zlata Blažina Tomić benefited from a grant from the Hannah Institute for the History of Medicine (now Associated Medical Services) in Toronto and the Croatian Academy of Arts and Sciences "Researching the Croatian Medical Heritage" project, which was co-financed by the Ministry of Science and Technology of the Republic of Croatia.

Zlata Blažina Tomić and Vesna Blažina

EXPELLING THE PLAGUE

Svuda ga jes puna slava, svud on slove
hrvatskih ter kruna gradov se svih zove.

Because it is known and praised everywhere
it is called the crown of all Croatian cities.

–Ivan Vidali, 1564, *Zbornik stihova XV i XVI stoljeća*
(Anthology of poetry of the fifteenth and sixteenth centuries)

Introduction

This is a study of the origins and early history of plague control measures in the Croatian city of Dubrovnik from 1377 to 1533. The inspiration for this study was drawn from the work of Mirko Dražen Grmek, who established that Dubrovnik, also known as Ragusa, was the first city-state in the world to develop the concept of quarantine legislation as early as 1377.[1]

Zlata Blažina Tomić began her research with the hypothesis that, over time, Ragusan patricians must have continued to refine and ameliorate their plague control measures. The archival sources retrieved in the State Archives of Dubrovnik confirmed that in 1390, thirteen years after its quarantine legislation, Dubrovnik had established the first recorded Health Office, responsible for the implementation of plague control regulations issued on a regular basis by the city Councils. The founding and development of the Health Office in Dubrovnik constitutes the core of this research, with a particular emphasis on the disastrous 1526–27 plague.

The first author of this work, Zlata Blažina Tomić, has analyzed all the extant sources in the State Archives of Dubrovnik concerning plague containment regulations, from 1377 to 1533, during the years of the most frequent plague epidemics in Dubrovnik. The records of the deliberations of the three Councils governing the Ragusan Republic, namely, the Major Council (Consilium Maius), the Minor Council (Consilium Minus), and the Senate (Consilium Rogatorum) were consulted, as were the earliest documents collected in the *Reformationes*, the *Liber omnium reformationum*, and the legislative books known as the *Liber viridis*, and the *Liber croceus*, supplements of the Ragusan Statute of 1272. Many of these regulations are here transcribed, translated, and published for the first time. Present-day research in the State Archives of Dubrovnik has been possible due to the outstanding diligence of the Ragusan notaries, chancellors,

and scribes who industriously and assiduously registered, classified, and preserved archival materials over many centuries. From 1272 until 1808, the
Ragusans meticulously documented all the activities of their government and
carefully preserved all the records.[2] These sources make it possible to recreate
the life of this maritime Republic with all its perils and frustrations, as well as
its triumphs and accomplishments.

Zlata Blažina Tomić discovered the manuscript *Libro deli Signori Chazamorbi, Sanitas, Series 55, vol. 1, 1500–1530* while sifting through the legislative documents in the State Archives of Dubrovnik. Without any doubt, this
document is the most significant sixteenth-century archival source concerning
plague control measures, particularly during the calamitous 1526–27 plague
epidemic. Health records from the Ragusan medical series Sanitas exist only in
fragments for other periods, but this one, which covers the period from 1500 to
1530, has been preserved in its entirety. Therefore, the value of this only extant
manuscript, a rare health record of a plague stricken city from the first quarter
of the sixteenth century, becomes even more compelling. It registers the activities of the health officials who, in the fifteenth century, were also known as
Signori Cazamorti.

Chiselled into the cloister wall of the Franciscan monastery in Dubrovnik,
a soul-stirring inscription still stands:

Lord Almighty,
oh death you destroy everything
in 1527 with the cruel pestilence.
Life is a journey,
days are fleeting.

These words encapsulate all the suffering that the people endured during the
1526–27 plague epidemic. A 1391 Senate regulation forbade the use of monasteries as plague hospitals. However, in 1527, the Franciscan monastery was
used for this very purpose and the dead were buried in the common grave in the
cloister.[3]

The 1526–27 plague was certainly the most devastating epidemic that struck
Dubrovnik since 1348. The loss of more than twenty thousand lives launched
this city-state on a dizzying demographic downward spiral from which it never
recovered. The plague control measures adopted in Dubrovnik to combat this
disastrous epidemic are described and analyzed in the latter part of this work.
Although by 1527, a culture of plague control measures had been part of

government policy for 150 years, Dubrovnik was not able to avoid this lethal plague upsurge. A variety of reasons may have been responsible for such a turn of events.

In times between plague outbreaks, the health officials mostly controlled the arrival of travellers and goods into the city. However, the arrivals were most conscientiously registered at the peak of the plague epidemics. The individuals entering the city had to take an oath confirming that they had arrived from places not afflicted with plague. If the health officials discovered that the travellers had tried to conceal the fact that they had arrived in Dubrovnik from infected places, confinement in quarantine as well as fines and punishments were imposed. During plague years, the health officials implemented the plague protection legislation and even served as trial judges in cases against persons who had contravened the health regulations. The punishment was most often a monetary fine, sometimes physical torture (the "jerking" of the rope, a version of the *strappado*) or, in the rarest of cases, even death by hanging. Moreover, the health officials were empowered to burn the houses and the belongings of plague victims. They were given wide-ranging executive and judicial powers but the government did not hesitate to threaten them with fines if they did not implement the decisions of the Councils promptly.

The trial records of the Health Office abound with real people: the health officials and the Councils tried to contain the epidemic while physicians, surgeons, barbers, and priests coped with the diseased and dying. This unique material gives the historian a rare opportunity to reconstruct events of everyday life during plague epidemics and to recapture the emotions, attitudes, and behaviour of common people, such as laundresses and gravediggers, otherwise rarely mentioned in archival sources. As can be expected, these individuals felt intimidated by the health officials, but in their own way, they tried to protect their rights. To understand their testimony, it is necessary to read between the lines. Often their violations of health regulations proved to be strategies of survival. What may have looked like a transgression to the health officials turned out to be the desire of common people to improve their lot under extraordinary circumstances: make some money, feed their families, and take care of their sick without interference of the authorities.

The Ragusan government invested large amounts of money in the deployment of unprecedented plague control measures. In the process, it gathered an enormous amount of information about its citizens. This led to an increased governmental control of Ragusan citizens. The manuscript *Libro deli Signori Chazamorbi* reveals that the plague control measures had a tremendous impact on all social groups in Dubrovnik: the health officials, the Councils, the Church, the physicians, the surgeons, and the commoners. Secular authorities in Dubrovnik dominated the Church. As far as plague control measures were concerned, the health officials and the Senate always had the last word, and, all social groups, including the clergy, had to obey them. The health care professionals in Dubrovnik were supervised by the health officials and included university-educated physicians, surgeons, plague doctors, pharmacists, barbers, travelling empirics, as well as laundresses and gravediggers. In the chapters that follow, the role of the health care professionals during plague outbreaks is analyzed and their relations with the secular authorities and the Church are scrutinized.

All the activities of the health officials demonstrate that they firmly believed in the communicable nature of plague and acted accordingly. Although the plague was always referred to as an "infection," at that time this term referred to the tainting of the environment. It did not have the same meaning it has today. The expressions "miasma" or "corrupt air," often mentioned by physicians as causes of plague, have not been encountered in Ragusan archival documents.

This study seeks to answer some essential questions about the establishment and development of plague control measures in Dubrovnik: Why did the city take this unusual step of introducing quarantine? What were the contributing factors that made Dubrovnik the first city to establish the Health Office? Why did the Health Office become permanent in Dubrovnik when it was still non-existent or temporary in other cities? How did it evolve over time? What was the impact of the Health Office on the social, cultural, political, and economic life of the city? Were there any watershed years in the implementation of plague control measures? Finally, was Dubrovnik successful in combatting plague?

It is impossible to consider the medical history of Dubrovnik apart from the wider social, cultural, economic, and, above all, political forces at work in this early period because all these factors were inextricably intertwined. It has to be pointed out that the officials governing the Mediterranean cities developed the plague control measures – not the health care professionals. Therefore, the principles of the rulers, as well as the type of government, played a crucial role in the development of plague containment. The Ragusan accomplishments in this field can only be evaluated with an understanding of the Ragusan intellectual profile that includes its philosophy, its form of government, and the functioning of the Ragusan society. The Ragusan attitude towards plague control was conditioned by its geopolitical situation, its economy based on trade, as well as its aristocratic, republican, and Christian values. The situation of Dubrovnik at the point of contact between the Christian and Islamic worlds, as well as between the Mediterranean and the Balkans, played a significant role in shaping its world view as well as its health policies. For this reason, the first chapter introduces readers to the history of Dubrovnik and thus lays the foundation for the subsequent chapters, which focus on the history of plague control measures in the city.

In presenting the history of Dubrovnik, we have concentrated on those aspects of the Ragusan society that lead to a better understanding of the development of plague control measures. Thus, in order to explore the larger significance of the Ragusan experience, the study of plague control measures has been integrated with the unique characteristics and particular circumstances of mediaeval and Renaissance Dubrovnik.

In a republican city-state, with a strong sense of belonging to the community and a fierce feeling of independence, the role of government was to look after the common good. That included keeping the population healthy and free from epidemics. Over time, these ideas emerged as the basis of the republican political doctrine, and the protection against disease became synonymous with good government. It is, therefore, not by coincidence that early public health measures were developed primarily in aristocratic republics on both sides of the Adriatic Sea with their proclaimed ideals of liberty, stability, economic prosperity, longevity, and social tolerance.[4]

This study is focused on Dubrovnik and its rich archival records.[5] However, its revelations about state responses to plague epidemics add an important chapter to the world history of plague control measures in the mediaeval and early modern periods.

I
History of Dubrovnik

Non pro toto libertas venditur auro.
(Liberty should not be sold for all the gold in the world.)
–Inscription on the Lovrijenac Fortress in Dubrovnik

WEALTH, FREEDOM, AND DIPLOMACY

Dubrovnik, also called Ragusa in the past, was an aristocratic city-state that wielded enormous power in the Mediterranean. Flourishing maritime and caravan trade, as well as shipbuilding and shipping, contributed to its incredible wealth (see Figure 1.1). In his work *Opis slavnoga grada Dubrovnika / Situs aedificiorum, politiae et laudabilium consuetudinum inclitae civitatis Ragusii* (Description of the illustrious city of Dubrovnik), written in 1440, Diversis, an educated eyewitness and reliable chronicler, reports on the rapid development and the economic prosperity of this bustling city.[1] During the years that Diversis spent in Dubrovnik, the whole city was an enormous construction site (see Figures 1.2 and 1.4). "Ceaselessly trading, Ragusan citizens, the patricians as well as commoners, become miraculously wealthy. Rare are the merchants in any other cities who are as rich … Therefore, all who can afford to do so build magnificent homes, the gentlemen and their spouses wear luxurious, splendid clothes made of silk or wool. The ladies' garments are richly adorned with precious stones, pearls, silver and gold," notices Diversis.[2] Not forgetting the merchandise exported on Ragusan vessels, he identifies an astounding array of goods that are brought to the city every day by land and by sea, for trading or for consumption by its citizens (see Appendix B).

Dubrovnik was skilful at protecting its freedom by astute diplomacy and sophisticated political mediation between East and West. It was also successful at developing a remarkable reputation as a peace-loving, stable, prosperous, and socially tolerant republic that lasted for many centuries despite the most dangerous of circumstances.[3] Diversis explains that "the Ragusans send their diplomats, who convince with nice words and bring presents for the one

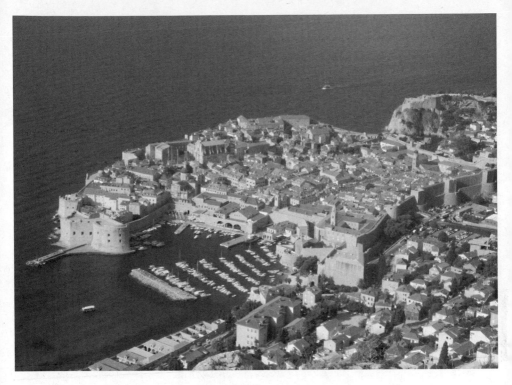

Figure 1.1 Panoramic view of Dubrovnik, 2013

who provokes, and for those of his advisers who seem to have his trust, in order to soften his heart, temper his appetite and vouch for peace and friendship."[4]

The patricians personified the Ragusan Republic. This small group of people imprinted their values on the city and shaped its identity. In order to defend their privileges, the patricians protected the freedom and statehood of that small segment of the Croatian territory united under the flag of St Blaise (Sveti Vlaho).[5] In every sense – territorial, political, ethnic, and cultural – the Ragusans considered themselves to be part of Dalmatia, a coastal region inhabited by Croats. Citizens of other Dalmatian cities therefore enjoyed special status in Dubrovnik. Ragusans were multilingual: they spoke Croatian, Ragusan (an old Romance language), Latin, and Italian, and most foreigners visiting this busy port city spoke at least one of these languages.[6] While it is difficult to trace with certainty the precise balance between Slavic and Latin-Romance languages in Dubrovnik at particular times, toponyms and personal names demonstrate that by the thirteenth century, the city was mainly Slavic.[7]

The notion of *libertas* (freedom) varied over centuries but it always remained a fundamental political value and a tool that gave legitimacy to the patriciate.[8] Diversis emphasizes the dispersal of executive power and its

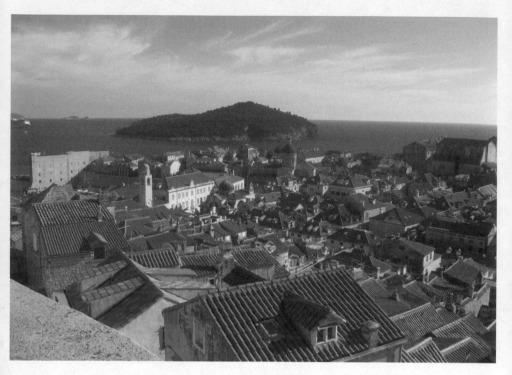

Figure 1.2 View of Dubrovnik from the city walls, 2013: Church of St Blaise (centre), the Cathedral (right), and the Jesuit Church (extreme right); Old Port (left) with the fortress of St John; Lokrum in the background with the islets of Mrkan and Bobara in the distance (left)

limitation in the Ragusan system of government that guaranteed real authority to the patricians as a group. The Ragusan concept of power abhorred personal domination and guarded against it at all costs. Diversis describes it as a "rule of citizens, free and equal who alternate in power; a rule where several officials, whose power is limited by city laws and statutes, as well by the decisions of the patricians, are elected to the same office."[9]

GEOGRAPHY, TERRITORIAL EXPANSION, AND POPULATION

Encircled by massive mediaeval walls and precipitously perched on a rocky promontory above the Adriatic Sea, Dubrovnik occupies a narrow coastal strip at the southern end of a long string of Dalmatian islands. Mount Srđ (Sergius), 412 metres, dominates the city from the north and is part of the Dinaric chain of Alps that extend along the entire length of the Dalmatian coastline. In the vicinity of Dubrovnik, there are only two openings in the mountain wall permitting access into the interior: one, located northeast of the city, winds its way up the Brgat (Vergatum) Pass and then continues into Popovo polje (field) and the town of Trebinje in Herzegovina; the other, located further northwest, begins at the mouth of the Neretva River and offers access into Herzegovina and from there into Bosnia and Serbia. These routes played a crucial role in the development of Ragusan trade with the hinterland.

Because of the prevailing currents and favourable winds, as well as the protection to vessels provided by the islands, ships, sailing south from Venice into the Mediterranean, preferred the Dalmatian side of the Adriatic. Seafarers stopped in Dubrovnik to get provisions, change crews, and repair their vessels before heading into open sea. The geographical situation of Dubrovnik thus offers major advantages for both maritime and overland traffic.[10]

Astarea, the original Ragusan territory, stretched about ten kilometres northwest to Zaton and ten kilometres southeast of the city all the way to Župa. It also encompassed the island of Lokrum, Koločep, Lopud, and Šipan in the immediate vicinity of the city. In the thirteenth century, the territory was expanded with the acquisition of Lastovo, the most remote island of the Ragusan jurisdiction. The Pelješac Peninsula, also called Stonski Rat, and the town of Ston, of crucial value for defence, were acquired in 1333.[11] To secure its northwestern border and protect the navigation in the Pelješac Channel, Dubrovnik built massive walls around Ston.[12] The island of Mljet was acquired after a peasant uprising against the Benedictine abbot in 1345.[13] Diversis reminds us that "while almost all other peoples strive by war, by force, by the sword, by arms and by deception to increase their dominions, the Ragusans have expanded their jurisdiction peacefully and in a friendly fashion."[14] In 1399, they bought Primorje, situated north of Dubrovnik; in 1419, they bought the eastern part, and in 1426 the western part of Konavle, the agricultural region south of the city.[15] These acquisitions from neighbouring rulers were not always as friendly as Diversis put it. Dubrovnik was ready to go to war over Konavle. The effort was financed with public money and the land was distributed to the citizens: three-quarters to the patricians and the rest to commoners.[16] With the inclusion of Konavle, the territorial expansion of the Ragusan Republic was concluded (see Figure 1.3). This 135-kilometre strip of coastline, together with the islands, would remain under the control of Dubrovnik until 1808.[17]

During the 1990s, Croatian researchers made available more accurate estimates concerning the population of the Ragusan Republic in the fourteenth, fifteenth, and sixteenth centuries. Their data, based on scientific evidence, refer to the period before 1673, the date of the first surviving population census.

Figure 1.3 Map of the Ragusan Republic, 1426–1808

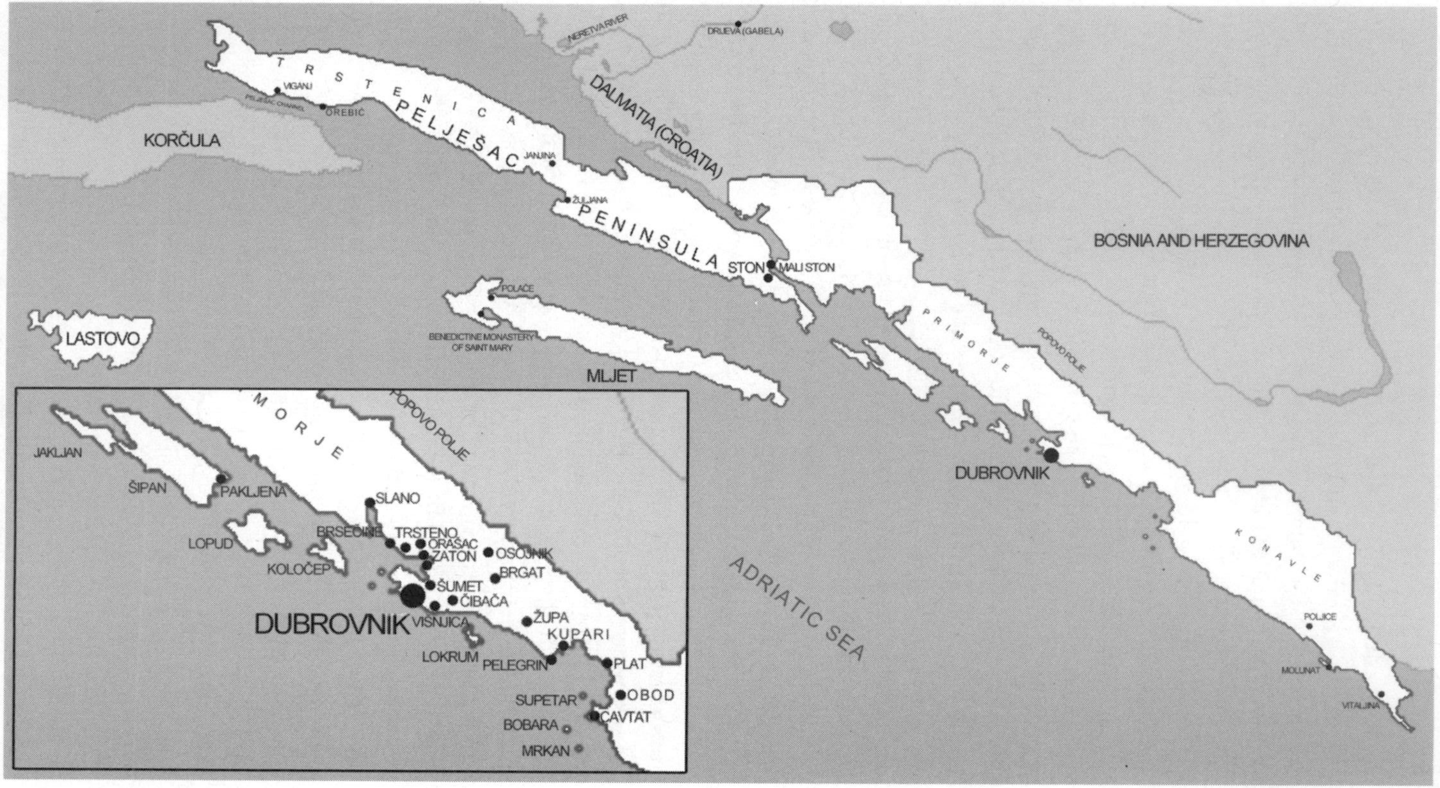

Their evaluation of the population of the city of Dubrovnik is based on the comparison with the population density of other Dalmatian urban centres and with the appraisals of chroniclers and historians. The researchers concur that the city of Dubrovnik, without the suburbs, must have had about three thousand inhabitants at the end of the thirteenth century, and no more than that at the end of the fourteenth due to the devastating plague outbreak in 1348 (see Chapter 2, p. 46); there were five to six thousand dwellers within the walls, and up to nine thousand, counting the suburbs, in 1498, with the numbers declining in the following centuries. The largest population growth occurred in the second half of the fifteenth century when, due to Ottoman expansion, the Ragusan Republic accepted a large number of refugees from Bosnia and Herzegovina. All through its history, Dubrovnik also provided political asylum to many individuals from neighbouring countries.[18] According to the most recent estimates by Nenad Vekarić, the Ragusan Republic had 88,548 inhabitants in 1498, but only 65,022 in 1536 due to the disastrous plague outbreak in 1526 (see Chapter 6); there were 40,000 in 1630s and only 26,000 in 1673 after the catastrophic earthquake of 1667.[19]

GOVERNMENT, ELECTIONS, AND LEGISLATION

The foundation of Dubrovnik remains shrouded in mystery.[20] Recent archaeological research has demonstrated that the site of the city has been inhabited since antiquity. The Dubrovnik harbour could also provide shelter and water needed by the mariners.[21] During the archaeological excavation after the earthquake of 1979, under the present cathedral of the Assumption of St Mary, Josip Stošić discovered the walls and foundations of the Romanesque cathedral built between 1131 and 1157.[22] Under that cathedral, he found another church – a Byzantine basilica built in the seventh to eighth centuries with frescoes from 1060. In 1992–95, during the restoration of the Church of Our Lady of Sigurata on Prijeko Street, stone fragments of an early Christian church from the sixth century were found.[23] With these findings, the date of the establishment of the city was pushed back several centuries.

Except for some brief interludes, Dubrovnik remained under Byzantine protection from 1000 to 1204.[24] Between 996 and 999, Pope Gregory V elevated the Ragusan bishopric to the rank of archbishopric with metropolitan authority. By this promotion, the Ragusan ecclesiastical jurisdiction was considerably enlarged.[25] According to the recent re-creation by Željko Peković, the first

Figure 1.4 Map of Dubrovnik, 2013

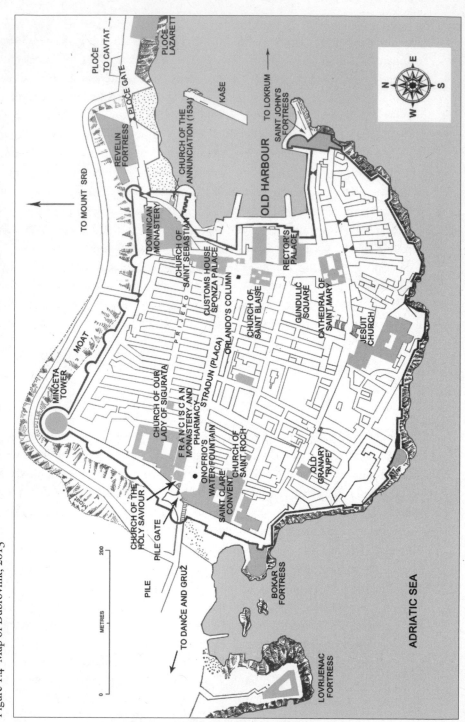

cathedral of Dubrovnik (998–1022) was the early pre-Romanesque church of St Peter the Great, which was torn down in the fifteenth century.[26]

Extant trade treaties from the twelfth and thirteenth centuries, the period when documentary sources concerning Dubrovnik became more frequent, are preserved in the State Archives of Dubrovnik. They reveal that the trade contacts with Italian cities of Molfetta (1148), Pisa (1169), Ancona (1188), Fano (1199), Monopoli (1201), Bari (1201), Termoli (1203), and Bisceglie (1211) multiplied rapidly. In 1190, a treaty was signed with Rovinj in Istria. In these treaties, the city is usually referred to as Ragusium, Ragusa, *communitas Ragusii* or *civitas Ragusii*. However, the term *Dubrovčani*, the Croatian name for the inhabitants of Dubrovnik, is used for the first time in the 1189 treaty with the Bosnian Ban Kulin.[27] Furthermore, in 1153, the Arabic geographer El Idrisi, describing the eastern Adriatic coast, stated, "Ragusa is thirty miles distant from Ston. It is inhabited by Dalmatians, resolute and audacious people who possess fast ships. Ragusa is the last city of Croatia."[28]

Over time, Ragusan merchants established a vast network of diplomatic and trade channels so that they could deal effectively with friend and foe alike. They tried to avoid conflict by using the influence of their overlords or the pope. In other circumstances, they offered money or favourable trade contracts. However, in the eleventh century, Byzantium was weakened by the irruption of Seljuk Turks (1071) and could not offer any real protection to Dalmatia. Therefore, the cities of Zadar, Šibenik, Trogir, Split, Kotor, and Dubrovnik took the matter into their own hands and organized their independent political life. Since some belligerent rulers depended on Dubrovnik for their trade exchange, they often made concessions and thus, even war, did not close the door to commerce. After a protracted period of internal disorder in Serbia, its ruler, Stevan Nemanja, planned to penetrate the Adriatic coast. He besieged Dubrovnik but failed to conquer it. Finally, both parties signed a treaty in 1186 granting Ragusans free trade throughout Serbia. In 1192, the Byzantine emperor Isaak III Angelus issued a chrysobull to Dubrovnik allowing Ragusans free trade in his empire. Dubrovnik had become a serious commercial partner, a supplier of raw materials from the hinterland and from the Dalmatian coast in exchange for manufactured goods from Italy. It was thus ready to become a point of contact and to begin playing a role in East-West relations.[29]

It so happened that the Ragusans had to deal with Damjan Juda, their count who had overstayed his welcome and had ruled for two years instead of only six months. He behaved like a tyrant and intimidated his opponents by bringing soldiers into the city. Wanting to get rid of him, some Ragusans invited the Venetians to help. Although the count and sometimes the archbishop provided the only Venetian presence in the city, Ragusans only grudgingly accepted the Venetian rule that lasted from 1205 to 1358. The count acted as the head of the commune with the archbishop countersigning the most important documents. In other respects, Venice left a lot of room for Ragusan self-government and ambition to grow. Dubrovnik adopted the Venetian political model of an aristocratic republic and modified it according to its own needs and customs.

A remarkable improvement in the legislation and administration of Dubrovnik took place when the Ragusan Statute Book was promulgated in 1272. It is a codification of all laws previously scattered in various books and composed mainly of Dalmatian law – a kind of Roman substratum – and Slavic customary law, with additions of commercial and maritime regulations utilized in the Mediterranean countries.[30] In the Statute, public and private interests were carefully balanced to achieve an overall civic harmony. According to the subjects dealt with, the Statute is divided into seven books. The seventh book, for example, determines all the regulations concerning maritime shipping law. In 1358, the Statute was enlarged by the addition of the eighth book dealing with enactments on diverse matters.

In 1277, the Ragusan Customs Statute was adopted.[31] In 1301, the first book of consolidated Council minutes – the *Libri reformationum* was started while the *Liber omnium reformationum* covered the Council decisions from 1335 to 1410. After the Treaty of Višegrad in 1358, a new book of statutory laws was started.[32] The structure of the Ragusan legislation and government was established early and lasted for centuries.

Venice introduced restrictions on Ragusan maritime trade but it did not impose any taxes on the goods exported from the hinterland. That gave the Ragusans the opportunity to develop overland trade. Even when the powers that dominated the Balkans changed, the Ragusans could always rely on the wealth of knowledge and valuable connections in the Slavic hinterland that they had acquired. Trade rivalry in the Mediterranean led to generally strained political relations with Venice while commercial and personal relations, based on mutual interests as well as social and cultural similarities, flourished over the centuries.[33]

The power of the Venetian count was limited. His decisions had to be confirmed by the Ragusan Councils that continued to govern the commune. In the early days, the count appointed the Minor Council and then they jointly appointed the members of the Major Council and the other organs of government.[34] The Major Council began to emerge in 1235 and the Senate in 1252. From 1293, the members of the Minor Council were appointed from the ranks of eminent nobles. The authority of the Major Council grew. Also, nobles were almost exclusively appointed to perform diplomatic missions to the Slavic rulers of the hinterland. In 1332, the ranks of nobility were "closed" and the Ragusan patriciate was formed. Their names bore the honorific titles Ser and Donna.[35] At that time there were seventy-eight noble families.[36] From then on, only the male aristocrats participated in political life and could vote in elections. Diversis, writing in 1440, quotes the names of thirty-three surviving noble families and states, "Only the legitimate sons descended from these lineages are noble and no one else."[37] One of the reasons for the "closing" of the ranks of the nobles after 1332 may have been the need to have a reliable list of noble families for the distribution of land on the Pelješac Peninsula, which was bought in 1333.[38] With this decision, the nobles limited their reproductive chances and became more sensitive to demographic catastrophes (plague, earthquakes) than the rest of the population. Inevitably, the proportion of the nobles in the general population had to diminish over time.[39] Nenad Vekarić considers that with the closing of the noble ranks, the aristocrats had sealed their own fate that eventually brought about the downfall of the Ragusan Republic.[40]

The political decision of 1332 was supported by the marriage practice: the nobles mostly married among themselves. However, the actual "biological wall" was erected on 19 March 1462 when it was decided that the patricians were not allowed to marry commoners. The penalty for not respecting this regulation was the loss of aristocratic title and of all aristocratic privileges.[41] From then on, the patrician men entertained extramarital relationships with plebeian women but married only patricians. This rule created the strictest social rank endogamy in all of Europe. The Ragusan patricians distanced themselves equally from patricians in many other cities and countries. In order to keep their status, they were allowed to marry only patricians from Dubrovnik, from other Dalmatian cities, or from Venice.[42]

In 1358, the combined Hungarian and Croatian armies of King Louis I of Anjou (1342–1382) defeated the Venetians in Italy and Dalmatia. With the Treaty of Zadar, signed on 18 February 1358, Dalmatia came under Croatian-Hungarian rule. Officially, Dubrovnik was part of Dalmatia but it was unclear what its position was in the new scheme of things. On 28 February 1358, the

Ragusan Major Council broke off its relations with Venice and accompanied the Venetian count to the ship that took him home.[43] Then, after a two-month preparation to decide on the position to adopt, the Ragusans dispatched to King Louis I a five-member diplomatic mission lead by Ilija Saraka, the highly respected archbishop of Dubrovnik. Demonstrating their diplomatic skills, the Ragusans took advantage of this moment in history to become masters of their own fate. With the Treaty of Višegrad (Hungary), agreed on 27 May 1358 and confirmed by the Ragusan Major Council on 18 July 1358, Dubrovnik became de facto independent: its territory and its self-rule were guaranteed.[44] The city was freed from Venetian domination while the attention of their new protector, a powerful military and political player, was concentrated on central European affairs. The king of Hungary, Croatia, and Dalmatia was a distant overlord who had no mighty fleet in the Adriatic. The obligations of Dubrovnik towards the crown were minimal, while the king, together with the *ban* (governor) of Croatia, had promised to defend the city against its enemies. Moreover, if the king were at war with the neighbours of Dubrovnik, the Ragusans would be allowed to continue trading with those countries. The Treaty of Višegrad thus became the cornerstone of the Ragusan Republic and the starting point of two centuries of tremendous growth and outstanding accomplishment.[45] The Ragusan coat of arms as we know it dates from that time.[46]

After 1358, instead of a count, Dubrovnik elected a rector as head of state. A new rector was elected every month and could not be re-elected for another two years because Ragusans wanted to make sure that there would be no accumulation of power in one man. The duties of the rector were honorific and ceremonial.[47] The commune of Dubrovnik came to be known as a republic after 1358.[48] The ultimate authority of the republic was vested in the Major Council (Consilium Maius). All the adult male patricians were members of this assembly that elected the rector, the Minor Council (Consilium Minus), the Senate (Consilium Rogatorum), and most of the government officials, including the ambassadors. The patrician youths had to learn to read and write in order to be accepted into the Major Council.[49] To become successful merchants, young men studied arithmetic, reading and writing, some Latin and some Italian. The public school for boys was first mentioned in 1333. Girls were educated at home. The level of their education depended on the philosophy of their parents. For example, Benedikt Kotruljević (Benedetto Cotrugli) was a merchant and diplomat, who, in 1458, wrote the book *On the Art of Trade and the Perfect Merchant*. He is credited with the first description of the double-entry book-keeping system. Kotruljević had five daughters and, although the society frowned upon it, he gave all of them an excellent education.[50]

The rights and duties of the other two Councils – the Minor Council and the Senate, and of the rector – were determined by the Major Council that usually delegated some of its powers to these bodies. The Major Council formulated laws and regulations and determined policy but most of its time was occupied with elections. In the fifteenth century, there were about fifty or sixty positions to be filled every year. The state apparatus consisted of about 160 patricians.[51] David Rheubottom has drawn up a list of 270 men who sat on the Major Council from 1455 to 1490.[52] The Minor Council was made up of eleven members: six members directly elected by the Major Council and five justices of the Criminal Court. It met three times a week and elected certain officials. Its role was to advise the rector and to act as the executive body of the state that carried out the decisions of the Senate. One of its important functions was to elect the health officials (see Chapter 4).[53]

In the fifteenth century, the Senate had forty-five members. It consisted of eleven members of the Minor Council, eleven previous members, twelve rectors sitting for eleven months after their term of office, five civil judges, and a number of other members elected directly by the Major Council. The minimum age for the Senate was set at thirty. The Senate had the power to decide on all financial matters and, most importantly, on foreign affairs. It also acted as the Supreme Court of Appeal. Over time, the Senate accumulated a lot of power.

The governmental obligations of the patricians were indeed demanding and left little time for family business, trade, and private affairs. Some consider that the commoner merchants were in a more advantageous position because they enjoyed the same high standard of living but they were not burdened with the obligations of the state and could devote all their time to commerce. Although the patricians were not always eager to perform their governmental duties, they accepted them because they understood that this was the price of their freedom and of their economic prosperity. They were well aware that they were better off than the patricians in other Dalmatian cities, and admittedly better off than anyone in the neighbouring countries. Moreover, there was always the pride of their noble rank and their unfailing devotion to the Ragusan Republic as their homeland (see Figure 1.5).

The Major Council had its own building next to the Rector's Palace where elections took place.[54] Indeed, if three officials were elected to exercise a function, two could not be from the same family. If one family member was

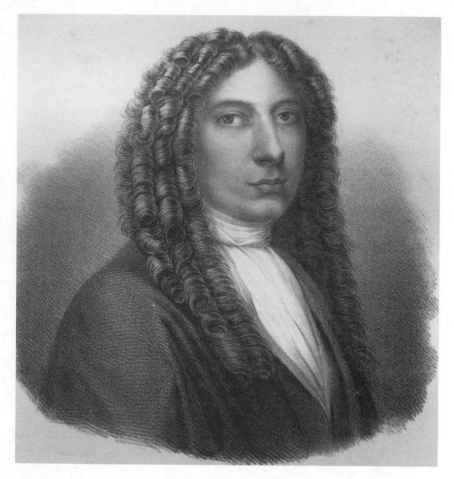

Figure 1.5 Ilija Lambrov Crijević (Cerva, Zrieva) (1463–1520), Ragusan patrician
and writer

proposed for election, his relatives had to leave the hall during the voting
process. A candidate had to obtain the majority of votes to be elected. Otherwise, the election process had to be repeated.

Interestingly, *scrutinium* – the direct nomination of candidates – was practised only for filling the vacancies outside the city, that is, positions in the local
administrative units (e.g., count of Ston, count of the island of Lastovo), certain missions abroad, along with some lower ranked offices.[55]

In the eyes of the patricians, order and precedence were of paramount importance. Generally, older men occupied the more senior offices.[56] However, the

actual career paths of patricians varied considerably. A patrician might occupy a senior position one year and a more junior one the next. Moreover, Ragusan offices were not professional but specific knowledge was required to perform them. Thus, a degree of specialization occurred: some individuals excelled in financial matters, others in judicial affairs or diplomatic service.

Due to the demographic crisis after the plague epidemics in 1348 and 1527, the age requirement for many offices was lowered (see Chapter 4, note 48). Men thirty years old already occupied the functions that their grandfathers had filled in their fifties. Except for the rector, most officials tended to be younger. In the fifteenth century, patricians in their forties and fifties were elected to the duty of rector. A hundred years later, no one became rector before the age of seventy. The basic political principles of the Ragusan Republic were prudence, pragmatism, conservatism, harmony, and moderation. Such a society preferred the experience of older men to the risk-taking of young people.[57]

RELIGION, THE CHURCH, AND THE CONFRATERNITIES

There is no doubt that Catholicism permeated all aspects of Ragusan life. The Ragusans were very devout. Their personal piety was never in question and was often remarked upon by foreigners.[58] Exquisite churches were built in the city and in the countryside, some of which were truly magnificent. Diversis describes many of them but most of his admiration is reserved for the Cathedral of St Mary the Great, built from 1131 to 1157.[59] He also depicts the elegant architecture of countless churches, monasteries and convents where priests, monks and nuns maintained a vibrant religious life that lasted for centuries.[60]

Belonging to the Catholic Church was of paramount importance for Ragusans. Because of the constant threat on the borders of the Republic, the Ragusans believed that, by pledging their allegiance to Catholicism, they would protect their freedom and independence. Their faith was also a way of expressing their affiliation with the Western world. Surrounded by peoples of other religions and foreign cultures, the Ragusans saw themselves as a "fortress of Christianity" – *antemurale Christianitatis* – defending not only their own state but doing an enormous favour to the whole Christian world by stopping the Ottoman Empire on their borders and assisting the Christians enslaved in that empire.[61] They therefore took both of these aspects of their identity very seriously.[62] Wherever they established their colonies on foreign soil, they built their churches.[63]

By the end of the fourteenth century, lay authorities had established full control of the Church.[64] The dominance of secular authorities had started with the 1272 Statute that did not treat the Church as a single organization with the archbishop at its head but instead made a difference between priests, monks, nuns, and the archbishop. The secular elite did not want the archbishop to get any significant income and made sure that it was enshrined in the Statute.[65] Furthermore, procurators of the cathedral were elected by the Venetian count and were solely responsible to him, and not to the archbishop, in matters concerning the financing of the construction of the cathedral. The judicial power of the archbishop was equally limited. In criminal cases, he was subject to the count's court as were priests, nuns, and monks. With some exceptions, they were all treated like other citizens of Dubrovnik.

The Ragusan Statute of 1272 reserves a more favourable position for the abbot of the Benedictine monastery on the island of Lokrum than for the archbishop of Dubrovnik. In case of a war situation, "when lay persons would not dare," the Benedictine monks from Lokrum were obliged to act as ambassadors of the commune of Dubrovnik. This shows the close ties of the Benedictines with lay authorities. Still, the authorities consistently encroached on the rights of the Benedictines on Lokrum and by the fourteenth century, the laymen were in a position to choose their own candidate for the abbot of the monastery. Their next step was to establish control over the finances of the monastery.[66]

Ilija Saraka became a particularly well-known archbishop of Dubrovnik mainly because he was willing to follow the Ragusan political program of territorial expansion and political emancipation. After the acquisition of Ston and the Pelješac Peninsula, he played an important role in organizing life in these territories. In 1345, Archbishop Saraka assisted the inhabitants of Mljet in their conflict with the Benedictine abbot, the feudal lord of the island. He reached an agreement and vouched for its application. By 1410, the state had taken over Mljet and integrated it into the Ragusan political system. All of these were valuable contributions of Ilija Saraka, but his moment of glory was definitely the negotiation of the Treaty of Višegrad that granted the independence of Dubrovnik.[67] However, he was the last archbishop to wield such political power. It is reported that, in 1361, on his deathbed, stricken by plague, he warned the Ragusans to never permit another archbishop to exert as much power as he had exercised. Strange as it may sound, on 29 August 1409, the Major Council prepared a law by which it forbade a Ragusan citizen to seek the position of the archbishop.[68] This was done out of fear that if their own citizen became head of the Church, he would wield too much power. Moreover, Ilija

Saraka suggested such a course of action because he wanted the archbishop to be answerable directly to the pope, without the interference of the king.[69] Since then, only foreigners could become archbishops of Dubrovnik.[70] The patricians did not want the archbishop to have any close connections with anyone in the city. From then on, lay authorities did everything in their power to curb the political influence of the Church. They interfered with the election of the prelates, meddled in the affairs of the Church, took over the management of the property of the Church, and controlled the development and the activities of the confraternities.[71]

Unlike monasteries, all the convents were situated within the city walls. The Benedictine nuns were the first to have a convent in the city that was registered in the documents of 1108. In the Statute, the legal and financial position of the nuns was worse than that of monks and priests.[72] The Statute also gave a father of an underage girl the right to send her to a convent against her will.[73] The income of the convents was much lower than that of the monasteries. In comparison with considerable amounts of money bequeathed to the monasteries, the sums reserved for the convents were symbolic.[74]

In some cases, until the convents accepted the decision of the government, they were held under siege, without food or outside contacts. In 1415, the Senate decided that the convent of St Clare belonged to the Republic and had to accept every patrician girl that the parents wished to send there. The punishment for the abbess who refused to accept a patrician girl was imprisonment and even banishment from Dubrovnik for five years. The Senate was adamant that this convent should not accept any commoners. This was against the principle of universality proclaimed by the Church. In 1422, the Senate decided that no foreigner could be accepted into any convent in Dubrovnik. If an abbess did not obey she would lose her position and would be banished from Dubrovnik.[75]

In legal and financial matters, the Statute favoured priests over monks.[76] It was considered that monks enjoyed better protection than priests. At the beginning of the fourteenth century, all monasteries had procurators elected by secular authorities. In 1460, the Republic took over the control of monasteries' revenues and distributed their income as it saw fit (see Figure 1.6).

The Treasury of St Mary was named after the patron saint of the city cathedral, the Virgin Mary, but there was no connection between the Treasury and the cathedral. It was a channel through which the government supervised the finances of hospitals, monasteries, churches, and confraternities. The authority of the Treasury extended not only to private benefactors and their pious bequests, but also to confraternities. Thus, a confraternity could not be named as

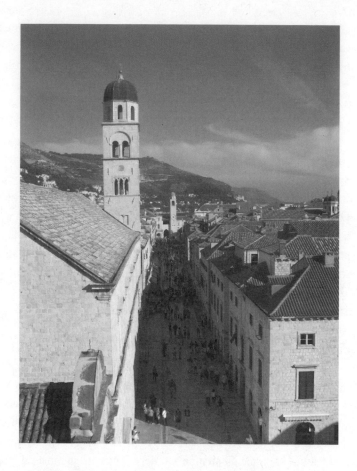

executor of a will: a layperson had to be designated or else the right of the executor would be passed to the Treasury.[77] The property of religious institutions
was administered by procurators. They could sell or lease the property of the
monastery to benefit the monastery and the state. In the latter part of the fifteenth century, only the patricians with more than twenty-four years of experience in the Major Council were eligible to become trustees of religious
institutions.[78]

The nomination of Church dignitaries belonged formally to the archbishop
and the pope but the government always promoted its own candidates using
every means at its disposal. On 23 November 1442, the Major Council decided
that the canon of the cathedral of Dubrovnik could only be a Ragusan patrician because "the patricians founded the city, built its cathedral and had to bear
the burden of maintaining the Republic." If anyone decided to vote for another
candidate, for example, a commoner, he would be banished from Dubrovnik

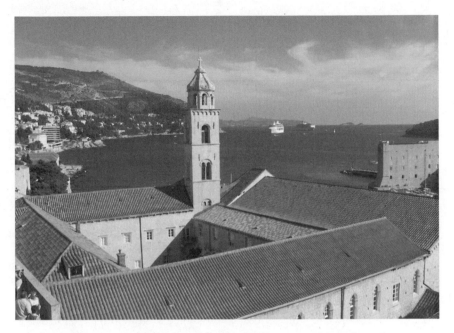

Figure 1.6 A. (Opposite) Franciscan monastery (left), Stradun, the main street in Dubrovnik and the city bell tower in the background. B. (Above) Dominican monastery, church, cloister, and belltower in Dubrovnik, built in the fourteenth and fifteenth centuries.

and his property would be confiscated. This decision could be changed only if the proposal received unanimous support of the Minor Council.[79]

The government considered the Church hierarchy as potential rivals for power and contemplated it with circumspection. The Senate, for example, never allowed the division of the city into parishes. St Blaise was the only parish church for the whole city while other priests were not responsible for a specific territory.[80] The patricians found it particularly difficult to accept that the Church offered equal opportunities to candidates from all social strata. In spite of their personal devoutness, the ruling elite always kept in mind that the Church represented an autonomous organization whose ultimate authority remained outside of the Republic.[81] This was the main reason secular authorities desired so ardently to have control over the election of Church dignitaries. The Church was uneasy about the limitation of its jurisdiction and especially about the right to grant asylum.[82] Such situations often led to tensions with the Vatican. Since Ragusans always emphasized their role as defenders of the Catholic faith in their part of the world, and they also managed to get the support of the

Hungarian-Croatian king, the Vatican had to tread lightly. This allowed the state
to continue its domination of the Church. The government scheduled the calendar of religious holidays and processions; it took care of the holy relics of the
saints, and especially of St Blaise, the protector and symbol of the Republic
(see Figure 1.7).[83] Indeed, the feast of St Blaise celebrated on 3 February was
the most solemn holiday of the Ragusan Republic and remains, still today, the
most important date in the Dubrovnik calendar. The image of the saint is ubiquitous – it can be found on all the city gates and all the fortifications of
Dubrovnik, on the official seal, and on the flag of the Republic.[84] St Blaise had
both a religious and a political meaning.[85]

Having complete control of the religious rituals was of paramount importance for the patricians – it gave them the opportunity to express the superior-
ity of their social class and a chance to promote the idea of social unity and
political loyalty.[86] In other words, the religious ritual was used to promote the
political ideology of the Republic: the myth of freedom and the myth of statehood.[87] In the procession for the feast day of St Blaise, the rector and the archbishop either walked together or the rector walked in front of the archbishop in
order to show the pre-eminence of secular authorities.[88] The symbolism of the
procession suggested that the rector inherited his authority from St Blaise, and
through the rector, as symbol of government, that authority was passed on to
all the administrative bodies of the Republic, that is, to the patricians. The heav-
enly protection of the established order thus found its ultimate confirmation in
the procession of St Blaise. Respecting the strict social hierarchy, the rector, accompanied by the physicians, marched in front of the archbishop. They were
followed by all the patricians, the abbots, priests, and monks carrying other
relics.[89] The most prestigious commoners – members of confraternities –
marched next. The rector and the archbishop were preceded by men responsible for the security of the Republic – farmers and sailors from the islands who
marched with their weapons.[90] They were followed by artisans, even butchers,
marching two by two, and carrying their burning candles. In front of the military men marched the musicians. Every citizen had his or her own place in the
procession that reflected his or her position in the community. All of this contributed to the exceptional self-esteem of the Ragusans and the vision of a
united community.[91] Such a political ideology also motivated the government
to work for the common good, which included health protection and plague
control measures (see Chapters 3 and 4).

The Ragusan confraternities, which were, first of all, religious associations,
also contributed to the idea of a united community. Their role was to take care

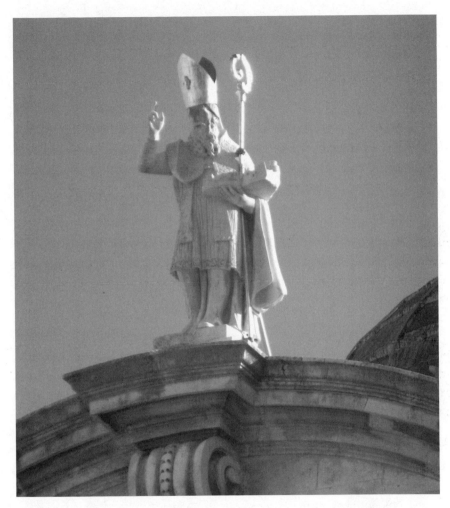

Figure 1.7 St Blaise holding the model of the city, Church of St Blaise, Dubrovnik

of a particular church or devotion. In the villages, the principle of membership was geographical: all the inhabitants of a community became members of the confraternity. Outside the city, the confraternities also played a policing role on their territory: their geographical coverage often coincided with a *kaznačina*, a local administrative unit in the countryside.[92] As such, they were obliged to lead a moral, religious, and charitable life. That meant being regularly present at religious services and helping less fortunate members. Mutual assistance and companionship were the primary roles of the confraternity. Members were usually of modest means.[93]

In the fifteenth and sixteenth centuries, professional confraternities in the city became craft guilds. Their role was to regulate the activities of their craftsmen and to try to achieve not only as much autonomy as possible but also a monopoly in their own sphere of activity. However, all the decisions of the confraternity had to be confirmed by the Minor Council. Otherwise, they were considered null and void. The government punished notaries, chancellors, or scribes who entered into the statute a secret decision of the confraternity. Decisions unpopular with the authorities could lead to the prohibition of the confraternity. The Minor Council kept a close watch over these associations and, if necessary, interfered directly.

The most distinguished confraternities were founded by wealthy tradesmen. Officially founded in 1432, the Antunini, members of the confraternity of St Anthony, trading in the West, were the most affluent merchants in the city. Many of them had surpassed the patricians in their wealth. The Lazarini, the confraternity of St Lazarus, formed in 1531, represented the merchants dealing with the East. Under the watchful eye of the authorities, these two groups soon became the most influential commoners in Dubrovnik. In their lifestyle, they imitated the patricians. Mostly as a reward for contributions to public good, the Senate could propose eminent citizens for membership of the Antunini. They were allowed to participate in governmental duties as chancellors, notaries, and secretaries, and they were granted the status of elite citizens. Having earned the trust of the patricians, the Antunini always remained loyal to them, craving more the recognition of their status than political power.[94] The Ragusan model of dealing with the prestigious commoners provided the Republic with a stable social organization that lasted for centuries.[95] The patricians feared that the political activity of the commoners would lead to the formation of political parties, which, as was shown in other Dalmatian cities, would ruin the political unity of the Republic.[96] The Ragusan confraternities were thus never allowed to achieve the degree of autonomy and political involvement that was possible, for example, in some Italian cities.

HEALTH CULTURE AND SANITATION

With a relatively small population and phenomenal wealth, Dubrovnik was willing to improve the living conditions of its citizens by investing in cleanliness and sanitation. In fact, the government made it a priority. The authorities always had the common good on their mind. It was part of their Christian ideals and of their aristocratic republican identity. Sanitary conditions in Dubrovnik were comparable to that of the most advanced Mediterranean cities. Some public health measures were already present in the Statute Book of 1272.[97] To secure law and order, and to prevent public drunkenness at night, there was a regulation in the sixth book requiring all taverns to close after "the third bell," approximately three hours after sunset.[98] The Statute also mentions social benefits for sailors. In the seventh book, there are two regulations concerning the rights of the sailors who fall sick while at sea. Whether they were sailing for shares (*ad partem*) or for pay (*ad marinariciam*), the laws provided full payment during their sickness.[99] In the eighth book of the Statute, pharmacists (*speciarii*) were ordered to weigh medicines on a big scale and were not allowed to keep in their shops a small scale that served for measuring silver, gold, and pearls only.[100] This is the first time the pharmacists are mentioned in Dubrovnik. They sold medicinal herbs and also many other items.[101]

The lepers are mentioned in the sixth book. They are ordered to move further away from the city. The leper hospital was founded as early as 1306.[102] Care for the lepers and their isolation was a forerunner of the later concept of isolation of the infected during plague epidemics (see Chapter 4, p. 107).

The Statute contains a number of decisions concerning street planning. New streets were laid out in straight lines. In 1296, there was a devastating fire that destroyed a good part of the city. Since the early 1300s, it was decided to construct all houses alike in facing rows. This type of built environment was to become the characteristic of Dubrovnik.[103] Between 1406 and 1412, 175 wooden houses were torn down because of a fire hazard and replaced by stone houses.[104] At the same time, it was decided to regulate the drainage of water from the streets. In 1415, the first garbage collection was organized. In 1436, a sewage system was planned to carry all the waste into the sea.[105]

THE RUPE GRAIN DEPOSITORY AND THE AQUEDUCT

In 1410, the Rupe (literally *holes*) were dug out in limestone for the purpose of storing grain in an underground depository and ensuring wheat reserves for the Republic in case of famine, trade interruption, or an enemy siege.[106] From 1548 to 1590, a massive, new, three-storey Rupe building was erected with fifteen silos dug up to nine metres deep in the rock.[107]

In 1436, Onofrio Giordano de la Cava, architect and chief engineer, and Andreucio de Bulbito de Tramonte, building contractor, both well-known masters from the region of Naples, were hired to build an aqueduct at the cost of 8,500 ducats. Completed within sixteen months, the aqueduct stretched from Šumet, twelve kilometres north of the city, all the way to the Minčeta fortress within the city walls. From there, it was split into two canals: one going west to the Franciscan monastery and to the great fountain that Onofrio de la Cava would build in 1441; and another one, running east along the northern city walls and supplying water to the tanners, the Dominican monastery, and the small fountain constructed at the same time and adorned in the 1460s with sculptures by Pietro di Martino from Milan (see Figure 1.4).[108] Both fountains are still operational to this day (see Figure 1.8). Diversis reports enthusiastically that "Dubrovnik is a city with abundant drinking water, from a source eight thousand steps away, which flows into the city piously, magnificently and liberally."[109] The water supply was also crucial for the development of the textile workshops in the western part of the city (see Chapter 9, note 16).

These early measures illustrate a major preoccupation of the Ragusan authorities with cleanliness and hygienic living conditions for all citizens. No wonder Diversis and many other discriminating European visitors observed that Dubrovnik matched the finest cities of the day.

TRADE, SHIPPING, AND SHIPBUILDING

The Ragusan accomplishments in diplomacy, culture, or plague control measures would not have been possible without the abundant financial means created by both caravan and maritime trade. Diversis provides the detailed description of the extraordinary variety of goods that were imported to the city and exported to other countries (see Appendix B and Table 5.1 in Chapter 5 for the origin of merchants and their goods).

Because its maritime trade was limited during the Venetian rule, Dubrovnik was forced to expand its trade with the Balkan hinterland. Salt was an item that all stockbreeders in the interior needed and Dubrovnik held an almost exclusive monopoly on salt trade. Ragusans also brought garments, fabrics, and luxury items from the West. On the return journey to the Adriatic coast, they transported precious metals, especially silver from Srebrenica in Bosnia and from Novo Brdo in Serbia. Lead was obtained from Olovo in Bosnia.[110]

In the thirteenth, fourteenth, and fifteenth centuries, precious metal production in Serbian and Bosnian mines had developed on a large scale: copper, iron, and mercury were also extracted. At its peak, Srebrenica produced five to

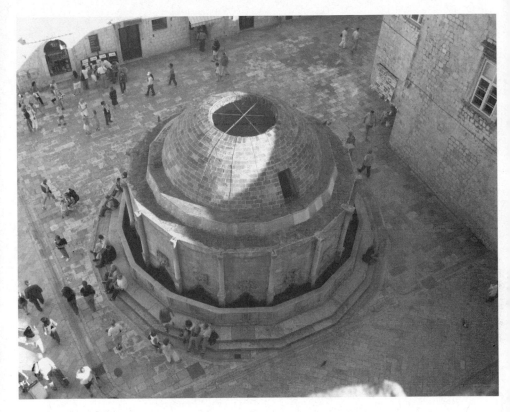

Figure 1.8 Onofrio's water fountain in Dubrovnik, built in 1441

six tons of silver while Novo Brdo churned out nine tons per year.[111] At the same time, no other European mine could produce more than three tons of silver a year. The Ragusan patricians and some commoners owned the mines and acted as investors, customs officials, and wholesale traders.[112] Their influence was ubiquitous. They controlled the mines, carried the metals by their own caravans to their own port in Dubrovnik, and shipped the ore to the West in their own vessels.[113] They became incredibly rich, just like the Bosnian and Serbian rulers who could thus afford to buy the manufactured luxury goods that the Ragusans brought from Italy.

The metals, the hides, and the wool were brought to Dubrovnik from the hinterland by caravans of pack horses, sometimes over three hundred, and in the sixteenth century even one thousand horses strong, accompanied by over two hundred men. As they descended into the port of Dubrovnik, where the goods were transferred onto Ragusan ships that carried them to Italy, the sheer size of the caravans presented an incomparable sight.[114] If the weather and the winds cooperated, the journey across the Adriatic could take about twenty-four hours.

In the commercial and mining centres of the Balkans, the Ragusans developed their colonies, which were run according to Ragusan laws. A consul, usually a Ragusan patrician appointed by the rector and the Minor Council, and two judges governed the settlement, which utilized the Ragusan currency as basis for exchange. Each community also had a church and a priest. Srebrenica, Novo Brdo, and Drijeva were among the earliest Ragusan colonies, established in the 1370s and 1380s. Other important commercial centres included Nikopol, Niš, Priština, Smederevo, Skopje, Kruševac, and Timişoara. When the Ottomans took over the Balkans, they prohibited the export of silver altogether and imposed an artificially low price on it. From then on, the Ragusans could only export the much cheaper lead, which was bulky and heavy to transport, wood for shipbuilding, grain, beeswax, cheese, fur, leather, and meat. The virtual monopoly that they held on the export of salt in Drijeva (Gabela) on the Neretva Delta continued to be a major source of income (see also Chapter 8).[115] In the 1460s, there were almost thirty Ragusan colonies in the interior of the Balkans. By the sixteenth century, there were only six left: Belgrade, Sarajevo, Sofia, Prokuplje, Novi Pazar, and Provadija. Not only did the Ragusans amass personal fortunes but their state profited from the tariffs on the trade and the monopoly on the salt and wine trade, all of which helped fill the Republic's coffers.[116]

In the 1560s and 1570s, the Ragusan Republic had between 170 and 200 ships with the carrying capacity of about 33,000 tons. More than 5,000 sailors were employed on those ships.[117] To a large extent, the Ragusans owed their prosperity to the ships on which they sailed.[118] With a large fleet of trade ships, the Ragusans became a major trade, shipping and shipbuilding power in the Mediterranean (see Figure 1.9).

In 1443, the Ragusans sailed to England for the first time to buy wool and woollen cloth. The English had never seen a ship as huge as the Ragusan carrack.[119] They coined the English word *argosy*, a corruption of the word *Ragusa*, to describe any large sailing ship. The Ragusan carrack could have a capacity of six hundred to eight hundred tons, but it only needed a crew of sixty to eighty sailors.[120] With the Portuguese and the English, the Ragusans were considered to be among the most accomplished shipbuilders in Europe. The appearance of Ragusan ships can be deduced from the stone relief carvings that adorned the private homes and the palaces in the fifteenth century and also by the votive paintings commissioned by the sixteenth-century captains. Those paintings often showed a ship in the storm, the person who asked for protection, the saint to whom the demand for protection was addressed, and a votive inscription.

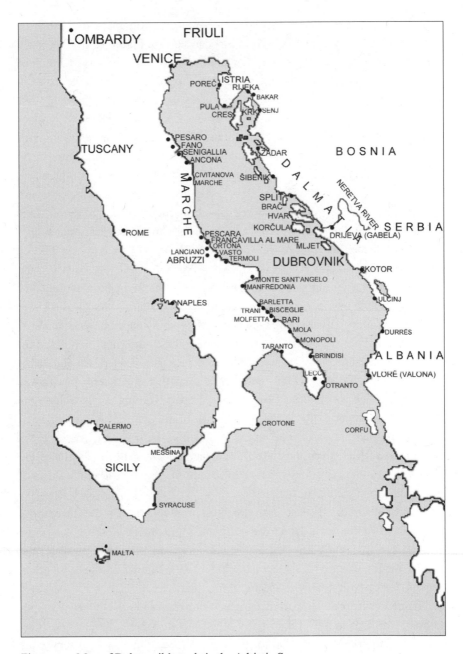

Figure 1.9 Map of Dubrovnik's trade in the Adriatic Sea

The oldest votive painting from Dalmatia depicts the Annunciation. The artist is the famous Ragusan painter, Nikola Božidarević (see Figure 1.10). The painting was commissioned in 1513 by captain Marko Kolendić for the Church of St Nicholas on Lopud. The central predella of the painting shows a luxuriously furnished carrack, moored in the bay of Lopud and flying the white flag of St Blaise, under the benevolent protection of Our Lady and St Nicholas, protectors of sailors, depicted in the medallions. This painting is an extraordinary source of information for the study of the Ragusan merchant sailing ships in the sixteenth century (see Figure 1.11). In the Church of Our Lady of Sigurata in Dubrovnik, there is a votive painting of a ship from the middle of the sixteenth century, which is generally considered to be from the workshop of Frane Matijin. It depicts a sailing ship with three masts in a storm and the figures of sailors in it who lift their arms in prayer towards the figure of Our Lady on a cloud holding baby Jesus (see Figure 1.12). In the sixteenth century, there is also the painting of the Ragusan galleon on the predella of the Franciscan church altar in Slano and the painting of a sailing ship above the altar of Our Lady of Šunj on Lopud. Sailors' silver votive tablets as well as ship-shaped objects, made of silver, also enlighten us about the appearance and the outfitting of the Ragusan ships. The oldest preserved votive tablet is the one from Lopud, which depicts a sailing ship in the waves with a votive inscription that says that the pledge was given and grace was solicited by captain Stjepan Nikolin Usrijenac and his crew on 26 February 1595 (see Figure 1.13). In the Dominican monastery in Dubrovnik, there is also the silver incense dish in the shape of a carrack, the so-called *navicula*, from the sixteenth century, showing all the details of the ship with a lot of precision – the bow even ends in a figurehead in the shape of a dolphin head (see Figure 1.14).[121]

Unfortunately for the Ragusans, the most profitable trade routes were those that were also the most dangerous – Egypt, Syria, and the Black Sea ports, which were frequently affected by plague outbreaks. Although aware of the danger, the Ragusans could not stop trading with the Middle East because grain, crucial for their survival, was imported from that region.[122]

To ensure the protection of its merchant ships and sailors, Dubrovnik maintained consulates in most major ports of the Mediterranean. Since the earliest times, an important destination for the Ragusans was the island of Sicily, the source of their grain.[123] At the peak of the so-called golden age of Dubrovnik in the sixteenth century, the Republic maintained almost sixty consulates in the Mediterranean.[124]

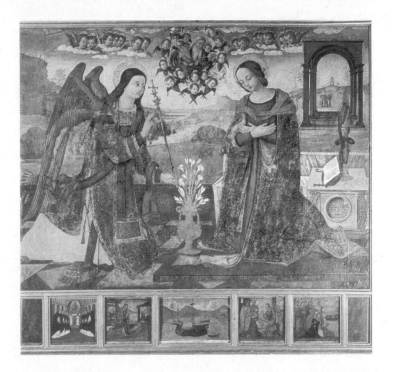

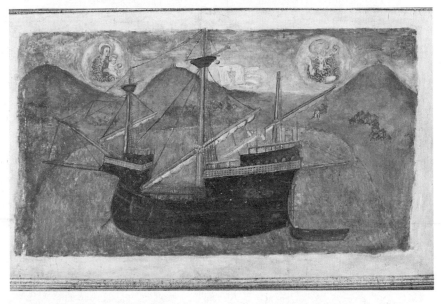

Figure 1.10 *Annunciation* by Nikola Božidarević, 1513, votive painting donated by captain Marko Kolendić to the Church of St Nicholas, Lopud

Figure 1.11 Marko Kolendić's ship in the Lopud harbour, the central predella of the *Annunciation* by Nikola Božidarević, detail, 1513

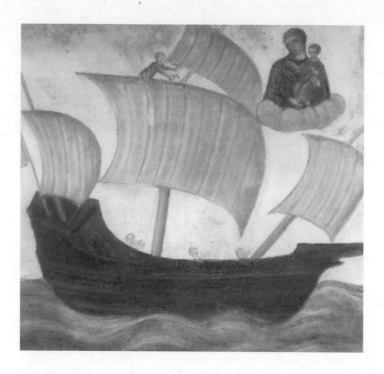

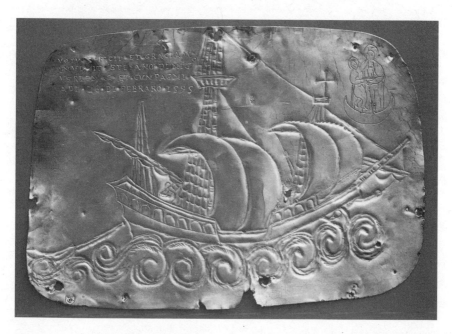

Figure 1.12 Votive painting of a ship in the storm, Church of Our Lady of Sigurata, atelier of Frane Matijin, Dubrovnik, sixteenth century

Figure 1.13 Silver votive tablet of captain Stjepan Usrijenac, 26 February 1595

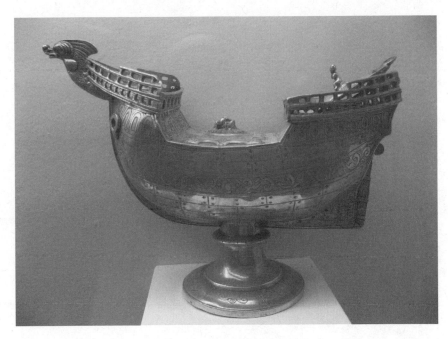

Figure 1.14 *Navicula*, silver incense dish in the shape of a carrack, sixteenth century

The Ragusans also built warships mainly for defence against the pirates but these ships also took part in many international battles where their presence was greatly appreciated. Since the fourteenth century, the harbour of Dubrovnik was equipped with the Great Arsenal with four berths for its men-of-war.[125] At the same time, to make it even more secure, additional fortifications were erected in the port. The Kaše breakwater was constructed at the entrance and the port was closed off with a chain (see Figure 1.4).[126] Judging by the dimensions of the berths, Antun Ničetić concludes that the Great Arsenal housed the biggest ships in existence at that time.[127] Soon after 1500, the most famous Ragusan painter, Nikola Božidarević, created a triptych for the Bundić family chapel in the Dominican church in Dubrovnik. The painting shows clearly what the Arsenal looked like at the beginning of the sixteenth century. St Blaise, holding a model of the city, is depicted on the left panel of the triptych. The harbour is depicted as full of ships and securely protected by the chain and the breakwater (see Figure 1.15). The painting itself can be dated by the observation of the exact stage of reconstruction of the Great Arsenal.[128] The Republic also had another arsenal in Mali Ston with three berths for big ships. The Ragusans possessed the most significant arsenals on the Dalmatian coast.

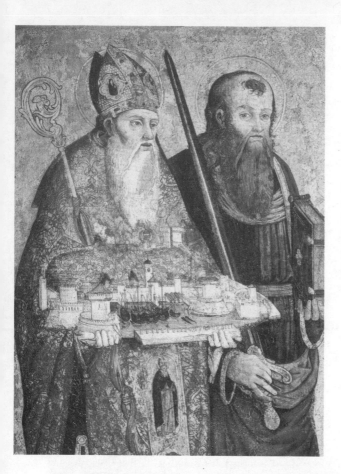

Figure 1.15 Model of the
city of Dubrovnik held by
St Blaise, left panel of the
Bundić family triptych,
painting by Nikola
Božidarević, ca 1500

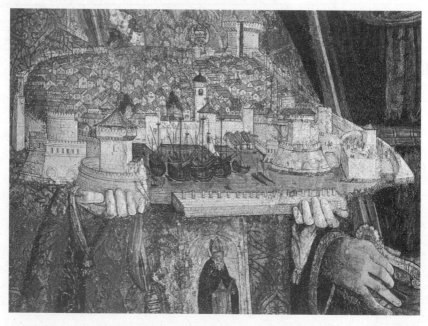

RELATIONS WITH THE OTTOMANS

In the fifteenth century, the Ottomans conquered large portions of the Balkan hinterland. Because they realized that the Hungarian-Croatian king would no longer be able to protect them, the Ragusans viewed these events with increasing trepidation. Small and vulnerable, they found themselves cut off from Dalmatia, threatened by Venice in the Adriatic Sea and by the Ottomans on land. In 1453, alarmed by the fall of Constantinople, they decided to spend thirty thousand ducats to strengthen their massive fortifications.[129] When the hope of a decisive joint action of the Christian states against the Ottomans petered out, the Ragusans were forced to take it upon themselves to find an understanding with the Porte. Although they viewed the prospect with little enthusiasm, they cautiously initiated a series of negotiations with the Ottomans in order to achieve a rapprochement.[130]

In 1458, the negotiations were concluded with an agreement by which the Republic retained its freedom and its self-government while its merchants were allowed to trade freely by land and by sea in Ottoman-controlled lands. Moreover, a highly favourable 2 percent rate of customs dues paid on Ragusan goods was obtained. The Ragusans reached this agreement as a result of their considerable diplomatic virtuosity and thus ensured the continued prosperity of the Republic in the centuries to come in spite of its most dangerous neighbourhood. In return, the Republic agreed to pay the tribute to the sultan, which began with smaller sums and slowly increased until it reached the sum of 12,500 ducats a year in 1481, the sum that Dubrovnik continued to pay until the end of the Republic in 1808.[131]

In 1463, when Bosnia came under Ottoman rule, followed by Herzegovina in 1482, the Ottoman Empire became the Ragusan Republic's only neighbour on land. This was a momentous event in Ragusan history. In the fifteenth century, the Ragusans responded by fortifying their city and building impregnable city walls within a very short time. Little by little, however, the initial resistance of the Ragusans was replaced by a pragmatic attitude towards the Ottomans. Moreover, the pope granted Dubrovnik a special permission for trading with the Ottomans.[132] The Ragusans thus managed to achieve a tacit double alliance with both the Ottomans and the Christian world. This was definitely one of the greatest achievements of the Ragusan diplomacy.[133]

Every year, the Ragusan diplomats (*poklisari*) travelled to Istanbul to pay the tribute (*harač*). In order to gain access to vital information and make friends, they utilized this occasion to establish contacts with the Ottoman officials, especially those of Bosnian descent.[134] On these difficult trips, the Ragusan emissaries were accompanied by their interpreters – the dragomans who had studied the Turkish language and customs. Moreover, since the access to the highest officials of the empire often depended on the skill of the Ragusan interpreters, it was important for them to entertain friendly relations with the sultan's dragoman.[135]

In Dubrovnik, the dragomans were in charge of the Turkish Chancery where the Ottoman documents for which the Republic showed great concern were archived and classified.[136] Owing to their hard work, and exceptional care of the Ragusan government, many inventories have been preserved. Some Ragusan dragomans whose expertise was held in high esteem by foreign governments are known to have worked for the French, Austrian, or Venetian representatives in Istanbul.[137]

Not only did the Ragusans have to win the favour of the mighty Porte, but they waged daily diplomatic battles on the Bosnian front, negotiating with an army of unpredictable Turkish officials, from *beylerbeys* to captains, *kadis* (judges), pashas (higher rank dignitaries), and local *aghas* (civilian or military officers). The Ragusan diplomatic efforts in Bosnia focused on the Bosnian *beylerbey* and the Herzegovinian *sancakbey*, the highest Ottoman dignitaries posted in the immediate vicinity of Dubrovnik, who wielded considerable influence at the Porte. A decree of the sultan was not valid in the Bosnian *eyalet* (province) and the Herzegovinian *sancak* (district) unless it was confirmed and reissued by the above officials.

The Ragusans found themselves in an almost absurd situation. Although they had paid the tribute to the sultan and had presented his ministers with costly gifts, they still had to redouble their efforts in their dealings with the Bosnian Ottoman officials on whose good will they depended. These provincial governors acted independently of Istanbul in many matters, which was not necessarily a good thing for the Ragusans. These officials often imposed additional, arbitrary customs duties and taxes, openly disregarding the orders from the Porte. Thus, regardless of the privileges granted by the sultan, peace, freedom, and prosperity of Dubrovnik still depended on the whims of the Ottoman officials in Bosnia and Herzegovina. Not to mention that a whole series of daily issues had to be settled with the Ottoman officials on the lower level: free trade along the border, loans, lease of arable land and of pastures to Ragusans, refugees and migrants in pursuit of work, crimes committed by Ragusans and Ottomans, and, of course, the regulation of the border crossings in times of plague.[138]

The Ragusans therefore relied primarily on their ability to develop a personal relationship with each individual and shower him with gifts, money, and favours. Each newly appointed official received a "standard" gift of four pieces of finest fabric (silk or velvet), candles, sweetmeats, sugar, marzipan, and spices. These were given in a formal ceremony that was part of the Ragusan diplomatic protocol.[139] The assistants of Ottoman dignitaries also received gifts. Watches, citrus fruit, writing paper, rose-petal liqueur (*rozolin*), Ragusan Malvasia wine, and cash were added to the above list in the eighteenth century. Many Ottomans demanded specific items or services, which, as might be expected, they were granted. A few days later, when current issues were discussed during a secret ceremony, the same official received a special or "secret" gift. Out of fear that their special gift would become standard, the Ragusans kept it as secret as possible, preferably with no witnesses present other than the dragoman. As Robin Harris put it, "Dubrovnik had honed its diplomatic skills in contacts with the Ottomans over centuries. As a result, it had achieved an extraordinary insight into the Turkish mind and tastes. It had established friendly relations with a succession of local Ottoman officials, whom it invited to the theatre and even on occasion showed around the cathedral to the strains of dance music played on the organ."[140] After the battle at Mohács in 1526, when the Croatian alliance with Hungary had ended and the kingdom was partitioned, the fate of Dubrovnik became increasingly dependent on and intertwined with the Ottomans.[141]

For many centuries, Dubrovnik, as an independent state, successfully played the role of bridge between East and West. Armed with self-confidence, sophisticated diplomacy and enormous wealth, the Ragusan Republic was able to turn its dangerous position at the crossroads between the Mediterranean and the Balkans, as well as between the Christian and the Islamic worlds, to its advantage.[142] The Ragusan patricians carefully nurtured the foreign policy doctrine of the Republic based on the image of a small, but significant, trade-oriented and at the same time neutral and peace-loving Republic.[143] From this small group of people emerged, in the longest lasting independent state on the territory of present-day Croatia, an astounding concentration of renowned statesmen, diplomats, scientists, and artists.[144] Political stability and economic prosperity laid the ground for other achievements in the realms of culture and plague control measures that hold unique value for Croatia, Europe, and the world.

2

The Plague Phenomenon and Plague Epidemics in Dubrovnik

Plague pandemics are ranked as the worst catastrophes to ever strike humanity. They appeared cyclically over many centuries and claimed millions of lives in Asia, the Middle East, the Mediterranean, and Europe. The appearance of plague had wide-ranging political, social, and economic consequences. Many historians consider that the first plague pandemic in the sixth century brought about the end of late antiquity.[1] Mirko Dražen Grmek argues that plague mortality may have left a demographic void in Dalmatia that was filled by the Slavs.[2] The second plague pandemic, later named the Black Death, was particularly virulent.[3] Between 1347 and 1350, it wiped out at least a quarter of the population of Europe, if not more.[4] Mediterranean port cities, where ships arriving from the Levant docked, suffered the most.[5] Unfortunately, those ships were loaded with infected goods and full of rats with their fleas. Trade ships and war galleons carried the plague to the ports of the Western Mediterranean while trade caravans and armies spread it further into the interior of the continent.[6] In 1347, the causative agent of plague was still unknown. It took another 547 years for the plague pathogen to be discovered.[7] Plague recurred in virulent onslaughts since 1348 and became endemic in the Mediterranean and Western Europe, remaining a constant reality of life of the early modern world for over 350 years.[8]

The fact that the Ottoman Empire, with which the Ragusan Republic shared a land border since 1463, did not have any organized plague control measures, was a constant source of concern for the citizens of Dubrovnik. Still, it seems that all major plague onslaughts had arrived on an infected ship, either directly from the Ottoman-controlled territories, or indirectly, via an Italian port city.[9]

Luckily, in cities such as Milan, Venice, Dubrovnik, and others, secular authorities, surgeons, and chroniclers, trusting their experience based on observation, came to the conclusion that plague is a communicable disease. These beliefs were instrumental in the development of plague control measures even though the mechanism of disease transmission remained a mystery for many centuries. Was it the patient himself or the corrupt humours that were poisoning the ambient air?[10] Was it through contagion – the idea that a disease could be transmitted from one person to another by contact? Or was it infection – the concept that a disease was caused by some agent that taints the environment or objects?[11] The idea that each disease could be caused by a unique agent became prevalent only in the nineteenth century.[12]

Plague is an extremely infectious disease with a very high mortality rate. It is primarily a rodent infection, a disease of the rats, as well as of many species of wild rats and sylvatic rodents (gerbils, marmots, prairie dogs, and squirrels). In humans, it is overwhelmingly a by-product of rodent infection, transmitted by an insect bite. The course of plague is thus determined by a very complex ecosystem involving a triad of hosts. The rat flea, *Xenopsyla cheopis*, lives on the rat as an ectoparasite and usually becomes infected by biting the infected host. Showing signs of septicaemia, the infected rat is able to withstand enormous concentrations of the plague bacillus.[13] When the flea sucks in the infected blood of the rat – its host – the bacteria in the flea's gut multiply with great speed and eventually form a solid mass in the proventriculus, which becomes obstructed.[14] At the same time, the flea feels extreme hunger and thirst, and, with frequent new bites, tries to satisfy its needs. When rats die of plague and become cold, their fleas are forced to seek the blood of other hosts, including humans. Unable to pump blood into its stomach, the flea then regurgitates the rats' bacteria-loaded blood into the tissues of its new host and becomes a vector of plague transmission to humans. Plague incubation in humans lasts from one to a maximum of seven days. When Alexandre Yersin identified the plague bacillus in 1894, he noticed a lot of dead rats in the affected area of Hong Kong. He suspected that rats were involved in the disease transmission but it was his colleague Paul-Louis Simond, also from the Pasteur Institute, who discovered the mechanism of the plague bacillus transmission from rat to flea to humankind. In Karachi, on 2 June 1897, Simond wrote, "I felt an indescribable emotion at the thought that I had just uncovered a secret that had tortured man since the appearance of plague on earth."[15]

When a blocked flea bites a new human victim, a small swelling appears on the site of the fleabite. This area can subsequently become necrotic – dead tissue blackens to produce a carbuncle or necrotic pustule, often called a "carbone" in many historical accounts.[16] Soon, egg-shaped swellings, the so-called buboes – hence the name bubonic plague – form near lymph nodes as a reaction to the multiplication of plague bacteria. The buboes, reaching the size of one to ten centimetres, usually appear on inguinal, axillary, and/or cervical lymph nodes. They become inflamed and unbearably painful. As the lymph nodes try to drain the infection, the buboes become full of pus. In historical accounts, there is often mention of buboes being incised and drained by physicians or surgeons to relieve the pain. On the first day, the patient develops high fever accompanied by headache, chills, and exhaustion. Because of toxins released into the blood, neurological symptoms appear on the second day. The patient becomes delirious. Death ensues between the third and the fifth day. If not treated, the mortality rate is estimated at between 60 percent and 90 percent, depending on the virulence of the bacteria. If the virulence is high, bacteria multiply very quickly. The so-called septicaemic plague, caused by blood poisoning, develops in the space of a few hours. In such cases, there is no time for buboes to develop. Death occurs within a few hours. If left untreated, mortality is almost 100 percent. Even with pharmaceutical products available today, it is very difficult to influence the course of the disease in such a short time span.[17] The pulmonary or pneumonic plague is another form of the disease in which buboes have no time to develop as the infection spreads directly from human to human through respiratory droplets. This is the reason why pneumonic plague is the most dangerous form of pestilence. If left untreated, the mortality rate is close to 100 percent.[18]

Rapid passage from health to death convinced the fourteenth-century subjects of the dangerous nature of this disease. Only a hasty retreat from the infected area could provide protection. The recommendation of the physicians was to flee fast, as far as possible and return as late as possible – *fuge cito, longe et tarde revertere*.[19]

A more accurate picture of mediaeval and early modern plague epidemics can be achieved only by multidisciplinary collaboration of many specialists. Still, contemporary notions of plague epidemiology have to be applied with great caution to epidemics in history. In spite of all the knowledge gained, it is still not possible to fully explain some aspects of historical plagues such as virulence, immunity, spreading, cyclical repetition, or even the disappearance of plague. Paul Slack and Stephen Ell state that one should not look for a single factor in the disappearance of plague as several may be at work: mutation of the organism, immunity of the rats, improvements in hygiene. They add that human action definitely played an important role in the disappearance of plague.[20] Peter Christensen firmly believes that public health measures and health officials were instrumental in eradicating plague from Europe. He notes that quarantine was in some cases ineffective because it was half-heartedly applied but that there were many instances where it was quite successful.[21] According to Alfonso Corradi, the basic principles of the quarantines were right but difficult to implement. If they failed, it was because their purpose was not well understood and all members of society did not cooperate to the same degree. Moreover, people used their cunning and invoked their privileges to stand above the law.[22]

Samuel Cohn also presents a vigorous argument in favour of the effectiveness of plague control measures in Italy in comparison with Northern Europe where they were not implemented.[23] Gunther E. Rothenberg argues that since the Austrian sanitary cordon, one of the largest and longest lasting public health measures ever undertaken, had been established, there were no more outbreaks of plague in Austria and Central Europe.[24] To summarize, various authors have tackled the disappearance of plague and have come up with an assorted list of answers, but most of them firmly believe that plague control measures ultimately freed Europe from plague. This disease remains a very complex phenomenon that demands more research.[25] An approach that combines historical sources with scientific research, especially in epidemiology and molecular biology, should benefit scholars on all sides of the plague debate.[26]

Since the 1950s, plague has been successfully treated with antibiotics, thus considerably reducing its morbidity and dramatically lowering its mortality to about 10 percent. Ideally, in an epidemic outbreak of plague, the goal should be to vaccinate as many people as possible. However, an effective and safe vaccine has not yet been developed. Several vaccines have been tried with more or less success. The main complaints were the short-lived protection of the vaccines and major adverse effects, which led to a gradual decline in their utilization. Furthermore, the immunity acquired by vaccination seems to be antibody-mediated and short-lived. It does not confer protection against a second attack. Although many questions regarding immunity to plague remain unanswered, long-term immunity appears to be cellular. The plague bacterium is taken up by the host cells and continues to live inside the cells in some tissues after the acute illness, thus giving lifelong immunity. This is the type of immunity that was acquired by mediaeval and early modern plague survivors. Persons who were treated with antibiotic drugs since the twentieth century may not have acquired this long-lasting cellular immunity. In Madagascar, in 1995, the first multi-resistant strain of *Yersinia pestis* was isolated from a patient suffering from bubonic plague. The resistance involved all the antibiotics recommended for plague therapy.[27]

THE PLAGUE EPIDEMICS IN DUBROVNIK

The accounts of the plague outbreaks in Dubrovnik that we recount in this book were gleaned from the Ragusan chroniclers – the Anonymous, Nikola Ragnina, and Serafino Razzi – as well as from archival and other sources.[28]

The second plague pandemic of 1347 devastated the majority of Mediterranean ports. The Dalmatian port cities of Zadar, Šibenik, Split, and Dubrovnik suffered serious plague epidemics and catastrophic demographic losses.[29] The Ragusan chronicler Nikola Ragnina writes, "The outbreak began on 15 January and lasted seven months, and it can be said that it lasted three years, in two ways. In the first five months the symptoms were continuous fever and spitting blood – those patients died within three days; the second type was accompanied by fever and abscesses in the armpits and the inguinal area – those patients died within five days. It was highly contagious, especially if one stood close to an infected person; and even from looking at each other, the people caught it. There was no remedy for it and all died, except at the end, those who had mature buboes. Seeing that the physicians could not defend them, the citizens decided to flee the city and purify the air with fire. When the scare was over, they were not eager to return."[30] In 1348, Dubrovnik suffered the greatest demographic loss of its whole thousand-year history.[31]

Stjepan Krivošić estimates that about fifteen thousand inhabitants lived in the district of Dubrovnik at that time.[32] On the basis of the number of the patricians usually present at the meetings of the Ragusan Councils the year before the plague in comparison with 1348, Krivošić maintains, without estimating the number that had died, that the mortality must have been lower than the losses reported by the chroniclers because patrician families had survived and their continuity was assured. Among the *casatae*, the enlarged nuclear families, 75 percent had become extinct and only 25 percent of the *casatae* were newly formed.[33]

Gordan Ravančić analyzed the 311 testaments from 1348 preserved in the State Archives of Dubrovnik. Most of the wills were written from January to May, with an apex in April 1348. This led Ravančić to conclude that the epidemic must have reached its most virulent climax in that period of the year. The archival documents demonstrate that in 1351 all the testaments from 1348 were still not executed. The decisions of the government testify to the massive flight of the population from the city. On 12 April, the Major Council ordered all Ragusans to return to the city before the following Wednesday. The Ragusans were also forbidden from leaving the city or its district but merchants were exempt. The same order had to be repeated in July. On 13 April, the Minor Council permitted the return to the city of all Ragusans who had left because of debts. This order had to be repeated in June. On 30 May 1348, the Major Council decided that from that date on, due to the great number of people who had died in Dubrovnik during the deadly plague outbreak, the age of entry into the Major Council would be lowered from twenty to eighteen. On the same day, the craftsmen were invited to come to live in the city, exempt from taxes for five years: three came in May, seven in June, ten in July, two in October, and one in December.[34] Immediately after the epidemic, as a result of major demographic losses, the prices of grain, salt, and wine were increased and stayed high in the 1350s; the wages of labourers and craftsmen were also higher.[35]

The 1348 plague outbreak had the potential of influencing the wealth (re)distribution in Dubrovnik to some degree. Due to high mortality, some individuals inherited considerable fortunes from several families. In 1348, two patrician women, Phylippa Menčetić (Mence) and Nicoletta Gučetić (Goce), were the only heirs of both their natal and their husbands' families. Phylippa Menčetić invested her fortune and managed to increase it while Nicoletta Gučetić decided to leave it all to one particular convent. Such concentration of great wealth in only one person was frowned upon by the Ragusan Councils. The usual pattern in wills was to distribute the charitable bequests among a number of monasteries and convents, with convents getting only a tiny proportion of what the monasteries received. (Compare the testament of Angelo de Leticia in Appendix C.)

The legality of Nicoletta's second husband's will was challenged by Francho de Basilio, her second husband's sister's son. Nicoletta was brought to trial, imprisoned, and eventually exiled from Dubrovnik for allegedly falsifying her second husband's testament, something that was never proven. Her troubles were probably exacerbated by her unwillingness to look after the next of kin first.[36] The other factor that sealed her destiny was her desire to leave this sizeable fortune to only one convent without considering monasteries. Notaries preparing the wills usually reminded the testators of their duty and proposed a formula according to which charitable gifts were distributed among several churches, monasteries, and convents in keeping with the Ragusan tradition. Later plague upsurges created similar awkward situations in which the Ragusan Councils intervened.

If plague was the expression of "the wrath of God" against a city or state, and not only against individuals who had done something wrong, then there was a possibility that the community could build up a pool of shared merits to keep the epidemics at bay. The Church considered that protection should be sought in God's grace, through prayer and repentance for one's sins; participation in religious processions and material assistance of priests, nuns, and monks; charity to the poor; bequests to churches, monasteries, and convents; and construction of votive churches dedicated to Virgin Mary and intercessory saints against the plague, above all St Sebastian and St Roch.[37] Even if the attitude of the Church towards plague was different from that of the state, its dignitaries had to obey the pragmatic public health measures of the secular government just like any other citizen.

Under these circumstances, the perception of God was changing. God was viewed as a distant judge who needed to be placated with the assistance of intercessory saints.[38] Everyone participated in this effort: the government and the individuals. The Senate, for example, used to start a new session by first donating some money for charity. In their testaments, individuals used to leave a significant part of their personal estate to the Church and for various charitable purposes. It was customary for the notary to remind the testator of his or her duty in that regard.[39] In quite a few wills the testator left a bequest for a priest to go on the donor's behalf on a pilgrimage to Rome, the Holy Land, or another shrine, usually in Italy, and pray there for the salvation of the donor's soul. It was also customary to leave an amount of money for a thousand masses to be celebrated for the salvation of one's soul (see Appendix C).[40]

In times of plague, votive offerings, a centuries-old tradition in Dubrovnik, became even more frequent because it was believed that such donations could ensure the grace of God and the protection against plague. A new votive Church of St Blaise, nicer and bigger than the old one, was built at a cost of forty thousand ducats.[41] Among the testaments of 1348, the will of Angelo de Leticia stands out (see Appendix C). He leaves one hundred *hyperperi* for the erection of a Church of the Annunciation of the Virgin Mary to be built on Mount Krstac (Cresta), on the way to Ombla, and he wants it to be constructed as fast as possible (see Figure 2.1). From the wording, we can tell that the testator is in a hurry. Angelo de Leticia does not forget to include the necessary income for the

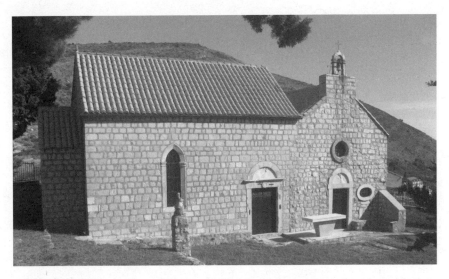

Figure 2.1 Church of the Annunciation in Gruž (right), votive church against the plague built in 1348, bequest of Angelo de Leticia. The church on the left side was added by the patrician family Sorkočević (Sorgo) in the sixteenth century.

upkeep of the church. He commands that his vineyard in Župa be given to that church in order to provide a permanent income for the priest who will serve there. The testator asks the priest of this church to celebrate two holy masses a week for his soul. The degree to which life was threatened during the plague outbreak is best illustrated by the fact that Angelo de Leticia named six executors of his will in the hope that at least two would survive. And should they all die, God forbid, he asked the highly respected treasurers of St Mary to be his executors.[42]

Virgin Mary was considered humanity's most powerful intercessor against the plague. According to the wishes of Angelo de Leticia, the Church of the Annunciation of the Virgin Mary, built in the Romanesque-Gothic style with a semicircular apse, was thus erected on a steep hill just above the port of Gruž, after the 1348 plague outbreak. This church still dominates its surroundings as a compelling visual guideline in the Ragusan urban landscape.[43] After this first votive church, the whole settlement on this escarpment in Dubrovnik came to be known as Nuncijata – Annunciation in Ragusan speech. It was believed at that time that justice was wholly localized in Christ, while mercy became the exclusive domain of the Virgin. Mercy was the source of her immense appeal: she constantly set herself against God's punitive intentions as well as against the strict accounting of divine justice, Mary is therefore presented as an omnipotent source of compassion, ceaselessly responsive to the needs of the faithful.[44]

Angelo de Leticia was a wealthy Ragusan landowner who left a considerable portion of his personal estate to his wife, his son, and his grandson. Nor did he forget the illegitimate son of his son. Another sizeable part of his estate was distributed for charitable purposes. The offerings of Angelo de Leticia have historical significance. He left a donation of 1,100 *hyperperi* for the construction of the bell tower of St Mary the Great, the cathedral of Dubrovnik, and additional sums for the construction of three churches, that of St Blaise, St Stephen, and St Peter the Great. Angelo de Leticia also bequeathed sums of money to the Franciscan and Dominican friars and other monasteries. Very small, symbolic amounts were entrusted to convents but appreciable amounts of money were assigned for hundreds of holy masses to be celebrated for the salvation of his soul.

This was related to the idea of purgatory. It was believed at that time that after death a person could still be saved if his soul was purged of sin. Purgatory was considered to be that intermediate state in which souls were prepared for the final judgment. In this process, the testament played an important role. The time of purging could be shortened by good deeds and charitable donations. Everyone, therefore, tried to prepare the transition from this world to the next as best he or she could. Thus, we find that, in the wills, individuals tried to give back whatever was unjustly taken, pay off their debts, straighten out injustices, and, in general, make peace with the people around them. Through the notion of purgatory, the Church gained a new source of power and a new source of income. At the same time, the faithful were offered hope and their fear of the fateful moment of death was diminished.[45]

We owe another outstanding work of art of that period to a bequest at the time of plague. In his will, composed on 3 March 1348, Šime Paskvin Rastić (Resti), a Ragusan patrician, left eighty *hyperperi* for a painted crucifix to be hung in the Dominican church in Dubrovnik.[46] A masterpiece of that era, the painted crucifix with Our Lady and St John on separate panels, has been attributed to the Venetian master Paolo Veneziano (ca 1333–1358). He probably painted it during his stay in Dubrovnik in 1352 (see Figure 2.2). However, it was only in 1358 that it was placed in the church as a votive offering against the plague.[47]

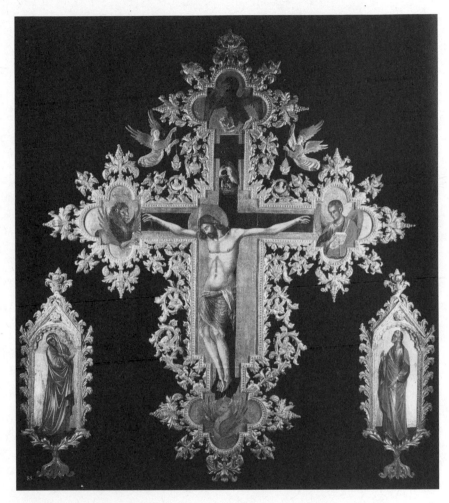

Figure 2.2 Painted Crucifix with Our Lady and St John by Paolo Veneziano, 1352, bequest of Šime Paskvin Rastić (Resti), 1348

Before the end of the fourteenth century, there were eight more plague on-slaughts in Dubrovnik. In 1357–58 and 1361, according to chroniclers, plague originated in Alexandria. Judging by the number of testaments (305), the 1361 outbreak seems to have been quite deadly. When plague was not prevalent, there were around thirty testaments a year.[48] Twenty-five hundred people per-ished "from fever and anthrax carbuncles" (*con febre et carboncoli antraci*), including Ilija Saraka, the highly respected archbishop of Dubrovnik.[49] In 1363, many citizens left the city, although the Rector Marin Menčetić (Menze) had instituted regulations against flight from the city.[50] In May, news about the epidemic in Apulia and Marche regions of Italy reached Dubrovnik, forcing the authorities to forbid travellers from those regions to enter the city and its district. Likewise, Ragusans were not allowed to travel to those regions.[51] From 1371 to 1374, Dubrovnik suffered several plague attacks. Ragnina claims that twenty-five thousand people died during that time.[52]

The 1390 plague prevalent in Rome seems to have reached Dubrovnik in spring 1391. Ston was practically empty. Andrija, the chancellor of Ston, stayed to guard the gate of Ston and to perform the duties of those who had fled. On 5 February 1392, Andrija Ragnina, the count of the Ragusan islands, who lived on the island of Šipan, was allowed to live on another island until the plague had subsided on Šipan or until told otherwise by the Minor Council.[53] In 1397, the Pelješac Peninsula was affected by plague.[54] In 1399, there were a few cases of plague in the city.[55] From their experience since 1348, the Ragusans had learned that plague was a recurring phenomenon. The first quarantine legislation was therefore promulgated in 1377 and the first plague officials charged with enforcing it were elected in 1390 (see Chapter 4, p. 109).

The new century started with a renewed plague upsurge that lasted two years.[56] In May 1400, the Venetian Senate, having concluded that Dubrovnik had denied the Venetian ships access to its port when plague was prevalent in Venice, decided not to admit Ragusan ships and refugees who were fleeing the plague epidemic.[57] Trade bans as retaliatory measures against commercial rivals created serious internal problems for cities affected by plague. What is even worse, from the sixteenth century onward, such measures were often used as instruments of foreign policy.[58] Chroniclers cited high mortality figures. Due to the epidemics, the number of Ragusan patricians in 1400 was 30 percent lower than in 1350.[59]

On 1 May 1416, because of plague, special measures for governing with only a few patricians present in the city were adopted. Five patricians were elected to govern and to find another twelve to fifteen patricians who willing to stay in the city with pay. When the plague abated on 29 June, the feast day of Sts Peter and Paul, the Major Council ordered a solemn procession to be held every year on that day at the church of these apostles and a holy mass to be celebrated in the presence of the rector and the Minor Council.[60] The physician Jacobus de Gondovaldis was present in Dubrovnik at that time. He advised the Senate to concentrate on prevention by isolating the infected.[61]

On 5 May 1422, by the decision of the Senate, the Ragusans were forbidden to travel to plague-infected ports on the western side of the Adriatic and

Valona (today Vlorë in Albania). On 8 May, special regulations were adopted for governing the city if only a few patricians were present. The measures that were adopted were similar to those in 1416. However, they proved unnecessary. The Councils never left the city during the summer of 1422 because the plague outbreak proved milder than expected. The infected were sent to Mrkan (St Mark), the islet of St Peter, and to the three major islands – Koločep, Lopud, and Šipan. By the end of September, all were allowed to return to the city.[62]

In 1427, plague struck the island of Lopud, which was kept under surveillance for another year. On 24 October 1427, the patrician Marin Nikolin Gučetić (Goze) was designated to supervise two ships that sailed around Lopud to make sure that the inhabitants of Lopud did not come in contact with anyone from anywhere else.[63] To relieve the food shortage, a ship was allowed to dock in Lopud but only to throw food items to the shore and no one was allowed to disembark. The infected were sent to the islet of Ruda in the vicinity, and the healthy were allowed to move to Dubrovnik within eight days. After that period, they had to either return to Lopud or leave the territory of the Republic, escorted by a Ragusan ship, which was to make sure that they did not stop anywhere within the Republic. When the plague outbreak in Lopud abated at the end of November, the inhabitants quarantined on various tiny islands were allowed to return home under the escort of a ship. In Dubrovnik the stores were closed for three days. People were asked to fast and hold processions every day for the extinction of the plague.[64]

Three years later, on 27 November 1430, the Senate adopted special regulations for governing if only a few patricians were present in the city during the plague onset.[65] The physician Jacobus de Gondovaldis, who was serving in Dubrovnik at that time, advised the authorities to burn the belongings of those who had died of plague.[66]

In 1431, plague was present on the island of Koločep. A ship was sent to sail around the island and prevent contact with the outside world. It stayed there all summer and the inhabitants were not allowed to leave the island to earn a living. The government, therefore, gave them a loan of fifty *hyperperi* and delivered grain and oil to the island. On 18 January, the authorities decided to build a house for the persons quarantined on the islet of St Peter to protect them from the elements. It was to be ten metres long and four metres wide, divided into two parts, each of which was to have a door, windows, and a chimney.[67]

Plague assaulted the city in April 1437 and declined in force by the feast of St John the Baptist, which is celebrated on 24 June.[68] This plague outbreak, as well as the plague control measures that the Ragusan government undertook, are described in detail by Diversis, who became sick with plague and survived (see Chapter 4, p. 119–21). From 1400 to 1450, despite plague epidemics, and due to generally positive economic and political trends, the population of Dubrovnik had doubled.[69]

In 1456 to 1459, plague was again constantly present somewhere on the territory of the Republic. Several times, after having adopted special regulations for the defence of the city, and a number of sanitary measures, the Councils had to leave the city and met in Gruž. When plague struck again in 1457, a votive Church of Our Lady at Danče, in an area of Dubrovnik just outside the city walls, was erected.[70]

In 1459, since the Ragusans thought that plague had reached their city by sea, they put special guards at the entrance to the Dubrovnik harbour. A captain from Lopud was accused of bringing plague on his ship. On 9 August 1459, the Major Council debated whether this ship should be burnt. The sentence was to serve as an example to other citizens and to warn them about avoiding such situations. However, the majority of the councillors decided that the Lopud ship should not be burnt.[71]

The Republic was again tested in a cruel way by plague onslaughts from 1464 to 1466. Considerable financial means were spent to combat plague and defend the territory of the Republic. For the protection of the harbour, an armed galleon was situated near the city. This plague onrush was even more of a challenge because it occurred at a time when the Ottomans had conquered Bosnia (in 1463) and it was feared that they could attack Dubrovnik.[72] The government spent four hundred ducats for the maintenance of the sick and six thousand ducats for the defence of the city. The quarantine compound at Danče was built at that time.

During the 1466 plague epidemic, at the entrance to the city, close to the Dominican monastery, a Gothic Church of St Sebastian was erected. According to Nikola Ragnina, as soon as the construction of the church had started, the plague became extinct.[73] The church, which had to be built close to the entrance to the city so that St Sebastian could prevent plague from entering the community, was built by Mihoč Radišić and Vlatko Dešković (see Figure 2.3). The perception of plague as "God's arrow" gave the incentive for the veneration of this early Christian saint who was tortured during the reign of the Roman Emperor Diocletian. St Sebastian, usually shown as a young man wearing only a loincloth, became a patron saint against the plague because his body was pierced by arrows that did not kill him. His body was wounded but he was still alive. St Sebastian acted as a living "lightning rod" drawing the plague arrows

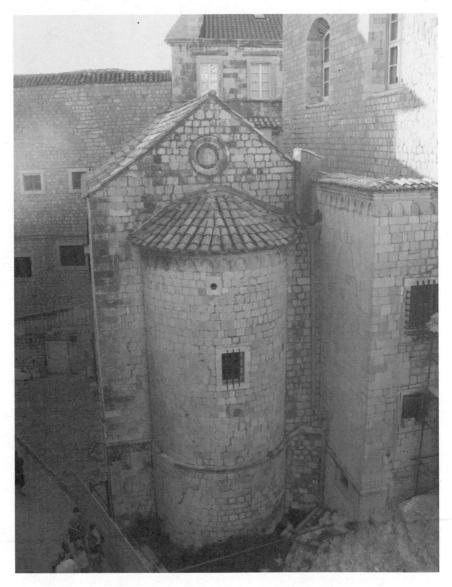

Figure 2.3 Church of St Sebastian, built in 1466 near the Ploče gate in Dubrovnik

away from people and "grounding" them harmlessly in his own flesh (see Figure 2.4).[74] According to legend, it was sufficient for a believer to see St Sebastian's image and be certain that on that day he or she would not die.[75] This saint's genuine suffering for his faith was thought to recommend him to God.[76]

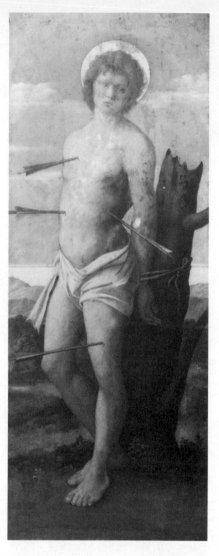

Figure 2.4 St Sebastian by Girolamo Santacroce, polyptych of the Church of St Mary of Špilica on the island of Lopud, detail, sixteenth century

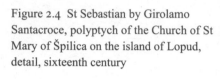

After fifteen years of reprieve, Dubrovnik was again infected by plague in 1482. To protect the lives of citizens, the authorities adopted a whole range of strict plague control measures and numerous regulations concerning the defence of the city (see Chapter 4). Since the patricians designated to govern the city had little desire to linger in the infected city, shifts were organized to allow the patricians to take turns of duty. The order of presence, the number of patricians required, and the length of time needed were clearly spelled out for each group. The Councils met in Gruž. The soldiers responsible for the defence of the city were allowed to spend time on the boats in the harbour instead of remaining within the city walls.[77]

In 1497, plague spread to Dyrrachium (today Durrës) and Valona (today Vlorë) in Albania, and further to Macedonia and Thessaloniki. In 1500, the plague continued its spread to Italy and Germany, all the way north to Cologne. On the Croatian coast, it ravaged Istria, Senj, and Zadar.[78] When, in the same year, people from all over Europe gathered in Rome for the celebration of the Christian jubilee, the danger of infection was evidently increased. The Ragusan pilgrims returning from Rome brought back to Dubrovnik a mild plague outbreak.[79] Upon their return home, they were questioned and confined to their houses (see Chapter 5). In 1517, a fever was present in the city, but it turned out not to be plague.[80]

To prevent the penetration of the disease, votive churches were always situated at the entrance to the city. The people craved protection and they certainly needed hope. Thus, in the fifteenth and sixteenth centuries, a considerable number of chapels and churches of Annunciation were built in Dubrovnik and its surroundings. At the beginning of the sixteenth century, the patrician family Sorkočević (Sorgo) attached on the left side of the Church of Annunciation in Gruž, a bigger chapel in the Gothic style, and added its coat of arms on the windows and the portal. The original three-part altar painting of the Annunciation has not been preserved.[81] However, the following exceptionally valuable artefacts are still present: a Renaissance stone altar from the sixteenth century and a rare figurehead from an eighteenth-century ship in the shape of a likeness of the Madonna with Christ, which became an object of devotion. In the past, the confraternity of St George administered the church. In 1897, the owner of the church was Pero Mihov Lujak, who added a new religious element to the architecture – a grotto with a sculpture of Our Lady of Lourdes. It is one of the oldest and the most beautiful grottos in Dubrovnik and its surroundings.[82]

The lethal plague outbreak that struck Dubrovnik in 1526–27 was certainly the most tragic since the first epidemic in 1348. It caused the demographic loss of more than 20,000 people that Dubrovnik could not replace in the centuries to come.[83] There were 38 testaments in 1526, 188 in 1527, and 46 in 1528.[84] The vertiginous multiplication of testaments in 1527 is a telling indication of the high level of mortality in that year.

LIBRO DELI SIGNORI CHAZAMORBI, SANITAS, SERIES 55, V. I, 1500–1530

The plague control measures adopted in Dubrovnik to combat this calamitous epidemic will be described and analyzed in the second half of this work (see Chapters 6 through 9). By the year 1526, the tradition of plague containment had been part of government policy for 150 years, and yet, the city could not

avoid this plague eruption. Zlata Blažina Tomić gleaned the most valuable information about this epidemic from the only surviving book kept by the health
officials, the manuscript *Libro deli Signori Chazamorbi, Sanitas, Series 55, v.
1, 1500–1530*. While health books for other periods have been preserved only
in fragments, this one is complete (see Figures 2.5 and 2.6).

In comparison with the fourteenth and fifteenth centuries, the archival
sources concerning the plague control measures in sixteenth-century Dubrovnik
are not so plentiful. One of the reasons is surely the fact that the books of the
health officials contained in the medical series Sanitas no longer exist. In that
context, the exceptional value of *Libro deli Signori Cazamorbi* has to be appreciated. This manuscript has never been analyzed before, probably because
of its intricate palaeographic characteristics. Its cursive script, extremely difficult to decipher, may have been the main reason that it lie ignored in the
archives for almost five centuries. The late Zdravko Šundrica, the expert
archivist of the State Archives of Dubrovnik, to whom we owe our deepest
gratitude, accomplished the tremendous task of transcribing the manuscript
from mediaeval Latin.

The manuscript offers a day-after-day, month-after-month, and year-after-
year record of the actions of the health officials in the first thirty years of the
sixteenth century. It chronicles everyday events in the lives of Ragusans of
every social class, sex, and age group during the times when plague was not
rampant as well as during a major plague outbreak in 1526–27. It relates the
suffering of the citizens from the plague as well as their subdued resistance to
public health measures.

The manuscript consists of two parts: the *A recto*, the front part, and the *A
tergo*, the back part of the book.[85] The whole document contains 236 folios.
The two sides of the book have a completely different content. The *A recto* consists of 101 leaves or 202 pages. In it, the health officials recorded the arrivals
of people and goods in Dubrovnik, by land and sea, and the sworn statements
of travellers who, under the threat of fines and imprisonment, vouched that they
had not visited any plague infected areas (see Chapter 5). Conceptually, the *A
tergo*, which consists of 135 leaves or 270 pages, constitutes the most important part of the book because it contains the original scribal notes of the trial
proceedings conducted by the health officials against those who had contravened the public health regulations, especially during the deadly 1526–27
plague epidemic (see Chapters 7, 8, and 9).

Four unnumbered leaves are inserted between the folios 97v and 98. They
contain a letter, dated 13 September 1528, addressed by the health officials to

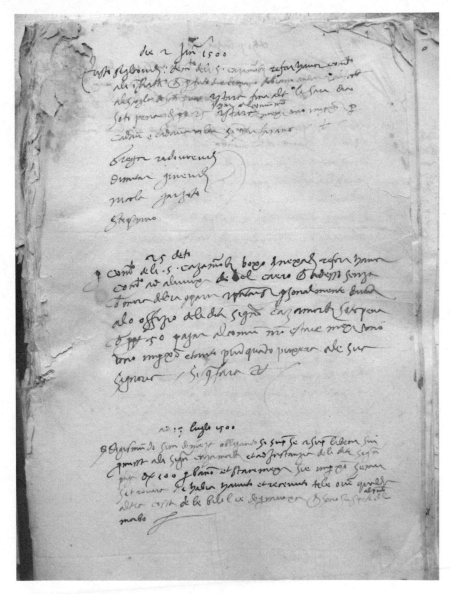

Figure 2.5 Facsimile of the manuscript *Libro deli Signori Chazamorbi, Sanitas 55, v. 1, 1500–1530, A tergo*, f. 1

the patrician Rafael Nikolin Gučetić (Goze) from Mljet. In it, the health officials order Rafael Gučetić to go by boat from Mljet to Zaton, and from there, because of the plague outbreak in Zaton, to transport several families to an islet close to Mljet.[86]

The *A recto* part of the book was written by five different scribes and chancellors while the *A tergo* part was recorded by six different hands. Rinaldo is

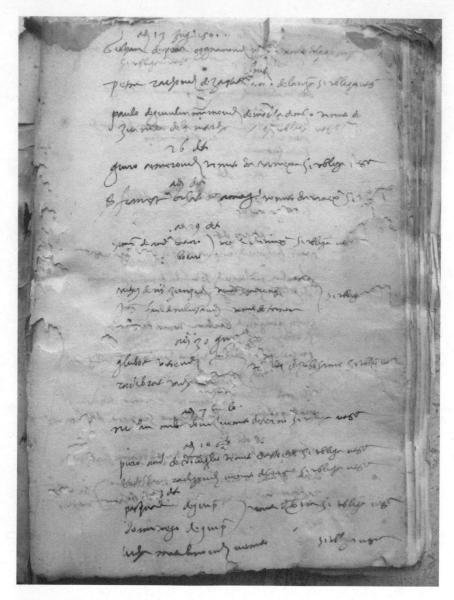

Figure 2.6 Facsimile of the manuscript *Libro deli Signori Chazamorbi, Sanitas 55, v. 1, 1500–1530, A recto*, f. 1

the only scribe who has signed his name, albeit in an abbreviated form – *R-do*.[87] Depending on the region of his origin, each scribe wrote in his own Italian dialect and sometimes added local Croatian expressions from the Ragusan speech – often spelled the Italian way, as the scribe had heard them.

ST ROCH AND OUR LADY AS INTERCESSORY SAINTS
AGAINST THE PLAGUE

The plague outbreak of 1526 ushered in the era of a new intercessory saint
against the plague. Following the Black Death, the paintings of the fourteenth
century were macabre and pessimistic.[88] However, in the sixteenth century,
hope and healing were more prevalent than fear and suffering. The paintings
showed not only how people coped with the plague but also how they expressed
their deepest hopes for health and salvation.[89] At the end of the fifteenth century, St Roch (ca 1295–1327 or ca 1348–1376–79), who was probably born in
Montpellier, became a new saint invoked against the plague. As a young man,
he went on a pilgrimage to Italy, where he helped care for the plague-stricken
patients. In Piacenza, he became sick with plague. When he felt the first symptoms of plague, Roch withdrew into the forest not to spread the disease. The dog
of a generous nobleman brought him food and thus helped him to survive. All
biographies of St Roch mention this episode because, by that time, the attitude
towards plague was changing. It was no longer considered "God's wrath" but
a disease that could be controlled with pragmatic plague control measures.[90]
When Roch recovered, according to one version, he returned to Montpellier
where, accused of spying, he ended up in prison and died. According to another version, he ended up in prison in Voghera, Italy, and died there. A confraternity of St Roch was established in Venice in 1478, and Venetians acquired
his remains in 1485. Building of a church dedicated to St Roch was begun in
Venice in 1489.[91] From then on, his cult spread quickly all over Europe. He became a symbol of a saint who had triumphed over plague and offered a promise of cure.[92] In paintings and sculpture, St Sebastian and St Roch often appear
together, sometimes accompanied by other saints such as St Cosmas and St
Damian, St Anthony the Abbot and St Vincent Ferrer, all helpful against the
plague. To ensure survival, the intercession of powerful protective saints whose
cult promoted reassurance, such as St Roch, was sought.[93]

St Roch is usually shown dressed as a pilgrim, carrying a staff, accompanied by his dog and by an angel who healed him. The saint always shows the
bubo on his thigh, his symptom of plague.[94] Vanzan Marchini maintains that the
cult of St Roch was chosen by the state of Venice with an educational goal in
mind: to teach people about the symptoms of plague (febrile face, hallucinat-
ing eyes, and the inguinal bubo) and to alert them to the danger of pilgrims,

travellers, and beggars. The government wanted the people of Venice to imitate the behaviour of St Roch who had chosen to die alone in the woods rather than transmit disease. The dog that brought him bread every day saved his life. The cult of St Roch was to help authorities persuade people to enter the lazarettos to be treated, but also to protect the community. The dog represents the public handout that the government provided until the patient's reinsertion into society. The depiction of the life of St Roch became the central tool of the campaign of information and of sanitary propaganda of the newly created Venetian Health Office.[95]

In Dubrovnik, the calamitous plague eruption of 1526–27 gave the impetus for the construction of new votive churches as well as offerings of votive altar paintings. There were also expressions of increased devotion. On the 1 January 1527, the Minor Council decided to donate money to eight convents, two monasteries of mendicant orders, the Church of St Mary the Great, and the Church of St Blaise. These donations were for holy masses to be celebrated so that "God may illuminate our government in order that we may govern this year in peace, health, humility always in fear of God and in the grace of God." It was also decided that throughout the year 1527, mass should be celebrated every Friday in the Church of St Blaise and every Saturday in the Church of St Mary and all the alms collected should be used for "our health and prosperity."[96]

In 1527, a small Church of St Roch was built in the Boninovo area of Dubrovnik, outside the walled city, in a street that once bore the name of St Roch but that today is a blind alley off the Ante Starčević main artery. On the gable hidden by the vegetation, one can still read "St Roch pray for us" (*Sante Roche ora pro nobis*). The text below this plea states that the church was built in 1527 and renovated in 1855.[97] In 1527, 16 August, the feast day of St Roch, became a state holiday in Dubrovnik.

The chapel of St Roch, added to the Church of our Lady of Šunj, built in 1488, was erected by Thomas Pidelli on the island of Lopud. The arched ceiling of the church bears the inscription: "Here Thomas Pidelli constructed a chapel to the divine Roch in 1527" (*Hoc tibi dive Roche Thomas Pidelli condidit sacellum 1527*). A sculpture and a painting of St Roch previously adorned this chapel. The sculpture of St Roch was later removed from the chapel but it can be seen in the Lopud Parish Museum. In the past, another chapel of St Roch existed on the northern side of Lopud.[98]

On 29 May 1533, Dubrovnik suffered the last major plague flare-up that penetrated the city walls. The Senate adopted the usual measures in times of plague, ensured the protection of the state, and issued specific orders to the health officials concerning the infected and their homes. Two galleons and one *fusta*, a fast ship, were armed for the defence of the city.[99] The quorum was reduced in all the Councils (see Chapter 6). The government decided to build the Gothic-Renaissance Church of the Annunciation in the space between the Dominican monastery and the city walls, close to the Ploče gate.[100] According to tradition, the church, with the angel of the Annunciation on the gable of its portal, was built on the spot where the house of the first victim of that plague outbreak, burned down by the authorities, used to stand (see Figure 1.4). For people dreading the onslaught of plague, the angel on the gable of the church portal, with his hands folded in prayer, conveyed hope that they would be spared. Petar Andrijić, the famous stonemason, finished the ornamentation of the church in 1534. This indicates that the construction of the church was begun as soon as the plague had started diminishing (see Figures 2.7 and 2.8).[101] On 2 October 1533, all the special plague control measures were revoked and all the public officials, including the courts, resumed their duties.[102] After that, there were smaller plague flare-ups for another twenty months.

The decision to build a Renaissance Church of St Roch in the city was made in 1535.[103] The construction was begun in 1540 or 1542 and lasted for fourteen years. Roko Fasano, an esteemed apothecary who came to Dubrovnik from Padua and stayed until the end of his life in 1598, was one of the founders of the confraternity of St Roch in 1558. As prior of the confraternity, Fasano was very active in securing the construction of the Church of St Roch in the city (see Figure 1.4).[104] The goals of the confraternity were to provide moral education of their members; mutual assistance to members who fall sick; assistance to poor young women in getting married; preparation and accompaniment to the gallows of those sentenced to death. The confraternity had two nurses whose duty it was to visit the sick and administer drugs.

The 1540 plague epidemic lasted three months, according to the chroniclers. However, it may have been some other communicable disease and not plague. One thousand ducats were spent to combat the epidemic and one galleon and two fustas were armed for the defence of the city.[105] The plague epidemics in the first half of the sixteenth century caused a major population drop. By 1550, the number of inhabitants in the Republic had dropped to approximately 53,000 and the number of patricians to 1,565.[106]

In mid-sixteenth century, Girolamo Santacroce (ca 1480–1556) painted St Roch in tempera on wood panel for the Franciscan Church of St Mary of Špilica

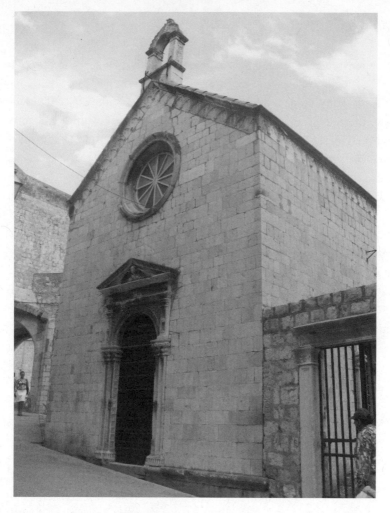

Figure 2.7 Church of the Annunciation near the Ploče gate in Dubrovnik, built as a votive church against the plague in 1534

on the island of Lópud. This painting belongs to the central part of the polyptych that includes St Sebastian and other saints. St Roch is shown standing outdoors and showing his plague bubo on the thigh.[107]

The altar painting, in the Church of St Roch in Grgurići near Slano, dates from 1586 and was probably painted by Marten de Vos (1532–1603), a Dutch painter from Antwerp. The Ragusan patrician Tonko Matkov Gradić (Gradi) ordered the church and the altar painting as a votive offering against the plague (see Figure 2.9). The painting shows, from the left, the donor with St Catherine, then St Roch with an angel on his left and a dog on his right side, and finally, the physicians St Cosmas and St Damian.[108]

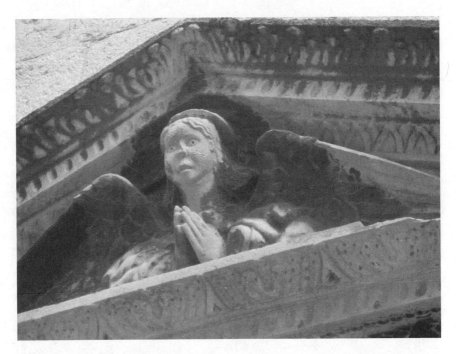

Figure 2.8 Angel on the facade of the Church of the Annunciation near the Ploče gate in Dubrovnik

In the Church of St Anthony the Abbot, in Mali Ston, there is an oil painting created by an unknown Venetian painter. It shows the Crucifixion, St Roch, and St Sebastian, with the priest in front and the faithful kneeling behind him. It was probably ordered as an offering against the plague. The elegant man, next to the priest, dressed according to the latest Spanish fashion, is probably the donor. Under the wood of the cross, there is a cartouche with the date 1588.[109]

At the end of the sixteenth century, Sante Peranda (1566–1638), a Venetian painter, disciple, and assistant of Palma Junior, probably created the votive painting of St Roch, in the parish Church of St Jerome, built in Pučišće on the island of Brač in 1576. St Roch is shown miraculously curing a sick man by gently touching his forehead. The powerful and upright saint is in contrast with the patient lying on his back. This contrast manifestly alludes to the frailty of human nature in comparison with the permanence and the eternity of the divine. In the background is a fortified city with a high bell tower that is assumed to be the city of Split. Next to the city is a deeply recessed Bačvice Peninsula

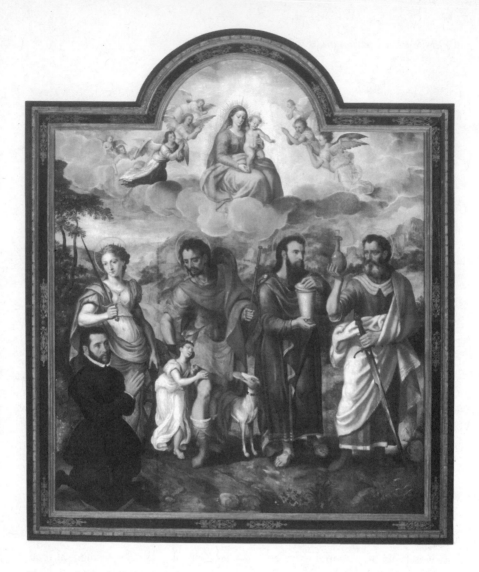

Figure 2.9 Altar painting by Marten de Vos, 1586, Church of St Roch in Grgurići near Slano. Votive painting against the plague donated by the Ragusan patrician Tonko Matkov Gradić

where groups of dying people are seen being transported and buried by the gravediggers. The Bačvice Peninsula is clearly identified as an inhumation ground. The painting unmistakably refers to the deadly plague epidemic of 1607 that lasted eight months and claimed more than half the population of Split. It is the only depiction of the burial of plague victims from that period. The painting demonstrates the power of the invocation of St Roch who, by his popularity, surpassed almost all the other protective saints in Dalmatia and other regions of Croatia.[110]

On 9 January 1691, there were several cases of plague at the Pile suburb among the women who took care of the children at the orphanage. This flare-up became known as *peste delle serve* because the plague was probably brought by the servants from Herzegovina.[111] The exchange place for goods from the Ottoman-controlled territory at Ploče, the so-called Tabor, was immediately closed down. The outbreak lasted until the beginning of May. That year, instead of on 3 February, the feast of St Blaise was celebrated only on 5 July, the day of the hand of the saint. Three votive processions were held in the city: most priests walked barefoot wearing ropes around their necks and thorn wreaths on their heads. The procession headed first for the Church of St Roch and then returned to the Church of St Blaise.[112] The last plague outbreak in the Ragusan Republic took place in 1784. It had spread from the Ottoman-controlled territory but it was limited to the village of Bani in Konavle.[113]

In the next chapter, the health culture of Dubrovnik will be explored. It includes monastic medicine, the establishment of pharmacies, the founding of the city hospital, and the hiring of physicians and surgeons. Ragusan plague control measures will be analyzed in Chapter 4 and subsequent chapters.

3

Health Culture: Pharmacies, Hospitals, Physicians, and Surgeons

In Dubrovnik, various institutions provided health care. Monasteries and their pharmacies offered it in the name of Christian solidarity. Religious confraternities also played a minor role but most of the health care was financed and organized by the government. The state established and funded the hospital. It also hired and paid for medical men who took care of all the citizens without any extra pay. Throughout its history, Dubrovnik was known for the state promotion of health care for all citizens.[1] This chapter discusses various sources of health care but it focuses on physicians and surgeons employed in Dubrovnik between 1280 and 1600.

The religious institutions of Dubrovnik were also a source of medical assistance.[2] The writings produced by the religious fathers often mention that it is wrong to disparage secular medicine but equally wrong to trust in physicians rather than in God. This was an attempt by the Church to harmonize the principles of classical medicine with monastic medicine.[3] Moreover, it is important to note that monastic medicine did not aim to cure but to care for the sick. Ragusans were fortunate to have five Benedictine monasteries close to the city that could all offer medical assistance. These monasteries also had gardens where monks grew medicinal herbs from which they made medicines.[4] Each monastery had an infirmary for the monks. To fulfill their Christian duty, they also accepted outside patients. Thus, the new emphasis on compassion led to Christian medical philanthropy.[5]

ESTABLISHMENT OF PHARMACIES AND HOSPITALS

The pharmacy of the Franciscan friars, the *aromatarium*, was founded in 1317 when their monastery was moved from a location at the Pile gate, outside the city walls, to its present site within the city. It occupied an area nine metres long and two metres wide. Every Franciscan monastery had to have a pharmacy to treat the monks but it seems that the one in Dubrovnik started serving the public very early.[6] Other monasteries also had pharmacies and the city hired pharmacists, too. Two pharmacists are mentioned in the early archival documents – *magister* Basilius from Bari in 1281–82 and *magister* Ghirardus from Piacenza in a testament from 1295.[7] They usually trained their sons to inherit their pharmacy and some of them stayed in Dubrovnik for several generations.[8] In 1301, the archival sources mention Marinus Marci, *speciarius* from Venice, and in 1318 the Minor Council asked *magister* Bonaventura to organize a well-stocked pharmacy so the population would not suffer from lack of medicines.[9]

The city hospital, one of the earliest in Europe, was founded on 30 January 1347 under the name the Hospital of the Commune (*hospedal del comun*). It was administered by government officials and funded by the public treasury for the benefit of the sick poor (*per beneficio dei poveri amalati*). At first, it was just a refuge or a hospice to meet the needs of the poor, especially of the impoverished widows or sick sailors far from home. In 1348, the government had to tear down six houses in the vicinity of St Nicholas Church to enlarge the hospital. During that same year, the authorities found a new location for the hospital close to the convent of St Clare and the western city gate.[10] The construction of the hospital took place from 1349 to 1356. Very little information survives from that period but it was recorded that, in 1389, the patrician Nikola Menčetić (Menze) gave a large sum of money for the enlargement of the hospital and the construction of a well inside the convent of St Clare. In 1407, the Minor Council gave permission to the hospital to create an opening in the city wall facing the sea to avoid any contact of the hospital waste with urban space. In 1410, the Minor Council decided to build the granary in the cellar above the hospital water reservoir.

The hospital pharmacy, established in 1420, was located in the building close to the convent of St Clare. In 1540, it was moved to Placa (Stradun), the main street, in order to serve as a city pharmacy. In the same year, the hospital was enlarged again and its name changed to *Domus Christi*.[11] Nowadays, only the entrance and a few surrounding walls survive from that period. The hospital building was probably rectangular in shape with eleven beds on the ground floor and another eleven on the first floor. While the old hospital primarily housed women, the new one cared for poor men who had curable diseases (*li poveri infermi di medicabile infirmita*). The new rooms had large windows to allow air and light to circulate freely. They seem to have been built according to the miasmatic theory of disease transmission. The hospital complex had a chapel and a kitchen for the poor, a garden for medicinal plants, and a wine cellar.

When the papal envoy Joannes Franciscus Sormano, bishop of Montefeltro, visited the hospital in 1573–74, the wards on the ground floor and the first floor each had an altar adorned with a religious painting and a large crucifix with two candelabra.[12] There was also a portable altar commonly used at the bedside of dying patients. The hospital priest was there to hear confessions, conduct prayer, and administer holy sacraments. Prayer and liturgy were part of the hospital routine. The papal envoy reports that the city physicians came to treat patients when summoned. The hospital thus provided therapy for both the body and the soul.[13] Three trustees, appointed by the government, administered the hospital. Although it did not involve a salary or other type of income, judging by the seniority of the patricians elected to this function, it was one of the most prestigious positions in the Republic.[14] The trustees had to receive patients upon their arrival, approve their admission, familiarize them with the hospital rules, and, when the time came, grant their discharge based on the recommendation of the physician. However, their main role was to administer the bequests for the hospital.

The *castaldo*, a commoner, was in charge of the daily administration of the hospital. He was supposed to visit the patients, oversee the administration of medicines, call the physician or the surgeon when necessary, organize the food supply, and supervise four male and five female servants. In contrast to Italian cities where hospitals were mostly financed by confraternities or private benefactors, in Dubrovnik, that role was reserved for the government. The Ragusan Treasury controlled charitable trusts and disposed of their funds. In this way, it could funnel funds to the institutions as it saw fit.

In his report of 1574, Bishop Sormano also described the other eight hospitals in Dubrovnik: St Peter's, a hostel for international pilgrims and a women's hospital, *in contratta Sancti Stephani*, both of which were operated by the confraternity of priests; the orphanage *Hospedal de Misericordia*, also one of the first in Europe, founded in 1432; St Theodore's women's hospital for poor patrician widows, for female unmarried patricians or women from respectable commoner families; three women's hospitals for the lower class poor – St John's *in contrata Sancti Iohanni*, a hospital *alle Pille*, outside the city walls, and a hospital in the southern part of the city; an institution *in contrata della Campana de Morti*, which provided accommodation only and where the poor had to work to buy food.[15] It has to be emphasized that these hospitals were never used to treat plague patients; they were housed in separate plague compounds built for that purpose (see Chapter 4). This was also the case in Italian cities such as Venice.

The orphanage was situated in a house opposite the Franciscan church and monastery on the main street. A baby could be anonymously deposited in a special wheel-like device and when the wheel was turned, the baby was delivered inside. These children were most often illegitimate. The authorities cared for them until the age of five and then gave them up for adoption. The government also provided dowries for the girls from the orphanage. In this very strict society, the attitude towards illegitimate children was tolerant. Everything was done to ensure the children's survival. While the main reason was compassion, perhaps it also had something to do with numerous patricians who had extramarital relationships with commoners. They often recognized their out-of-wedlock children and provided for them during their life and in their testaments. Generally, the illegitimate children of patricians did not end up living in poverty.[16]

As previously noted, the secular authorities in Dubrovnik dominated the Church and controlled the confraternities very tightly (see Chapter 1). Since the state was the main provider of health care, charitable institutions played only a minor role in providing poor relief in this city. Susan M. Stuard concludes that Ragusans trusted their civic authorities, which controlled every aspect of urban life. Health care in Dubrovnik was not a charity dispensed by confraternities as was the case in some Italian cities. Ragusans promoted urban welfare. The patricians who organized the health care were the first beneficiaries of the system but they also footed the bill.[17]

PHYSICIANS AND SURGEONS WHO SERVED IN DUBROVNIK

The status of physicians and surgeons in Dubrovnik was established during the Venetian protection period (1205–1358). What differentiated Dubrovnik from other Dalmatian cities was its growing economic prosperity. The thrifty Ragusan authorities were thus able to allocate considerable amounts of money for the salaries of communal physicians and surgeons. Venetian authorities used to send medical practitioners to the towns under their protection on the eastern Adriatic coast, including Koper, Pula, Cres, Osor, Zadar, Split, Trogir, and Kotor.[18] However, getting the services of a physician or a surgeon often depended on the capacity of the communes to pay for them.

The oldest Ragusan notarial documents reveal the names of four physicians who served in Dubrovnik from 1280 to 1300. First among them was *magister* Josephus in 1280, followed by *medicus* Pervoslavus in 1281, *physicus* Guillelmus in 1282, and *medicus* Johannes de Trevisio in 1283. Their names are mentioned in various deeds of sale but their professional contracts have not been preserved.[19] Since 1300, the names of physicians and surgeons with their professional title, their place of origin, and their salary are registered in the archival sources. From 1280 to 1600, there were seventy physicians and fifty-nine surgeons who served the Ragusans for a total of 129 professionals (see Table 3.1).[20] In the fourteenth century, Dubrovnik hired an approximately equal number of physicians (21) and surgeons (26), but in the fifteenth century the number of physicians (24) had doubled in comparison with the number of surgeons (12). These numbers indicate that, as more physicians became available, Dubrovnik made an effort to hire the more educated medical practitioners.

The years of service in Table 3.1 are based on the dates of contracts. However, many physicians and surgeons were present in Dubrovnik before their state contracts were signed and often after the expiry of their contract. They had their private practice and treated individual patients who paid for their services, as can be ascertained from the contracts between the physician and the private patient that have been preserved.[21] The physicians are sometimes mentioned as witnesses at the signing of notarial documents or in court. Some of them had married in Dubrovnik and stayed because of family ties. Others had developed various commercial activities in trade. Still others came to Dubrovnik and stayed for a while without ever becoming city physicians with a contract. They are not mentioned in Table 3.1. Most of the physicians and surgeons in the period of 1280 to 1600 were Italian, but five of them were Croatian – from Trogir, Kotor, Ston, and Dubrovnik; six were Spanish, two were French, two were Greek, and six were of Jewish origin.[22]

The sons of physicians and surgeons were often trained by their fathers to acquire the same skills. When looking for a physician, the first choice of the Ragusans always fell on the sons of medical practitioners who had already served in Dubrovnik: Thomasius de Stilo, who served from 1343 to 1347, was the son of Johannes de Stilo who had served in 1336; Petrus de Chamurata, who served

Table 3.1
Physicians and Surgeons Who Served in Dubrovnik, 1280–1600

NAME	PHYSICIANS	SURGEONS	SALARY	DATE OF CONTRACT	YEARS OF SERVICE
Josephus		magister	?	1280?	?
Pervoslavus (Prvoslav)	medicus		?	1281?	?
Guillelmus	physicus		?	1282?	?
Johannes de Trevisio	medicus		?	1283?	?
Marcus		medicus plagarum cirologus	8 Venetian pounds	1301–03, 1306, 1311	3
Mertacha		medicus plagarum	30 hyperperi	1301–13	5
Riçardus de Salerno	medicus fisicus		1302=140 hyperperi, 1313=9 V. pounds less 5 soldi	1302–05, 1313	5
Stefanus		medicus plagarum	8 V. pounds	1304–06	2
Ostesanus (Estesanus)		medicus plagarum	8 Venetian grossi	1304–06	2
Nicolaus de Marchia	medicus phisicus		70 hyperperi	1304	1
Petrus Marangius de Salerno	fisicus		400 hyperperi	1305–07	2
Bartholomeus		medicus in cirurgia cirologus	9 V. pounds	1313	1
Bonaventura		cirologus	1323=12 V. pounds	1319, 1323–24	3
Jacobus de Forlivio		medicus in arte cirologie	6 V. pounds	1319–?	1
Johannes		cirologus	9 V. pounds	1319	1
Guillelmus	physicus		?	1319–20	2
Thomaxius		cirologus		1321	1

Table 3.1
Physicians and Surgeons Who Served in Dubrovnik, 1280–1600

NAME	PHYSICIANS	SURGEONS	SALARY	DATE OF CONTRACT	YEARS OF SERVICE
Uguiccius de Padua	physicus, medicine professor		1322=13 V. pounds, 1329=20 V. pounds	1322, 1329	4
Garamons (Giramont)	medicus, medicine professor		12 V. pounds, 20 V. pounds	1322–23	2
Johannes de Anterminellis de Lucca	physicus, medicine professor		20 V. pounds	1323	1
Domenicus		cirologus	4 V. pounds	1323, 1332	2
Judeus	physicus			1324	6 months
Egidius	physicus		1329=14 V. pounds	1324, 1327–29	5
Johannes de Aquileia	physicus		1327=6 V. pounds	1324, 1327	14 months
Antonius	physicus		1329=6 V. pounds +20 hyperperi reward, 1333=7 V. pounds	1329, 1333	5
Benedictus de Fano		cirologus	8 V. pounds	1329, 1333	3
Johannes de Stilo		ciroicus	15 V. pounds	1336	1
Nicolaus Minor de Padua	physicus		8 V. pounds	1342, 1347	3 yrs, 6 mo
Thomasius de Stilo		cirusicus	12 V. pounds	1343, 1345	4
Menegellus de Venetiis		cirusicus	40 hyperperi	1345	1
Jacobus de Padua	physicus		1344=300 hyperperi, 1348=15 V. pounds, 1349=250 ducats	1344, 1348, 1349	5

Table 3.1
Physicians and Surgeons Who Served in Dubrovnik, 1280–1600

NAME	PHYSICIANS	SURGEONS	SALARY	DATE OF CONTRACT	YEARS OF SERVICE
Marinus		medicus cirogye	1346=10 V. pounds, 1358=200 hyperperi	1346–52, 1357–58	9
Nicolaus Maior	physicus		?	1347	2
Paternanus de Anchona		cyroicus	150 ducats	1349	2
Benedictus, olim Judeus	physicus		?	1355–56	2
Gerardus de Ravenna	physicus		1360=300 ducats	1357–58, 1360–64	6
Michael (de Lecce)		ciroycus	1356=300 hyperperi	1356–58, 1364–66	5 yrs, 4 mo
Cobellus		cirurgicus	1360=250 hyperperi, 1361=300 hyperperi, 1363=150 ducats	1360–63	3
Tadeus de Ferraria		ciroycus	?	1360	1
Christophorus de Benevento, earned a pension in Dubrovnik	physicus		1360=150 ducats 1363=200 ducats	1360–93, 1395–99	37
Gulielmus de Ravenna	physicus		1363=300 ducats	1361–66	5
Thomas ser Bone de Furlivio		cirosicus	1363=150 ducats	1363	2
Franciscus de Firmo	physicus		1366=150 ducats	1366	1
Bartolomeus		ciroicus	?	1366	1

Table 3.1
Physicians and Surgeons Who Served in Dubrovnik, 1280–1600

NAME	PHYSICIANS	SURGEONS	SALARY	DATE OF CONTRACT	YEARS OF SERVICE
Johannes de Tragurio (Ivan Trogiranin)		cerusicus	?	1375–80	4
Johannes de Aldoardis de Papia, earned a pension in Dubrovnik		cerusicus	1381=250 ducats, 1403=300 ducats	1376–1415	39
Petrus de Ricumbaldo de Barulo	physicus		1382=340 hyperperi	1381–84	3
Petrus de Venetiis		cyrugicus	1381=300 hyperperi, 1382=350 hyperperi	1381–85	4
Gregorius de Verona		cyrogicus	1384=450 hyperperi	1382–86, 1389–95	10
Albertinus de Chamurata de Padua	physicus		1390=400 ducats	1385–99	14
Dionisius		cirurgicus	1386=150 ducats	1386–88	2
Andreas de Pellagiis, de Barulo		cyrogichus	1396=400 hyperperi	1392–99	7
Baldessar	physicus		?	1399	1
Jacobus de Salgeriis de Padua	physicus		1402=320 ducats	1402–23	21
Urbanus		ciroichus	?	1403	?
Petrus de Bononia		ciroichus	1403=250 hyperperi	1403	1

Table 3.1
Physicians and Surgeons Who Served in Dubrovnik, 1280–1600

NAME	PHYSICIANS	SURGEONS	SALARY	DATE OF CONTRACT	YEARS OF SERVICE
Johannes de Ancona, quondam magistri Anthonii de Ancona		cyrugicus	1407=300 hyperperi	1403–21	18
Petrus de Chamurata, filius magistri Albertini de Chamurata	phisicus		?	1403, 1414–18	5
Bartholus de Squacialupi de Plombino	phisicus		1414=400 ducats	1409–14, 1420–25	11
Thomasius de Papia, filius magistri Johannis de Papia, earned a pension in Dubrovnik	phisicus		1422=300 hyperperi, 1424–28=400 hyperperi, 1429=500 hyperperi, 1453=440 hyperperi	1422–55	33
Johannes de Recanato		cirogichus	1412=300 ducats	1412–20	9
Jacobus quondam Castellani de Gondovaldis de Ferraria	artium et medicine doctor		1416=300 hyperperi, 1430=300 hyperperi, 1436=390 hyperperi	1416–30 rector of the school, 1430–36 served as physician	21
Johannes de Teolo de Padua, earned a pension in Dubrovnik		cirusicus	1424=225 ducats, 1431=220 ducats	1423–35	12

Table 3.1
Physicians and Surgeons Who Served in Dubrovnik, 1280–1600

NAME	PHYSICIANS	SURGEONS	SALARY	DATE OF CONTRACT	YEARS OF SERVICE
Johannes de Coronellis de Coneglano	phisicus		1430=1000 hyperperi	1427–35	8
Christophorus de Bonasiis de Padua	phisicus		1436=1200 hyperperi	1436–44	8
Johannes Mathias de Reginis de Feltro		ciroychus	1454=613 hyperperi	1436–54	18
Jacobus de Prothonotariis de Messina	medicine doctor		1437=200 hyperperi	1437	4 months
Georgius Spanus	medicus		1449=600 hyperperi	1444–53	9
Evangelista de Caversalis de Imola	medicus		?	1444, 1447?	1
Angelus de Contis de Venetiis	phisicus		1449=350 ducats	1449–55, 1459–60	7
Petrus Reginus de Feltro, filius magistri Johannis Mathiae		cirugicus	1455=210 hyperperi, 1461=350 hyperperi, 1484=150 hyperperi	1452–90	38
Bartholomeus		cirugicus	?	1455	1
Johannes della Dolce Calderia de Neapoli		cirugicus	1455=600 hyperperi	1455–57	2
Andreas Constantinopolitanus	phisicus		1458=500 hyperperi	1458	1

Table 3.1
Physicians and Surgeons Who Served in Dubrovnik, 1280–1600

NAME	PHYSICIANS	SURGEONS	SALARY	DATE OF CONTRACT	YEARS OF SERVICE
Johannes Franciscus de Tarvisio	phisicus		1460=1000 hyperperi	1460–63	3
Tadeus Ardoynus de Florentia	phisicus		1460=1000 hyperperi	1460–64	4
Johannes Petrus de Verona	artium et medicine doctor		1461=600 hyperperi	1461–64	3
Emanuel Marulla Grecus	phisicus		1467=700 hyperperi	1465–71, 1480	7
Johannes Cladus	phisicus et cyrogicus		1466=550 hyperperi, 1477=400 hyperperi, 1479=350 hyperperi	1466–79	13
Hieremias de Utino	artium et medicine doctor		1467=300 hyperperi, 1478=1000 hyperperi	1467–69, 1478–80	5
Hector Pindemonte de Verona	phisicus		1472=1000 hyperperi, 1477=995 hyperperi, 1478=990 hyperperi	1471–78	8
Gabriel de Galvano	phisicus		1477=200 hyperperi	1476–81	5
Johannes de Hyspania		cyrugicus	1482=500 hyperperi	1482–84	2
Hieronymus de Comitibus de Hydronto et de Urbino	phisicus		1482=300 ducats, 1489=250 ducats	1482–94	12
Michael de Catharo		cyrogicus	1483=250 hyperperi	1483–84	1

Table 3.1
Physicians and Surgeons Who Served in Dubrovnik, 1280–1600

NAME	PHYSICIANS	SURGEONS	SALARY	DATE OF CONTRACT	YEARS OF SERVICE
Jacobus Catellanus de Barchinonia		cirogycus	1486=400 hyperperi,	1486–1500	14
Pasqualis, medicus Stagni	medicus		?	1489–1506	17
Antonius de Victoriis, de Faventia civis Bononiensis	phisicus		1490–1516=300 hyperperi	1490–1516	26
Franciscus de Valentia	phisicus		1498=300 ducats	1497–1502	5
Bartholomeus de Vincentia		chirurgus	1506=500 hyperperi	1503–07	4
Johannes olim Jacobi Catellani		chirurgus	1505=150 hyperperi	1504–06	2
Jaymus Cattelanus de Villa Nova		cyrogicus	1506=500 hyperperi, 1508=370 hyperperi	1506–08	3
Hieronymus de Damascho		chirurgus	4–6 ducats per month	1506	5 months
Franciscus Marci Marcolinovich de Stagno		chyrurgus	?	1506–26	20
Ludovicus Florentinus		cyrurgus	1508=600 hyperperi	1507–08	2
Antonius Hispanus		cyrogicus	1510=400 hyperperi	1510–15	6
Andreas Montinensis a Mutino	phisicus		1514=800 hyperperi	1514–15	1
Bernardinus de Lovico (Luvigo)		chirurgus	1515=500 hyperperi	1515–27	12
Vincentius de Novaria		chirurgus	1518=500 hyperperi	1518–19	1
Cesar Tortus de Piceno	phisicus		1520=300 ducats	1520–23	4

Table 3.1
Physicians and Surgeons Who Served in Dubrovnik, 1280–1600

NAME	PHYSICIANS	SURGEONS	SALARY	DATE OF CONTRACT	YEARS OF SERVICE
Hieronymus Malipetrus de Padua	phisicus		?	1520–22	2
Jacobus Hispanus		chirurgus	1524=150 ducats	1524–25	1
Bartholomeus de Vegetiis Januensis	phisicus		1524=300 ducats	1524	1
Donatus de Mutiis	phisicus		1526=330 ducats	1526–36	10
Johannes Mednich (Ivan Mednić) de Catharo		chyrurgus	1526=200 ducats + 3 ducats for his 5 sons, 1527=200 hyperperi + 3 ducats for his 5 sons	1526–29	3
Jacobus Rizo		medicus pestis	1527=160 ducats for 6 months	1527	6 months
Mariano Santo	phisicus et chirurgus			1527–32	5
Bartholomeus Barisonus	phisicus		?	1527	?
Hieronymus Pavanellus		chirurgus	?	1527	?
Hieronymus de Verona	phisicus		?	1532, 1538	2
Ludovicus de Pisauro		chirurgus	1536=500 hyperperi	1536	2
Bartholomeus de Damianis	phisicus		?	1541	2
Isac Hebreus	phisicus		1543=170 ducats, 1552=200 ducats	1543–52	10
Johannes Andreas de Prato	phisicus		?	1550–55	5

Table 3.1
Physicians and Surgeons Who Served in Dubrovnik, 1280–1600

NAME	PHYSICIANS	SURGEONS	SALARY	DATE OF CONTRACT	YEARS OF SERVICE
Jacobus Pacinus	phisicus		?	1550–59	10
Cesar Buzzecharino de Pisauro	phisicus		?	1552–58, 1566	7
Amatus Lusitanus (João Rodriguez)	phisicus		?	1557–58	1
Johannes Baptista Vanutius (Vanucci)		chirurgus	?	1557	1
Abraham Hebreus		chirurgus	1558=150 ducats, 1568=120 ducats, 1571=150 ducats	1558–90	32
Bernardinus Paterna	medicine professor in Pavia, Pisa and Padua		?	1560	1
Aloysius Federici	phisicus		?	1566–78	12
Giosterius de Bassano	phisicus		?	1569–78	9
Gaspar Bazzo		chirurgus	?	1578–1602	24
Josephus Salama		chirurgus	1575=90 hyperperi, 1578=50 ducats, 1592=360 hyperperi	1575–92	17
Gaudenzio Mureto Gallus	phisicus		?	1584–87	3
Jacobo Riscarolo de Nizza	phisicus		1588=200 ducats	1588	1
Samuel Abeatar Judeus	phisicus		1588=200 ducats	1588–1607	19
Thoma Natalis Budislavich phisicus Ragusinus	phisicus		?	1580–1608	28
Nicolaus Rossus	artium et medicine doctor		?	1597–99	2

from 1403 to 1418, was the son of Albertinus de Chamurata who had served from 1385 to 1399; Thomasius de Papia, who served from 1422 to 1455, was the son of Johannes de Papia who had served from 1376 to 1415. Johannes Mathias de Reginis de Feltro served in Dubrovnik for eighteen years and died in the city in 1454. For the last two years, probably due to his advanced age and failing health, his contract stipulated that his son Petrus Reginus, who was a surgeon, had to work with him. After the death of his father, Petrus Reginus became a salaried surgeon and stayed in Dubrovnik for thirty-six years. His brother, Johannes Laurentius, was employed as chancellor of Dubrovnik. John, the son of the deceased master Jacob the Catalan – *magister* Johannes *olim magistri* Jacobi Catellani – practised in Dubrovnik from 1504 to 1506, four years after the death of his father whose contracts had been renewed for fourteen years.[23]

In the Ragusan Republic, the top physicians enjoyed a high social status. In his book, Diversis depicts the festivities of the St Blaise Feast Day, the patron saint of the city, celebrated on 3 February. This was the occasion of the most solemn yearly ceremonies in Dubrovnik when the rector and the councillors gathered in front of the Rector's Palace before the religious procession. According to the established protocol, the physicians were the first to be seated next to the rector and were followed by other dignitaries.[24] The rector thus formally honoured the physicians serving the Republic. They could be summoned to advise the Councils in questions regarding sanitation or epidemic control.[25] They could also be asked to participate in diplomacy. Their knowledge was expected to assist the councillors in making the best possible decisions. Diversis also describes the funerals of patricians and mentions that the rector and most of the patricians were present at the funerals of the city physicians, scribes, chancellors, and other foreign salaried employees who were held in high esteem.[26]

While physicians had university education, surgeons learned their trade by apprenticing for a number of years – usually eight – with an experienced surgeon.[27] Their formal education was more limited and they rarely had institutional connections to academic circles. Those who knew Latin could study at the universities.[28] Mariano Santo, for example, became a surgeon first and then decided to study medicine at the university. However, most surgeons could only use surgery manuals in the vernacular languages. Abbreviated manuals of Galen's anatomy or Celsus's *De Medicina* were found in their legacies. For example, in the surgery manual by Albucasis, surgical instruments were described and drawn in an understandable fashion. That aspect made it very useful for the students at the time. We have to keep in mind that translations of erroneous terms and obscure phrases abounded. Surgeons tried to clear up the confusion in technical books by adding more information from their own observations to the classics. As well, they included new recipes for medicines, balsams, ointments, powders, and plasters. They also registered their descriptions of wound treatment, incisions of buboes, and other swellings. Surgical interventions were limited by the patchy knowledge of the anatomy and physiology of the human body. Surgeons relied heavily on their experience and manual dexterity. The absence of anaesthesia, the impossibility of stopping bleeding, frequent infections, and the use of primitive instruments seriously restricted the development of surgery. Alcohol was the only anaesthetic, bleeding was stopped by cauterization and later by ligature of the blood vessels, while infections were *terra incognita* until the appearance of Robert Koch in the nineteenth century.[29] Under those circumstances, mortality was high and surgeons limited their interventions to procedures with a lower risk. Therefore, medical empirics, itinerant craftsmen who were specialized in performing a particular operation, for example, couching for cataract, treating hernias, removing bladder stones, pulling teeth, setting broken bones and dislocations, performed riskier procedures.[30] Midwives assisted in childbirth. They were usually self-taught or trained by friends or family members.

At the time of the Black Death pandemic in 1347, medicine was based on the heritage of Hippocrates (ca 460–ca 370 BC), Galen (129–210/217), and Avicenna (980–1037), the latter referred to as Ibn Sina in the Arab sources. The curriculum of the physicians consisted of studying and debating the most important works of these classics. Hippocrates based his theory of the origin of diseases on the combination of the humoural theory prevalent in ancient Greece and his own miasmatic theory of corruption of the air by noxious vapours.[31] Diseases were not ascribed to external entities invading the body but to internal disarrangements in the proportions of the four humours (yellow bile, black bile, phlegm, and blood) that were strongly influenced by climate. To these, Galen added a new element – contagion. He pointed out that it was dangerous to be close to sick people who had a bad breath. Galen thought that the putrid breath of the patient tainted the air around the sick person and poisoned it for others. The theory of plague contagion consisted of an eclectic collection of presumptions with the addition, in some cases, of the empirical observation of the symptoms of the disease. Sorely lacking from these theories were the causative agent of the disease and the mode of infection.[32] Since there was no disease like it in the ancient sources that they had studied, physicians were bewildered by the plague. They quickly realized that their medical art could not cure plague, so they concentrated on giving people hope.[33]

During plague outbreaks, physicians usually asked for a leave of absence as soon as they had diagnosed plague. They knew very well how dangerous plague was and they systematically avoided serving in plague-stricken cities because they did not want to stay in the epicentre of the epidemic. The physicians were paid high salaries and were be able to afford an unpaid leave of absence, which they were usually granted because the infected cities were happy to reduce their expenditures during the economic downturn that the plague inevitably brought with it. Thus, escape clauses in their contracts were not even necessary. Nevertheless, there were sometimes exceptional individuals who chose to stay in infected cities. In Dubrovnik, Jacobus de Gondovaldis, who was helpful to the government with his advice during the 1416 and 1430 plague outbreaks, stayed in the city and survived both epidemics. Two other medical men were offered a leave of absence in 1457 and 1482 but bravely chose to stay and died of plague. Certain physicians who were helpful during the plague epidemic, such as Donato Muzi in 1526, were granted a leave of absence with full pay (see Chapter 6).

Moreover, physicians were highly educated individuals and it was important to protect them from dying of plague. At that time, physicians considered plague to be a major calamity, a horrific event, in the same category, for example, as an earthquake, and therefore, something that was definitely not within their jurisdiction. They did not feel qualified to fight it, so they preferred to leave. In their own words, plague made it impossible for them to practise medicine.

Their place was usually filled by plague doctors – *medici pestis* – who specialized in incisions of buboes. In the absence of physicians, plague doctors, empirics, and priests offered the assistance that the plague victims needed. In such moments, there were always a few charlatans and quacks who tried to take advantage of the crisis created by the plague upsurge and offered their services as plague doctors.[34]

RECRUITING PHYSICIANS AND SURGEONS

Dubrovnik used to hire abroad a number of salaried state employees, including the city notary, the chancellor, teachers, musicians, soldiers, craftsmen, and two physicians (*physici*), two surgeons (*chirurgi*), and a few barbers or barber-surgeons.[35] Several private pharmacists, known in Dubrovnik as *spičari*, were also present.[36] Since there was no medical school in Dalmatia, Ragusan authorities invested a lot of time, energy, and money into hiring qualified, reputable, and well-educated physicians and experienced surgeons. Through every possible channel – commercial, diplomatic, private, and ecclesiastical – they sought out the best available medical practitioners. The Major Council usually asked the Minor Council to send their representative, a *syndicus*, to Venice, Padua, or Bologna to recruit a candidate for a city physician or surgeon. When the right person was found, the *syndicus* had to attract the candidate to come and work in Dubrovnik.[37] If the candidate agreed, a contract, usually for the duration of one or two years, was signed. The physician would swear on the Bible that he would respect all the clauses of the contract. He thus became the official communal physician – *medicus salariatus* or *salariatus communis* – and he usually had to show up in Dubrovnik within eight to fourteen days. Sometimes the *syndicus* had to look for several salaried professionals at the same time. In 1380, Jakov Prodančić was sent to Ancona to locate a surgeon, a chancellor, and an artilleryman to defend the city.[38]

Occasionally, the process of hiring physicians and surgeons met with great difficulties, particularly during plague epidemics. Seeking help for afflicted Dubrovnik, the *syndicus* travelled from one plague-infected Italian city to another. His mission was not greeted with enthusiasm by the local people, who needed a surgeon as badly as did the Ragusans. That hiring a surgeon could prove to be an arduous task is evident from the orders given to three patrician agents, Martol Đurđević (Georgi), Miho Bobaljević (Bobali), and Vlaho Držić (Dersa), who were sent to Italy in 1359. Plague had been rampant in the two previous years and surgeons were in short supply. The Major Council anticipated that it would be difficult to attract them to Dubrovnik. The Rector Ivan Bunić (Bona) gave the agents complex orders. They were to go to Venice and try to engage *magister* Gracioto or *magister* Albertino from Mantua or *magister* Nicolo from Treviso. If none of these surgeons were available, they were to recruit someone else of the same calibre in Venice. Failing that, one of the agents, under the threat of a fine of one hundred *hyperperi* if he refused, was to go to Padua, and, if unsuccessful there, he was to proceed to Bologna, because the Councils were informed that there were good doctors in Bologna.[39] If one of the three preferred surgeons accepted to serve, he was to have a contract for two years with the annual salary of two hundred ducats. The same terms were to be offered to a candidate from Padua or Bologna, but he would have to be an experienced practitioner and be prepared to depart for Dubrovnik within fifteen days. In the following centuries, there were often difficulties in attracting the right person. On numerous occasions, it proved to be a long and arduous process.

When *magister* Uguiccius, *physicus* and professor of medicine from Padua, was hired again in 1329, his contract specified that, without extra pay, he would have to take care of all the citizens, male or female, including the archbishop and his relatives, the count, present and future, and his family, the chancellor and his family, and all the monks and nuns of Dubrovnik.[40] Such a formulation was included in all the contracts of communal physicians and surgeons.[41] It is significant that this service was provided by the state and not by various charitable organizations as in Venice or in Florence. In Italian cities, the communally salaried physicians often took care only of the poor while the well-to-do hired their own private physicians.[42] In Dubrovnik, by contrast, the civic authorities selected the medical men who treated the citizens of every social or economic class. In 1454, for example, the contract of the surgeon, Petrus Reginus de Feltro, stipulated that he had to treat the people in the city and outside of it, that he had to go to Ston and other places, wherever and whenever the authorities sent him, and he even had to serve on the galleys, if necessary.[43] This policy continued for centuries and contributed significantly to the stability and the cohesion of the social fabric in Dubrovnik. In contrast with Italian cities, the physicians and surgeons serving in Dubrovnik did not form professional associations to advance their interests because they were foreigners and few in number. Furthermore, the authorities did not look kindly upon any form of association.[44]

Economic circumstances played an important role in recruiting physicians. They were urgently needed at the time of plague epidemics. Unfortunately, during such times, the affected cities suffered from an economic downturn. Economic activity ground to a halt and the infected cities found themselves in total isolation. In such circumstances, it was difficult for the authorities to finance physicians' salaries. The physicians, on the other hand, were afraid that the city would not be able to pay, so, in their contracts, they insisted on being paid in advance. The physician Giovanni Ventura, who negotiated with the city of Pavia in 1479, is an illustrative case in point. His contract, signed on 6 May 1479, is kept in the local archives. From the numerous clauses that were crossed out or added, it is evident that the negotiations were long and painstaking. For its money, the city wanted to obtain as many services as possible, while the physician, who had to spend a year among plague sufferers thus risking his life daily, tried to ensure the best possible financial conditions for himself. The city demanded that the physician visit all the patients every day and as many times a day as necessary, while the physician insisted that he would treat only the plague patients. The contract also specifies that *magister* Giovanni would not ask the patients for any money unless the patients or their relatives offered it. The physician asked to be paid a two-month salary ahead of time. In the contract it was reduced to one month. He also asked to be paid for two months after the expiry of the contract. That, as well, was reduced to one month. He received a salary of thirty florins a month, free lodging, and living expenses. One clause stipulates that the physician will be awarded the citizenship of Pavia if the city is satisfied with his services. Finally, it occurred to the physician that he may not live to see the end of his contract and demanded that, if God forbid, he should perish while performing his duty, his inheritors would not have to return the money already received. It is not known what happened to this physician afterwards and whether his fears, that Pavia would not be able to honour his contract, were justified. At that time, for thirty florins one could buy forty grams of pure gold. Medical books in Lombardy cost six and a half florins. Thus, at a time when few physicians possessed more than twelve medical books, *magister* Giovanni could afford to buy almost five medical books for his monthly salary.[45] According to Brian Pullan, Italian cities had trouble financing their hospitals, lazarettos, and health boards as well as the recovered poor patients because these institutions were only partly financed from the city budget. The major part of financing came from religious confraternities, wealthy donors, and other charitable organizations. In times of need, banks used to approve low interest loans for the poor.[46]

PHYSICIANS' DUTIES

The main duty of the physician was to examine the patient, establish the diagnosis, and prescribe the medicines that were usually prepared and dispensed by pharmacists. In order to establish the diagnosis of plague, medical men examined the patient or the dead body. The autopsy was usually performed by the barber-surgeon or surgeon. If the physicians had already abandoned the city, a surgeon or a plague doctor was asked to establish the diagnosis. In 1331, the Minor Council prohibited physicians and surgeons serving in Dubrovnik from having any association or private business with the pharmacists. In the fifteenth and sixteenth centuries, *theriac*, a universal medicine against a whole range of diseases including plague, was most often prescribed. It consisted of twenty to eighty different substances with the addition of opium. It was sold in the form of electuary, a thick substance mixed with honey or syrup, or as small tablets.[47] Twice a year, the physicians had to examine the freshness and the quality of medicines held in the pharmacies, known in Dubrovnik as *spičarije*, as well as the prices that the pharmacists charged for them. Also, physicians and surgeons were not allowed to conduct any trade.[48] One reason for the prohibition against trade was to encourage the highly paid medical men to concentrate on their professional practice. But, more importantly, they were excluded from trade because they were foreigners.

From the beginning, trade had been the privilege of local patricians and commoners, a right they jealously kept for the citizens of Dubrovnik. However, there were exceptions. Because they wanted to keep a certain physician or surgeon in their midst, the authorities were probably more lenient in some cases, especially in the years that followed the Black Death when there was a scarcity of medical practitioners. Thus, *magister* Ivan from Trogir – Johannes de Tragurio – a surgeon who had served in Dubrovnik for five years starting in 1375, owned a ship in which he transported oil, wax, and building materials from Trogir to Dubrovnik as well as to places all over Dalmatia, Albania, and Apulia.[49] Petrus de Ricumbaldo de Barolo, a physician who served from 1381 to 1384, also owned a ship and was permitted to engage in trade. These may have been isolated cases but they show the flexibility of the Ragusan approach. *Magister* Thomas, *medicus salariatus*, and *magister* Johannes, *ziroicus* (surgeon), owned taverns in the city, as did some clerics and even the archbishop of Dubrovnik.[50]

In the city where merchants, caravan drivers, and sailors of so many different cultures met every day, the potential for violent conflict was inescapable and had to be controlled by the authorities. Physicians and surgeons, the latter more often, had to act as expert witnesses when citizens were wounded in fighting among themselves or with foreigners, especially the Turks who found themselves temporarily in the city. If anyone was hurt in those incidents, physicians or surgeons had to extend first aid and give their expert opinion about the nature and the gravity of wounds since the criminal responsibility of the offender depended on their declaration.[51] Thus, the criminal records for 1421–24 register the name of *magister* Thomas, physician, who testified in court eight times, and four surgeons – Johannes de Recanato, Johannes de Ancona, Johannes de Padua, and *magister* Thoma, who testified nine times in this period; in 1430–31, three surgeons – Johannes de Padua, *magister* Thomas, and *magister* Thomas *ciroy-cus* (surgeon) – testified seven times.[52] In Venice, medical men also had the same legal obligation to serve as expert witnesses in court.[53]

SALARIES OF PHYSICIANS AND SURGEONS

Table 3.1 indicates the range of salaries that the physicians and surgeons in Dubrovnik were paid from 1280 to 1600.[54] Until the 1340s, they were paid six to twenty Venetian pounds a year, the highest amounts paid to any foreigners as salaried employees in Dubrovnik. By comparison, in 1333, the head of the arsenal (*protomagister arsenatus*) was paid five pounds a year while the chancellor earned between fifty and one hundred *hyperperi* during that period. In 1373, farmers working in the vineyards, by contrast, made two and a half hyperperi per month and were only seasonally employed.[55] The contracts of physicians and surgeons included free lodging or an amount of thirty hyperperi for the residence. They were well paid not only in Ragusan terms but in comparison with other cities in Italy, France, and elsewhere in Europe. Physicians who had studied at the most prestigious universities earned up to four hundred ducats a year. These were Albertinus de Chamurata de Padua in 1390, Bartholus de Squacialupi de Plombino in 1414, and Christophorus de Bonasiis de Padua in 1436.

Diversis reports that it is not up to him to disclose the salaries of physicians, but he notices that the sums that they were paid were fit for the most illustrious among them. He adds that Ragusan citizens of every social class show particular respect for physicians and shower them with abundant honours.[56] It is worth mentioning that Diversis was also one of those well-paid state employees. In the 1430s, he earned a salary of 450 hyperperi per year. Gregor Čremošnik reveals the salaries of chancellors in the fifteenth century Dubrovnik with the mention that only physicians earned more. In 1450, the state chancellors had a salary of 350 hyperperi and the physicians anywhere between 500 and 1,200 hyperperi. Čremošnik observes that only the salaries of the bookkeepers of the state treasury (*racionati camere*), who earned 400 to 450 hyperperi per year, could compete with those of the physicians. All the other state employees earned considerably less.[57] Numerous testaments of physicians who had served in Dubrovnik confirm their considerable wealth.[58] Susan Mosher Stuard, who examined the purchasing power of the medical men in Dubrovnik, concluded that a physician or surgeon could support his family and still have a considerable amount left over.[59]

By the 1480s there was a considerable drop in the salaries of physicians and other salaried foreigners. Johannes Cladus, the physician who practised in Dubrovnik for thirteen years, had a salary of 550 hyperperi in 1466, 400 in 1477, but only 350 in 1479.[60] On 24 May 1478, the Major Council, decided to extend the length of the contracts of salaried employees including the physicians to save money. Thus, in 1482, Hieronymus de Comitibus earned 1,000 hyperperi for fifteen months, in 1484, 800 hyperperi for twelve months, and, in 1489, he earned 750 hyperperi for fourteen months.[61] In the following century, the salaries of physicians remained low and ranged between 150 and 200 ducats. In sixteenth-century Dubrovnik, only a few rare individuals were paid 300 ducats: Cesar Tortus de Piceno in 1520, Bartholomeus de Vegetiis in 1524, and Donato Muzi – Donatus de Mutiis – in 1526. On top of the 30 hyperperi for lodging, sixteenth-century contracts often included an amount of 30 hyperperi for unguents.[62] Vivian Nutton and Richard Palmer maintain that, in the sixteenth century, the influence and reputation of physicians and surgeons decreased because their numbers had increased. Katharine Park adds that the medical practitioners had to fight to regain their reputation, which was lost because of their inability to fight plague. Their flight from plague-infected cities since 1348 was not forgotten and elicited contempt.[63] In 1348, Florentine chroniclers Matteo Villani and Marchinone di Coppo Stefani lamented the greed and impotence of doctors during the first plague epidemic; gone was the superior ethic of charity and service of the medical profession.[64] In Dubrovnik, a text added at the front of the book of testaments from 1348 bemoans that "all the art of Hippocrates, Galen and Avicenna was of no use to the Ragusans against the divine decision."[65]

Surgeons were usually allotted free lodging and only half the earnings of the physicians. They also suffered a general salary reduction in the 1480s. For example, the surgeon Petrus Reginus de Feltro, who stayed in Dubrovnik for thirty-six years, earned 210 hyperperi in 1455, 350 in 1461, but only 150 hyperperi towards the end of his career in 1484.[66]

PENSIONS AWARDED TO PHYSICIANS AND SURGEONS

In the period specified in Table 3.1, seven physicians and five surgeons stayed in Dubrovnik for ten to nineteen years; four physicians and two surgeons were engaged for twenty to twenty-eight years; two physicians and three surgeons practised in Dubrovnik for thirty-two to thirty-nine years (see Table 3.1). The most famous ones stayed the longest. These data attest to the fact that Dubrovnik was an attractive city for physicians and surgeons, a city where they were well paid and treated with respect.[67] Furthermore, quite a number of them served until they reached old age, and the Ragusan authorities awarded them a pension as a sign of gratitude for their dedicated service. On 7 October 1399, after thirty-six years of service, *magister* Christophorus de Benevento, *physicus*, was awarded by the Major Council a pension of ten hyperperi per month for as long as he lived. This was the first pension approved in Dubrovnik for a medical practitioner. Unfortunately, the good doctor did not enjoy it for very long. He died in the spring of 1400. He was able to leave very generous sums of money, including houses, land, vineyards, and other valuables to his children, his servants, monks, and the hospital for the poor. It is obvious from his testament that he had amassed a considerable fortune in Dubrovnik. On 8 January 1392, his son Rusko Kristoforov was hired as a chancellor in the Slavic Chancery of Dubrovnik.[68] During his long and conscientious service of about thirty-nine years, *magister* Johannes de Papia, *cerusicus*, had considerably indebted the Ragusans. On 24 February 1415, he was given a pension of two hundred hyperperi "as remuneration for his merits and for the honour of our Republic."[69] Johannes's son, Thomasius, *physicus*, followed in his father's footsteps; in 1458, after thirty-three years of service, he earned the same pension as his father.[70] He must have been an excellent physician given that, in 1419, he earned the Ragusan citizenship.

Johannes de Teolo, *cirusicus* from Padua, served in Dubrovnik for twelve years, from 1423 to 1435. When in 1435, he was too old and too sick to work full time, he asked to work according to his capacity. Diversis reports that he was weak and spent most of the time resting at home. On 9 April 1435, the Councils granted him a yearly pension of fifty ducats. He died in Dubrovnik three years later.[71] Diversis relates that there were two physicians, "one more learned that the other," and two surgeons employed by the city.[72] Pensions for physicians and surgeons, in the form of an amount awarded for life, became current practice in Dubrovnik. Jane Stevens notes that in the sixteenth century doctors in Venice, Verona, and Padua often received a monthly amount for life. This provided a form of financial security and guaranteed an advantageous social status for their descendants for generations.[73]

TREATING FOREIGNERS FOR A FEE

The patients who came from neighbouring countries and were not citizens of the Ragusan Republic represented an additional source of income for physicians and surgeons who could charge them per service.[74] The fees for one ailment ranged from five to twenty ducats. In the presence of the notary, a contract was signed where the physician specified what he was going to undertake, but he did not guarantee that the patient would be cured. There were cases when the physician had to return the fees received if the treatment was not successful. Major surgery, which represented a higher risk, was often performed by travelling empirics, surgeons without formal training, often of Slavic or Greek origin. The contract usually protected them from being physically attacked by the relatives of the patient if the treatment was not successful.[75]

On 17 October 1365, surgeon Michael from Lecce made a contract with Radan Dubravčić to remove his bladder stone. The patient was to give the surgeon ten and a half hyperperi when the surgeon put in the patient's hand the stone that he had removed from the patient's body. If the patient was cured, he would owe the surgeon another ten and a half hyperperi. If the patient died, his heirs would not owe the second sum. This case has great historical significance in medicine because it is the first bladder stone removal recorded in the State Archives of Dubrovnik and on the territory of present-day Croatia. In the margin of the contract it says that the contract was cancelled by the decision of the parties. Thus, we do not know if this particular patient was treated, but we know that such operations were performed in Dubrovnik at that time.[76] On 29 January 1382, Obercho Chilloresa signed a contract with Strojislav Popović, a Vlach.[77] Obercho was to remove the Vlach's bladder stones. The contract stipulated that "if the patient died during the operation none of the patient's relatives, especially sons or brothers, would do harm to Obercho." It was not recorded whether the patient recovered, or if Obercho received his fee of sixty hyperperi, a princely sum for any medical procedure.[78]

RAGUSAN PHYSICIANS IN ITALY

There were also native Ragusan physicians whose career evolved in Italy. Dominicus de Ragusia de Bononia, *physicus*, born in Dubrovnik, probably studied medicine in Bologna where, in 1394, he became a member of the College of Philosophers and Physicians. In 1395–96 he taught astrology, in 1397, moral philosophy, and in 1398–99 and from 1415 to 1421, he taught medicine in Bologna. Judging by his salary, he must have been an esteemed specialist. From 1422 to 1425, he taught medicine in Siena. He died in Bologna in 1427 and was buried in the Church of St Francis where the physicians of Bologna used to meet. It seems that Galeotto from Dubrovnik, who also taught medicine in Bologna from 1438 to 1453, was his son.

Dominicus wrote several medical books, which can be found in the libraries of New York, Rome, and Florence. Among the fragments of a work held in Rome, a recipe for an electuary against plague was found. It seems that this recipe was part of Dominicus's work on the treatment of plague. In the fifteenth century, Godefrid, who had obviously appreciated Dominicus's works, quoted this fragment. The complete work has not yet turned up. All of Dominicus's works were manuals for his students, based on his university lectures.[79]

PHYSICIANS AND SURGEONS AS DIPLOMATS

Physicians and surgeons were quite a mobile group of professionals and it was not unusual for the more prominent ones to be "loaned" to the neighbouring rulers. They would obtain an unpaid leave of absence from the Republic but they would receive instead a royal fee from the ruler they treated. If the mission was of great importance for the Republic, the government continued to pay the physician during his whole trip, covered all his expenses, and added a reward. In 1387, for example, the Major Council decided to send the physician Albertinus de Chamurata to treat Đuro Stracimir Balša of Zeta (nowadays Montenegro). Albertinus was allowed to stay there for twenty days and on top of his salary he was promised two ducats a day and all expenses paid plus any gifts that he may receive from the patient.[80] In spite of that, physicians needed a lot of coaxing to undertake such a trip. Travelling at that time was not particularly easy or pleasant so the physicians offered various excuses – the roads were bad, the journey was dangerous, they were old and sick, or the climate was unhealthy. Consequently, it was necessary to send the physician with a considerable escort, including a patrician, who would hand the illustrious patient a message from the Senate. The escort also included several servants and armed soldiers for protection.[81] On 4 April 1395, Johannes de Papia, *medicus cerusicus*, was sent by the Senate to treat Dabiša, the king of Bosnia. He was paid forty ducats and his medical expenses were covered.[82] In 1420, Johannes de

Ancona, *cyrugicus*, was given a leave of absence with full expenses in order to be able to treat count Balša Stracimirović, the ruler of Zeta.[83] In 1424, the physician Bartholus de Plombino was sent to Bosnia under armed escort to treat the duke Vukmir Zlatonosović. In 1425, Bartholus had to undertake the arduous trip again to attend to the needs of the Bosnian grand duke Sandalj Hranić.[84] Many other Ragusan physicians treated foreign dignitaries and their families. Physicians also played other roles. Sometimes they served as witnesses when tribute was paid to other rulers or when state contracts were signed. They also acted as diplomats, especially in the latter part of the sixteenth century when native Ragusans became physicians educated in Italian universities.[85]

In 1442, when Isak, the Turkish high official fell ill, the Ragusans negotiated with Simon, the physician from Naples, who was sent to treat Isak. In 1445 and 1449, a Ragusan physician was asked to treat the count of Kotor. From 1445 to 1461, various physicians were sent on nine different occasions to treat *herceg* (duke) Stjepan, the Bosnian nobleman who had a bad leg. The Ragusan government covered all the expenses of three of those trips.[86] In 1463, Stjepan Tomašević, the last Bosnian king, was beheaded by the Ottoman sultan Mehmed II Fatih. After that, Bosnia came under Ottoman rule and the balance of power in the Ragusan hinterland changed dramatically. The Ottomans continually endangered northern Croatia and Hungary. On 12 December 1463, at the request of the Hungarian king, Matthias Korvin, the Ragusans sent the physician Johannes Petrus to treat the wounds of the soldiers on the battlefield.[87] In 1467, when the Ragusan Republic was requested to send a physician to treat the Turkish official Esebeg, it had to increase the physician's salary.[88] Since then, Ragusan physicians were often solicited to take care of the Ottoman dignitaries and their families in Bosnia. The Ragusans were fully aware that they were surrounded by the Ottomans on their land borders, and did not refuse such requests. By sending their physicians, not only did they show their benevolence and their loyalty toward their neighbours, but upon the physicians' return they received precious briefings concerning the political, economic, and health circumstances in those countries. In June 1493, the Ragusan government sent the illustrious physician Antonius de Victoriis from Faenza (Faventia), who used to teach medicine in Bologna, to treat Sulimanbašić, the Ottoman high official in Foča, eastern Bosnia.[89] A year later, another physician and a barber-surgeon were again required for Sulimanbašić. This practice of providing physicians and surgeons continued in the sixteenth century when physicians from Dubrovnik often travelled to Banja Luka, Travnik, and other parts of Bosnia at the request of the Bosnian *beylerbey* and the *sancakbey* of Herzegovina. The

Ottoman subjects also used to travel to Dubrovnik to seek treatment. As soon as they arrived, they were asked to sign a statement in the presence of the Ottoman *emin* declaring that, in case of death, the heirs of the patient would not sue the Ragusan authorities or the physician who treated the patient. The extant documents date from the eighteenth century.[90]

Lujo Đurašević studied medicine in Bologna with the support of the Ragusan government. As a person of particular confidence of the Republic, in 1547–48, he was sent to the court of Charles V as a diplomatic emissary on an exceedingly sensitive mission. He was to ask Charles V to let go, from his service, one of his confidential intelligence agents in Dubrovnik. That agent was Marin Stjepanov Zamagna, a member of an influential Ragusan patrician family, and as such, was not allowed to perform consular or diplomatic duties for a foreign country. Upon his return, Lujo Đurašević gave the government a detailed report of his negotiations. Such missions were of strictly confidential nature and if they were recorded in the archival books, they were found mostly in the secret documents of the Senate – *Secreta Rogatorum*. This collection exists only in fragments because, by the order of the Senate, parts of it were systematically destroyed for security reasons. It seems that Đurašević, who was definitely one of the most prestigious persons of his time in Dubrovnik, was not successful in his mission because the famous patrician continued to work for the Spanish until his death.[91] Đurašević died in Bologna in 1565 where he had taught medicine at the university. The inscription on his grave reads, "Aloysius Georgius ex Epidauro in Dalmatia 1565."[92]

Another native of Dubrovnik who studied medicine in Bologna with the support of the Ragusan government was Toma Natalis Budislavić (1545–1608). He belonged to a select group of physicians who performed diplomatic missions for the Republic. After his studies, he stayed in Dubrovnik for a while and then he went to Rome and from there to Constantinople where he treated sultan Murat III who suffered from asthma. As a reward for his work, the sultan gave him the duchy Bobane near Trebinje in Bosnia. After that, the physician went to Poland where he met the king Stefan Batory (or Stephen Báthory) (1575–86) who conferred on him a Polish aristocratic title while the Cracow bishop Piotr Marikowski bestowed upon him the title of dean of Cracow. In 1580, Toma Natalis Budislavić returned to Dubrovnik. In 1590, he was sent to Banja Luka to take care of Hasan Pasha Predojević, the Bosnian *beylerbey*. It seems that the pasha suffered from stomach problems and wanted the physician to stay with him all the time. The Ragusan authorities had trouble getting their physician back, even after he had been away for six months. When Toma Natalis finally returned to Dubrovnik, he continued sending the pasha medicines prepared by the local pharmacists Fridrik Ogerio, Ivan Bartolomej, and Ivan Markulin, who were paid by the Ragusan government.[93]

At the end of the sixteenth century, a movement for the liberation from the Ottomans developed among the Christians of Bosnia. During that period, Toma Natalis Budislavić often travelled to Banja Luka, Jajce, and other regions of Bosnia where he took care of Ottoman dignitaries. He used these occasions to establish contact with those who had organized the movement against the Ottomans, but he had to be extremely discreet. The Ragusans wanted to support the goals of their coreligionists but they had to be very careful. It is obvious that the Senate was involved in decisions concerning all the engagements of this physician and treated Toma Natalis Budislavić according to the status and rights of Ragusan ambassadors. In 1606, the Senate named him the bishop of Mrkan-Trebinje. In 1608, Toma Natalis Budislavić died in Naples. He left all his possessions to the foundation Collegium Orthodoxum Budislavum, which was to be founded in Dubrovnik. The foundation was to finance the studies of the students from his bishopric. From his bequest, the Ragusan authorities later supported native sons who studied medicine in Italy.[94]

When the territory of the Republic was in imminent danger, the government had to be pragmatic and drop the usual rules of not relying on foreigners. In such cases, the Ragusans did not hesitate to ask foreign physicians to intervene directly according to their instructions. In 1590, the Ottomans set their mind on conquering Gruž and Konavle, a considerable part of the territory of the Ragusan Republic. They also asked for an enormous sum of 150,000 ducats to be paid as a tribute, supposedly owed to the descendants of duke Stjepan Vukčić Kosača. The Ragusans sent the army to defend Konavle but they also tried to prevail through the diplomatic contacts of the Ragusan physician of Jewish origin, Samuel Abeatar. His relative, Daniel, was a highly respected physician in Constantinople who cared for the top Ottoman dignitaries at the Porte. The Ragusans asked both of them to intervene in their defence. By this combined military and diplomatic action, Dubrovnik was able to deflect the attack by the Ottomans and keep Konavle permanently. Later on, the Ragusan Councils asked Cardinal Paolo Emilio Sfondrati in Rome to intervene directly on behalf of Abeatar. Difficulties arose when the ecclesiastical authorities in Dubrovnik wanted to prevent the physicians of Jewish origin from treating Christian patients without the presence of at least one Christian physician. On

13 March 1597, four physicians serving in Dubrovnik wrote to Rome on behalf of Abeatar. Two of those physicians were Nicolaus Rossus from Sicily and Dominicus Lanceno from Bologna. In their letters they emphasized the virtues Abeatar possessed both as a physician and as a human being. The Ragusans prevailed in Rome and Samuel Abeatar continued performing his duties in Dubrovnik where he was highly respected because of what he had done for Dubrovnik and where he probably stayed until his death.[95]

The status of the physicians who travelled to the Balkans was unpredictable. It was never clear in advance what the outcome of the trip, in the diplomatic sense, would be. The contribution of the physicians to the maintenance of peaceful relations on the uncertain fault line between East and West, where Dubrovnik was often the only intermediary, was considerable. By securing medical treatment for dignitaries of neighbouring countries, Dubrovnik wisely maintained good diplomatic relations in the region, protecting its territory and its political as well as economic interests. It has to be pointed out that Ottoman officials in Bosnia did not have access to physicians and they did not employ them on a regular basis. The assistance of physicians from Dubrovnik was therefore even more precious.

However, as a Catholic country surrounded by the Ottomans, Dubrovnik had to tread very gingerly. The Republic sought the protection of the pope and tried to maintain as close relations as possible with countries of the Western Mediterranean, especially the Spanish, with whom it maintained a vivid trade exchange. The possibility of a subtle, covert diplomatic activity and even influence of the medical practitioners on the various rulers is inherent in the nature of their work, which requires complete confidence between the patient and his treating physician. The personal contact with the ruling dignitaries carried the potential of leading into the intricate world of diplomacy. On the other hand, there was also the underlying obligation of maintaining neutrality.

In 1584, the surgeon Gaspar Bazzo was sent to Banja Luka to treat the Bosnian pasha. After that strenuous trip, he asked for a two-month leave of absence to treat his sciatica. In his letter to the Senate, he mentioned that he was almost paralyzed by pain because of cold weather in Bosnia. He also asked for his Ragusan salary to be paid for that period because he had become sick while in the service of the Republic and because during the time of his sickness, he could not practise medicine. Both of his wishes were granted.

When Hasan Pasha Predojević became the *beylerbey* of Bosnia in 1590, he asked the Ragusan consul to be present at all times in Banja Luka to take care of communications, negotiations, and his special wishes. During his reign from

1590 to 1593, the pasha often asked for Ragusan physicians. The arduous trip to Banja Luka was made by the famous Toma Natalis Budislavić and several other physicians: Salamun Oefo and Jacob Danon, both of Jewish origin, as well as by the surgeons Joseph Salama and Mihajlo Squadro. Joseph Salama had married Zoe, the daughter of the famous surgeon Abraham Hebreus. Joseph's father-in-law, who was employed in Dubrovnik since 1558, had trained him and taught him his art. In 1592, he was sent to Banja Luka where he died.[96] Since both sides found it advantageous, from the fifteenth century until the end of the Republic in 1808, Dubrovnik regularly sent its physicians to treat Ottoman dignitaries in Bosnia.[97]

FAMOUS PHYSICIANS WHO SERVED IN DUBROVNIK IN THE SIXTEENTH CENTURY

The Ragusan Republic had an enlightened attitude towards the health of its population and invested a lot of money and energy into the organization of the Health Office, hospitals, and quarantine compounds during plague epidemics as well as medical care provided by physicians and surgeons. Still, descriptions of particular diseases and their therapy or descriptions of surgical interventions are scarce. In the sixteenth century, however, based on new anatomical and botanical knowledge, enlightened physicians tried new methods of treatment rooted in their own experience. First and foremost among them were Donato Muzi and Mariano Santo, Italian innovators who served in Dubrovnik. In their works, they left the descriptions of patients they had treated in Dubrovnik. In the latter part of the century, they were joined by Amatus Lusitanus, a famous Portuguese physician of Jewish origin.

On 28 May 1526, the Major Council decided to employ Donato Muzi – Donatus de Mutiis – as a community physician in Dubrovnik with a salary of 330 ducats.[98] His contract was renewed every year until 1536. Donato Muzi was born in Venice around 1490 and died around 1554, place unknown.[99] He started his medical studies in Padua but when the University of Padua closed between 1509 and 1517 because of the war between the Venetians and the French near Cremona, he decided to go to Bologna. Muzi, like many other students, took his final exam at the Venetian College of Physicians because its fees were much lower than those in Padua.[100] Muzi was critical of Galen and the ancients in general. Since his knowledge of Latin and Greek was very good, he re-examined what they had written and came up with his own criticism of

Galen's interpretation of fourteen aphorisms by Hippocrates. This was published in Zurich or Basel in 1547.[101] From the point of view of contemporary medicine, Muzi's criticism is entirely justified. He discloses that Galen's misconceptions are whispered about among physicians but never openly discussed because most people do not want to confront the celebrities who enjoy full public recognition. Muzi criticizes his contemporaries for blindly believing some classical authors and accepting as indisputable dogma that which is just a personal opinion of famous individuals. According to him, erroneous scientific explanations can be found even in the works of the most famous scientists.

Donato Muzi also describes the frequency of bladder stones as well as cystic echinococcosis, a parasitic liver disease in Central and South Dalmatia. He opposes Hippocrates's aphorism VII 55, in which a rupture of such a cyst is described as ending in death. Muzi doubts Galen's knowledge of the digestive organs and states that he has seen patients survive after an incision of the cyst. Muzi also criticizes Hippocrates's aphorism IV 79 in which he maintains that the presence of sand in the urine indicates the presence of bladder stones. Galen believes that stones can be deposited in the kidney but Muzi concludes that the presence of sand in the urine does not indicate the presence of stones in any urinary organ. Muzi maintains that he has often seen such patients in Venice and especially in Dubrovnik where he had "practised medicine alone for nine years." Muzi can be considered a reformer of classical medicine who left an abundance of precious data about the pathology in Central and South Dalmatia. However, his most important contribution to Croatian medical historiography is his description and diagnosis of plague in December 1526 (see Chapter 6).

The Ragusan archbishop Philippo Trivulzi asked Muzi to provide an opinion about treating arthritis from which his brother Pomponius, the governor of Lyon, suffered. At that time, turpentine resin was touted as efficient treatment for this problem. In his answer to the letter of Philipppo Trivulzi, Muzi stated that he doubted the efficiency of this medication and that he considered that it could be very dangerous for the stomach. He added that he did not know why some physicians used medications for which he, from his own experience, could not say were helpful. In his opinion, some physicians used such medicines at the moment when the patient was already getting better anyway so that the cure could be later ascribed to the medication. Muzi's letter was published in Lyon in 1534 as an addendum to the book *Gallicum Pentapharmacum* of the French physician Symphorien Champier.[102]

MARIANO SANTO

Mariano Santo was born in Barletta in 1488. He received his surgical training first in Naples and then in Rome where he continued his studies and became a doctor of philosophy in 1520 and a doctor of medicine in 1522. Although very successful and well-known in Rome, in 1526 he moved to Milan to become the physician of the Trivulzi family. When Philippo Trivulzi was named the archbishop of Dubrovnik, Mariano Santo followed him, first as his personal physician and later as a physician hired by the Ragusan Republic. Lavoslav Glesinger studied Mariano Santo's Ragusan days and was able to untangle several mysteries of his biography.[103]

At that time, an intense political battle was taking place between France and Spain for the dominance of Italy while all of Europe was threatened by Ottoman expansion. To everyone's surprise, in 1536 the French concluded an agreement with the Ottomans so that together they could counter the Spanish.[104] In Dubrovnik, squeezed between these belligerent superpowers, there were those who supported the French and those who supported the Spanish. Philippo Trivulzi was not only the representative of the francophiles in Dubrovnik but he was an agent of the French king François I. Trivulzi was the one who transmitted the correspondence between France and the French ambassador in Istanbul. The French representatives, who arrived in Dubrovnik on their way to, or from Istanbul, were wined and dined by Trivulzi in his palace. In spite of the repeated protests of the Ragusans who wanted to remain neutral in this conflict, Dubrovnik remained an important centre for the French diplomacy and its secret agents.[105] One of those diplomats who enjoyed the confidence of the Ottoman sultan Suleiman was the Spaniard Antonio Rincón, who worked for the French. He was in Dubrovnik at the end of May 1532 and from there he wanted to travel to Istanbul. Suleiman had gathered a huge army with the intention of marching on Hungary and from there, to Vienna. Antonio Rincón was sent to meet Suleiman, apparently to dissuade him from taking Vienna. However, it seems that Rincón's task was just the opposite. He was to beg Suleiman to attack Italy because the French King François I wanted to use this moment to conquer Genoa and Milan.[106] As it happened, Rincón became sick in Dubrovnik and could not continue his trip. He was obliged to send a message to Suleiman, who had already reached Belgrade, that he could not come. Suleiman answered that he would send his men to carry Rincón all the way to Belgrade. Still, Rincón stayed in Dubrovnik because he was in great pain caused by bladder stones. There he was treated by Mariano Santo, who had invented a new method of removing bladder stones, known in the history of urology as *sectio Mariana*. Santo's method consisted in removing the stone from the urethra and not cutting into the bladder as previous methods had done. Santo, who described his method in his work *Libellus aureus de lapide e vesica per incisionem extrahendo* published in Venice in 1522, also used more instruments that served to enlarge the incision, remove the stone, and clean up the bladder. It took most of the month of June for Rincón to recover in Dubrovnik. On 23 June 1532, the Senate decided to allow Mariano Santo to take a three-month leave of absence to accompany Rincón on his journey.[107] They arrived in Belgrade on 5 July where Rincón was received with all the honours, but Suleiman did not change his war plans.[108] Rincón returned to Venice via Dubrovnik without having accomplished his mission.[109] In his works, Mariano Santo discusses his trip to Belgrade and mentions that he observed the Ottoman surgeons using a lancet, a small, broad, two-edged surgical knife with a sharp point, to perform phlebotomies. He liked the instrument and made sure that he obtained one for himself.[110]

The last mention of Mariano Santo in Dubrovnik took place on 16 December 1532 when the Major Council decided not to renew his contract for another year with the same salary. On the same day, however, the Major Council renewed the contract of the physician Hieronymus de Verona for a year. Why refuse the famous Mariano Santo and confirm Hieronymus de Verona? Mariano Santo was a great innovator, an excellent surgeon, and an outstanding physician. He was against treating head injuries with rose oil and used the wine alcohol instead. He stopped bleeding from arteries by ligature instead of using cauterization. He considered the skull trepanation to be a useful intervention and instead of the hammer and chisel, he used the trepan. For a number of skin diseases, he used unguents with the addition of mercury, which he called *unguentum Marianum*. Because he had a good knowledge of both surgery and internal medicine, Santo had an advantage over other physicians and did not stop at measuring blood pressure and studying the colour of the urine of his patients. However, as a person of his time, he did not give up astrology and, just like his colleagues, prescribed nebulous recipes. He wrote twelve books, and, in some of them, he boasts how he cured his Ragusan patients after his colleagues had prescribed incorrect treatment. All his works teem with attacks on his colleagues, whom he mocked and criticized without pity. Therefore, he often changed his place of work and died in Rome in 1577. In Dubrovnik, he was constantly in conflict with other physicians. On numerous occasions, he also complained about the empirics, miscellaneously trained practitioners who he thought the Ragusans should have expelled from the city. Glesinger concludes that this aspect of his behaviour, rather than his professional work, may have been the reason that his contract was not renewed at the end of 1532.

AMATUS LUSITANUS

João Rodrigues, born of Jewish parents in Castelo Branco, Portugal in 1511 was known by the name Amatus Lusitanus. Although his family had embraced the Catholic faith before his birth, after his medical studies in Salamanca, which included medical botany, he was persecuted in his homeland and had to leave Portugal. Starting in Holland and Belgium, he travelled throughout Europe, before settling in Ferrara where he distinguished himself as professor of anatomy. There is reason to believe that while in Ferrara (1540–47), Amatus Lusitanus discovered and was able to demonstrate to his colleagues the existence of venous valves. In *Centuria* 1, curatio 51, he describes how he blew air into the lower part of the azygos vein and showed that the vena cava would not be inflated. It was not possible for the air to escape because of the venous valve. If air could not pass, blood, much thicker than the air, could not flow through either. Eventually, Amatus Lusitanus had to leave Ferrara and, after living in Ancona for a while, settled in Pesaro wherefrom he most probably left for Dubrovnik in the summer of 1556. He wrote seven books of *Centuriae* and in each he described the case histories of one hundred patients. In *Centuria* 6, he describes his patients in Dubrovnik by name, their symptoms, the diagnosis, and the therapy that he had prescribed. Amatus did not manage to become the Ragusan state physician. All his patients were private, mostly members of the illustrious patrician families and wealthy citizens. He also adds his comments for each case report. His recipes, which sometimes contained more than twenty ingredients, are also included. In the introduction to *Centuria* 6, he describes Dubrovnik as being "a small, but ancient city, like Venice, situated on the rocky coast of the Adriatic Sea, with southern orientation, and therefore exposed to southern winds in which people suffer more frequently from diseases in winter." Amatus Lusitanus advised the surgeons in Dubrovnik but he did not interfere with their interventions. Like other physicians of his time, he confused the disease with the symptoms and tried hard to rid his patients of the disorders they suffered. He travelled to Kotor and Hercegnovi and described the case histories of his patients there. After 1558, Amatus Lusitanus was no longer in Dubrovnik. In 1568, he died of plague in Thessaloniki.[111]

In this chapter various forms of pre-plague health care as well as the role of physicians and surgeons (1280–1600) have been discussed. The practice of hiring city physicians and surgeons, who provided medical care for all the citizens without extra pay, started in Dubrovnik as early as 1280, and continued for centuries. It has been demonstrated that most physicians preferred to avoid plague-stricken cities and, in those crucial moments, left the health care to surgeons and plague doctors. The next chapter will focus on the establishment of the Health Office, the most important government agency in the fight against plague.

4

Founding and Development of the
Health Office, 1390–1482

This chapter examines the development of plague control measures from 1377 to 1482. The chronological evolution of the plague legislation reveals that, gradually, during each new plague epidemic, more complex regulations, dealing with a large variety of issues, were promulgated. Thus, each plague outbreak represented a new milestone in fighting the epidemics and every time strict and more repressive measures were adopted. The 1390 addition of plague control officials to enforce and implement the quarantine legislation promulgated in 1377 constitutes the most important development in this period. Another milestone was reached in 1397 when the regulation, which prescribes the elections of plague control officials and lists their duties, was enacted. Then again significant additions to the plague control measures were adopted during the 1426, 1457, and 1482 plague attacks. Each of these moments marks a major watershed in the development of plague control measures towards a complex system of plague defence that will became useful again in 1526–27 during the worst plague attack to strike Dubrovnik since 1348.

Invisible to the human eye, plague followed the paths of maritime and overland trade.[1] Forced movements of great numbers of people during armed conflicts also favoured its spread. In comparison with other Dalmatian cities, Dubrovnik, as a community with a large international trade and a rather small population, suffered more frequent plague attacks that took an enormous toll in human lives. According to Lawrence Conrad, even more threatening than the mortality itself was, and still is, the challenge of the epidemic disease to the ideological structures that sustain all societies. The sense of origin, identity, purpose, and future of a society are all badly shaken and seriously disrupted by epidemics.[2] Combating plague therefore became synonymous with the survival of Dubrovnik and the defence of its territory. These new circumstances required an original way of thinking and a novel approach. The frequency of the recurring epidemics prompted the city fathers to draft the quarantine regulation in 1377. Not long after that, the first plague control officials were named.[3]

THE FIRST QUARANTINE LEGISLATION IN THE WORLD

On 27 July 1377, the Major Council promulgated the regulation under the title *Veniens de locis pestiferis non intret Ragusium vel districtum* (Those arriving from plague-infected areas shall not enter Dubrovnik or its district), which became known as the first quarantine regulation in the world. The original text of the regulation is available in the *Liber viridis* (Green book), which contains the chronological supplements (1358–1460) to the 1272 Dubrovnik Statute regulations. Due to its extraordinary historical importance, both the Latin original and its translation are quoted here:

> Veniens de locis pestiferis non intret Ragusium vel districtum. Eodem anno [1377] die XXVII Julii in Consilio Maiori congregato, ut est moris, in quo interfuerunt consiliarii XLVII, captum et firmatum fuit per XXXIV ipsorum quod tam nostrates quam advene venientes de locis pestiferis non recipiantur in Ragusium nec ad eius districtum, nisi steterint prius ad purgandum seu in Mercana seu in Civitate Veteri per unum mensem.
>
> Item per consiliarios XLIV eiusdem Consilii captum fuit quod nulla persona de Ragusio vel suo districtu audeat vel presumat ire ad illos qui venient de locis pestiferis et stabunt in Merchana vel Civitate Veteri, sub pena standi ibidem per unum mensem. Et illi qui portabunt illis de victualibus seu aliis necessariis non possint ire ad illos sine licentia officialium ad hoc ordinandorum, cum ordine a dictis officialibus illis dando, sub dicta pena standi ibidem per unum mensem.
>
> Item per consiliarios XXVIIII euisdem Consilii captum fuit et firmatum quod quicumque non observaverit predicta seu aliquod predictorum, solvere debeat de pena ypperperos quinquaginta et nichilominus teneatur predicta observare.[4]

On 27 July 1377, gathered in the Major Council, according to custom, in which forty-seven members were present, thirty-four Councillors voted in favour of the proposed regulation, which stipulates that those who come from plague infested areas shall not enter Dubrovnik or its district unless they previously spend a month on the islet of Mrkan (St Mark) or in the town of Cavtat, for the purpose of disinfection – *ad purgandum*.

Furthermore, forty-four Councillors decided that, under the threat of being sent into quarantine for a month, the residents of Dubrovnik are strictly forbidden to visit those who arrive from plague-infested areas and who will be confined on the islet of Mrkan or Cavtat. Those who dare bring food or any other necessities to the interned, without the permission of the officials designated for that function, will have to stay there in isolation for a month.

Furthermore, twenty-nine councillors decided that whoever did not obey the above decisions, would have to pay a fine of fifty *hyperperi*, and everyone would be obliged to observe it.

The goal of the Ragusan Major Council in adopting this regulation was primarily to stop, or at least to limit, the spreading of plague infection; second, the Council wanted to make sure that maritime and overland trade, even if considerably slowed down, continued, above all, to secure the vital import of grain. Mrkan, an uninhabited rocky islet, situated in the vicinity of Cavtat, became the quarantine location for those arriving by sea.[5] The town of Cavtat, more conveniently situated at the end of the caravan road, south of Dubrovnik, became the place of isolation for those arriving from the hinterland.

In 1377, Christophorus de Benevento, an eminent physician, was employed by the city of Dubrovnik, as were two surgeons, Johannes de Tragurio (Ivan from Trogir) and Johannes de Aldoardis de Papia (see Chapter 3). The Councils might have sought their advice when they prepared the quarantine legislation but there is no trace in the sources to indicate such a possibility.

Particular thanks are owed to Josip Đelčić (Gelcich), the head archivist of the State Archives in Dubrovnik, who was the first to transcribe and publish the text of the quarantine regulation.[6] Mirko Dražen Grmek, who later brought the Ragusan quarantine regulation to the attention of medical historians worldwide, also deserves special mention. Due to the research efforts of these two men, scholars who are interested in the chronology of plague control measures have become familiar with the conceptual originality of the Ragusan quarantine and its role as a precursor of public health legislation. Grmek emphasizes that, in order to arrive at the preventive isolation, a major leap of knowledge was necessary in the perception of plague: the notion of incubation and maybe also the concept of healthy carriers of disease had to be accepted. Quarantine, as we know, requires the isolation of apparently healthy individuals who could be potential disease carriers. In the legislation, the expression "all those arriving from plague-infected areas," implies the notion of healthy carriers – that is, whether they are healthy or sick at the moment of arrival, they have to be isolated. The sick were separated from the healthy, from their goods, and from their usual environment, but that separation was not the isolation of individuals in the modern sense. People were isolated in groups of healthy individuals, groups of sick persons, and groups of people who had been in contact with the sick (suspects).[7] The quarantine became necessary because a simple medical examination could not definitively exclude the diagnosis of the plague in apparently healthy subjects. Mirko Dražen Grmek notes that although the cities of Genoa, Messina, Lucca, and Venice sometimes used weapons to stop the infected from entering their city during the plague epidemic of 1348, systematically forbidding the entrance of all the ships arriving from plague-infected areas was never an option. Moreover, Grmek considers that the preventive quarantine legislation is one of the highest achievements of mediaeval medicine.[8] The plague incubation period lasts only one to seven days, but this fact was not discovered until the end of the nineteenth century. Since the fourteenth-century Ragusans had no way of knowing this, they imposed a much longer isolation period. The quarantine legislation was predicated on the idea that the government was justified in controlling the space and the movement of the few in the interest of the common good. The merchants accepted it and cooperated with the government.[9]

The shrewd Ragusan aristocrats and common citizens, all of them keen observers, soon learned from experience that the infection followed maritime trade routes, its source hiding in grain, wool, cotton, leather, and fur.[10] Although it was not detectable by the human eye, the Ragusans handling these goods were in constant danger of contracting plague. Already in the second half of the fourteenth century, they understood that there was a cyclical repetition of the plague epidemics every five or ten years. A recollection of the previous plague epidemic remained in the living memory of each generation.[11] At that time, Dubrovnik enjoyed rapid economic growth and it was developing into a major maritime trade power in the Mediterranean. Since the soil of the Ragusan Republic was not particularly fertile, food in quantities sufficient to satisfy the needs of all the citizens could never be grown locally. Thus, there was no choice but to continue unloading the grain – mainly wheat, millet, and barley – from Sicily or the Levant in the Dubrovnik harbour, and with every shipment a renewed danger of plague infection would arise.[12] Plague always came from the Levant. It was brought by infected ships, either directly from the Ottoman lands or indirectly, on a ship from one of the Italian port cities on the other side of the Adriatic.

The memory of the first plague epidemic in 1348, when the city ran the risk of becoming almost completely depopulated, was still fresh in the minds of the governing patricians (see Chapter 2, p. 46). Physicians, burdened by Galen's and Avicena's humoural and miasmatic theories, were not able to respond to plague. Because the patricians could not afford to risk chaos or panic in the city, they had to take the matter in their own hands. Therefore, they approached the protection of the city from cyclical plague epidemics in the same fashion as they faced the organization of defence of the state against enemies on land and sea.[13] That included a more rigorous discipline among the government officials of Dubrovnik. Anarchic and panicky flight from the city would not be allowed.[14] Although flight from the source of infection was considered the best reaction to plague, it represented a problem for the city fathers. If Ragusans were allowed to flee to their suburban villas or to the islands, who would stay to defend the city and provide services to the citizens, including the sick? Therefore, in a disciplined society such as Dubrovnik, only those who had no specific tasks to perform during a plague outbreak could leave the city. This included certain patricians as well as commoners.[15]

Moreover, the Senate would soon consider the establishment of a special office with extensive authority in the application of health regulations. In June 1390, the news that plague was rampant in Rome caused great concern in the Ragusan councils. On 21 June 1390, the Major Council directed the rector and the Minor Council to give authority to the plague control officials to forbid all those arriving from plague-infected areas to enter the city and to punish the violators as they saw fit.[16]

FOUNDING OF THE HEALTH OFFICE

On 24 June 1390, the Minor Council, with the authorization of the Major Council, elected three Officials Against the Plague, the patricians – Marin Krušić (Croze), Pasko Rastić (Resti), and Šimun Gučetić (Gozze) – and gave them the same authority that had been vested in their predecessors.[17] This formulation draws our attention to the fact that plague control officials may have been elected even before 1390. However, no record of their elections prior to 1390 has been preserved in the State Archives of Dubrovnik. The second paragraph of this regulation states that under the threat of being punished by the Officials Against the Plague, all those arriving from plague-infected areas have to stay away from the territory of the Republic for fifteen days. In this regulation they are called Officials Against Those Arriving From Plague-Infected Areas – *officiales contra venientes de locis pestiferis* and *officiales ad providendum super venientibus de locis pestiferis*, a descriptive phrase used for lack of a specific name.[18] This term was used in the fourteenth century to be later replaced by the terms the *Cazamorti* and the *health officials*.

On 17 July 1390, the Minor Council decided that all those who were returning from plague-stricken Rome had to be taken to the islet of Mrkan or to Molunat, south of Dubrovnik, with a warning that they were not allowed to stay anywhere except in Molunat.[19] This decision illustrates the implementation of the quarantine regulation of 1377. Constant danger of infection forced the Councils to name successors of the plague control officials before the end of their usual term. On 4 September 1390, the Minor Council thus elected as a new plague control team, the patricians Petar de Saracha, Nikola Menčetić (Menze), and Marin Martolov Bučinčić (Bucignolo). They were ordered to prevent those coming from plague-infected areas from entering the city and they were empowered to punish the violators in the same way as their predecessors.[20] The appointment of officials to enforce the plague control regulations definitely represents an important step forward in the fight against epidemics. It is also logical that the plague legislation required officials to implement it.

On 1 April 1391, the Minor Council ordered the Officials Against the Plague to prevent the ship owners and their crews, as well as all other persons, from going to plague-stricken areas between Budva and Ulcinj (present-day Montenegro), south of the Ragusan Republic. Likewise, persons from those infected areas were not allowed to enter Dubrovnik. New, more stringent fines were implemented and persons who did not respect this order could be punished with monetary fines of up to one hundred ducats.[21] In May 1391, the infection started spreading within the city walls. On 8 June, the Major Council adopted new measures of governing if only a few patricians should remain in the city.[22] On 22 December, when the danger of plague had subsided, this regulation was cancelled.[23]

On 8 January 1392, Matija Vitov Benešić (Benessa) was named Official Against the Plague, and Nikola Đurđević (Giorgi or Georgi) and Marin Petrov Bučinčić (Bucignolo) were elected to replace the other two plague control officials on 18 February 1392. The Minor Council instructed them to fine violators as they saw fit. If those contravening the health regulations did not pay their fines within a prescribed period of time, the Officials Against the Plague, who were given ever more authority, were even authorized to inflict corporal punishment such as lashing, branding, and cutting off of one ear.[24] This is the first time we encounter corporal punishment for violators of plague regulations. The behaviour of the plague control violators was putting at risk the lives of many other citizens, so the government felt justified in not showing any particular consideration for them. Increased authority of the plague control officials and severe punishment were probably the result of the violators lending a deaf ear to the regulations.

The regulation proclaimed on 11 June 1392 required those arriving from Ulcinj and other infected areas not to stay anywhere in Dubrovnik or its district, including the island of Mljet, for one month.[25]

The regulations of the Ragusan councils found in the archival series *Reformationes*, the main source of legislative decisions for this period, prove that the plague control officials were active even in the most poorly documented period of 1392 to 1395. While the consequences of the previous plague epidemics were still fresh in the memory of the citizens, the authorities were determined to further improve plague control measures. On 9 February 1395, the Minor Council elected three new Officials Against the Plague: Marin Krušić (Crosi), Matija Vitov Benešić (Benessa), and Theodorus Prodanello. They were given the same authority as the officials mentioned in the regulation of 23 October 1394.[26]

According to the short but significant regulation dated 27 September 1395, the Minor Council expanded the Plague Control Office by adding two more officials – Nalchus Prokulović (Procullo) and Volczo Vlahov Bobaljević (Baballio) – so that they could take turns with those previously elected. The two new officials also had the same authority as those elected earlier. According to the practice of the scribes of that period, the term *Caxamorti* appears for the first time in the margin of this regulation, as a subject heading for easier retrieval.[27] The term *Cazamorti* was common in the fifteenth century.

In the regulation dated 11 January 1396, the names and duties of five new Officials Against the Plague are listed. The Minor Council warns the elected individuals that they should perform their duties in the usual way with the customary authority vested in them. However, the monetary fines should be limited to one hundred ducats according to the regulation dated 23 October 1394.[28] On 12 January 1396, the Major Council decided to give the authority to the rector and the Minor Council to elect officials to deal with the persons coming from plague-infected areas, with persons receiving them and with those coming in contact with them, and to regulate the traffic between them as they saw fit. This decision was cancelled on the same day probably because its consequences seemed to reach too far.[29]

At the same time, the Officials Against the Plague kept an eye on the situation in other port cities. On 6 March 1396, they reported to the Minor Council that they heard from persons who had returned from Venice that plague was no longer rampant in that city. The travellers from Venice were thus allowed to enter Dubrovnik as they pleased.[30]

ELECTIONS OF THE OFFICIALS AGAINST THE PLAGUE

On 5 January 1397, the Major Council adopted a regulation known as *De ordinibus contra eos qui veniunt de locis pestiferis* (About the regulations against those coming from plague-infected areas). In it, previous decisions were repeated and new ones were added. It was decided that the Minor Council should elect the Officials Against the Plague. Furthermore, the Minor Council could decide to elect as many Officials Against the Plague as they saw fit – *tot officiales quot dicto minori consilio videbitur*. The aim was obviously to let the number of officials fit the level of danger from infection. The duties of those officials were to apply, enforce, and control the implementation of plague control regulations. They were authorized to punish the violators with previously established monetary fines. If the violators did not pay their fines within a prescribed period of time, the Officials Against the Plague were allowed to inflict corporal punishment as established in the regulation dated 18 February 1392. Moreover, they were to make sure that those coming from plague-infected areas did not enter Dubrovnik or its district, including the island of Mljet.[31]

The regulation of 5 January 1397, which prescribes the elections of plague control officials and lists their duties, constitutes an important milestone. The Plague Control Office was transformed from a regular but still ad hoc to a permanent office. From then on, the plague control officials would be elected in January with most of the public officials of the Ragusan state, as opposed to any time of the year as required by the circumstances. This regular January election period is in keeping with the Ragusan institutional history. For a while, officials for new functions were elected on an ad hoc basis, which allowed the Councils to evaluate the usefulness of the new office and modify its characteristics if necessary before deciding to keep it on a permanent basis. Thus, on 6 January

1397, Marin Bučinčić (Buccignollo), Matija Vitov Benešić (Benessa), Marin Ivanov Gradić (Gradi), Marin Crijević (Zrieva), and Theodorus Prodanello were elected as Officials Against the Plague by the Minor Council. The permission for these elections was granted by the Major Council the day before.[32]

Why did this office become permanent in Dubrovnik earlier than in other cities? Again, it was a result of the Ragusan institutional tradition. Primarily, once quarantine legislation had been adopted, officials were needed for its implementation. Second, the proximity of Dubrovnik to the Ottoman Empire – from where the plague arrived – made preventive measures an urgent matter of high priority.

In the second paragraph of the regulation dated 5 January 1397, the import of grain and other new merchandise is allowed but the import of used clothes and bedding from infected areas within the territory of the commune of Dubrovnik is forbidden. Persons arriving from plague-infected areas must remain in the quarantine on the islet of Mrkan or, for a month, in the (Benedictine) monastery (of St Mary) on the island of Mljet, or they have to stay outside of the Ragusan territory for the same length of time.[33] The citizens who dared travel to plague-infected areas were not allowed to return before spending two months in quarantine within the territory of the Ragusan Republic or remaining outside of the Ragusan territory. If they did not obey, they had to pay a fine of one hundred ducats.

On 28 January 1397, the Major Council forbade the transport of any goods –particularly grain, fruit, and clothes – from plague-infected areas within the Republic to the healthy areas, until such time as the infection had become extinct. This regulation dealt a hard blow to trade during the epidemics.[34] From these additions to the basic regulation of 5 January 1397, we gather that the growing danger from infection forced the authorities to decide on ever more restrictive measures to control the spreading of the disease. However, even in those months of crisis, trade continued with areas that were not affected by plague, thus softening the blow of economic losses caused by quarantine.

As fear of the plague epidemic grew, an addendum dated 25 May 1397 was appended to this regulation; the addendum stipulated that the violators who did not pay the fine, or did not offer a warrant, or did not find someone to vouch for them, would be punished by being branded on the face with four hot irons and would be expelled from Dubrovnik. If the warrantor did not pay the fine within a month, he would be thrown into prison and would not be freed until the fine was paid.[35] It is ironic that plague control policies that were designed to protect citizens also carried with them their own set of negative repercussions, often threatening the very existence of the people they were supposed to keep safe.

On 23 June 1397, the Minor Council, aware that the plague had spread to the Pelješac Peninsula, ordered guards to be posted there. Two boats were to be sent to Pelješac to prevent the citizens arriving from Dubrovnik from stopping in Viganj and other places infected by plague. This duty was to be performed by two men from Ston, according to the instructions that they had received.[36] The isolation of Pelješac was ended on 24 September 1397.[37]

The Officials Against the Plague had enormous authority vested in them. They acted within the framework of the plague regulations but when very serious violations had to be dealt with, the measures had to be previously approved by the Minor Council. However, when renewed plague outbreaks required even more rigorous protective measures and immediate action, the Officials Against the Plague received ad hoc orders from the Minor Council. The ever-growing authority of the Officials Against the Plague is evident in a whole range of heavy monetary fines and serious corporal punishments that they were empowered to inflict. The strict control of arrivals in Dubrovnik that applied to citizens and foreigners alike drastically changed the way of life and slowed down the economic activity (see Chapter 5).

The Senate showed caution in the initial regulations by making at least a limited circulation of goods possible. When this measure proved to be inadequate, the authorities ordered a complete cessation of the transport of goods from plague-infected areas. Punishment imposed on the violators was heavy-handed and only the most adventurous dared to contravene. Although the prerogatives of the Officials Against the Plague respected the regulations, they were threatening, unpopular, and most often contrary to the economic interests of the citizens. For example, the regulation of 7 October 1397 asks the Officials Against the Plague not to permit captain Benedikt Contareno and the crew from his two ships to enter the city harbour because they were suspected of being infected. After spending three days in Split, they were forbidden from entering Dubrovnik for a month, counting from the day they entered the Split harbour.[38]

On 13 January 1398, five Officials Against the Plague were elected in the first month of the year, the usual date for elections of most officials. This date indicates that they had become a permanent office. The elected candidates – Stjepan Sorkočević (Sorgo), Ursus Džamanjić (Zamagno), Nikola Ranjina (Ragnina), Klement Budačić (Bodaca), and Natalis Prokulović (Procullo) – were members of patrician families.[39] On 1 January 1399, five new Officials Against the Plague were elected to control those arriving from the plague-infected areas and those travelling from Dubrovnik to plague-infected areas – *contra euntes ad loca pestifera*.[40] Elected were Volczinus Bobaljević (Babalio), Nikola P. Pucić (Poza), Martholus Džamanjić (Zamagno), Ivan Jakovov Gundulić (Gondola), and Martinussio Baraba. On 15 October 1399, the Minor Council instructed the plague control officials to go to Obod in Konavle, a region on the southern border of the Ragusan state, and gave them the authority to implement the plague regulations as they saw fit. The Minor Council also approved their expenses.[41]

Based on the regulations promulgated from 1390 to 1400, it is possible to determine that plague control measures were applied during the whole period. On the basis of the books *Reformationes* and the Deliberations of the Minor Council examined until the year 1426, we have concluded that, with slight exceptions for the years 1392 to 1395 (the period for which the archival books no longer exist), the Officials Against the Plague were appointed every year, together with those who were to succeed them at the end of their term, or earlier, if their term was interrupted for justifiable reasons, or if they died during the epidemic (see Table 4.1).[42]

In the fifteenth century, the plague control officials were called *Officiales Cazzamortuorum, Signori Cazamorti*, or simply *Cazamorti*. The regulation dated 10 November 1413 orders the *Officiales Cazzamortuorum* to send into quarantine Marino Sasnić and Tomado Mihov from Župa, if, upon their return from Brindisi, they happen to have stayed in an infected place. If they did not obey, they would be punished with a fine of one hundred ducats and six months in prison.[43] A renewed increase in the severity of the penalties imposed indicates that this was not a lone case. It was obviously possible for the sailors on smaller ships, with a small crew loyal to the captain, to omit mentioning that they had stopped in an infected port, especially when they were eager to see their families after a long journey or if business interests were involved. Such occurrences were later investigated and severely punished (see Chapter 8).

On 28 June 1415, the Minor Council instructed the Cazamorti to have ready for fifteen days, at the expense of the commune, an armed boat to guard the islands from persons arriving from plague-infected areas.[44]

THE CAZAMORTI SERVING WITHOUT PAY

On 15 January 1426, the Major Council adopted the regulation that dealt with the elections of the Cazamorti.[45] The Major Council states, in no uncertain terms, that the Cazamorti are elected to serve without pay – *per angariam*.[46]

Table 4.1
Elections of Plague Control Officials in Dubrovnik, 1400–1426

YEAR	DATE	OFFICIALS ELECTED
1400	28 June	5
1402	archival sources missing	
1403	1 January	5
1403	28 June	5 commoner assistants
1405	archival sources missing	
1406	archival sources missing	
1407	6 January	5
1408	15 January	5
1408	28 May	2 replaced
1409	archival sources missing	
1410	1 January	5
1411	December	5
1412	27 December	6
1414	16 December	authority mentioned but there are no names
1415	30 April	5
1416	1 January	6
1417	1 January	5
1418	9 January	5
1419	5 January	5
1420	2 January	4
1421	1 January	5
1422	10 April	4
1423	23 December	5
1423	1 January	5
1425	15 January	5
1426	15 January	5

However, they were regularly granted some expenses incurred while exercising their duties, such as hiring a boat for their patrols.[47] At the age of twenty, which, in times of demographic crisis was lowered to eighteen, every male aristocrat automatically became a member of the Major Council and as such could be elected, in a secret ballot, to serve as *Cazamorto*, a duty that he could not refuse.[48] In general, hefty penalties, mostly monetary, were prescribed for refusing to serve in any capacity. In some cases, the violator, or even his whole family, could lose his aristocratic title, temporarily or permanently.[49] Such judgment was rarely passed because the patricians were careful to protect their ample privileges. They were aware that they had to serve as Cazamorti and fulfill this onerous, dangerous, and unpopular duty.[50] During plague epidemics, the patricians were burdened with greater responsibilities than other citizens. They were actually expected to risk their lives to ensure the survival of the Republic.[51] In 1426, the Cazamorti had to serve without pay.[52] However, thirty-one years later, the circumstances would force the authorities to start remunerating them.

The 15 January 1426 regulation stipulates that members of the Minor Council or the Civil Court should not be elected to serve as Cazamorti. This was in accordance with the general principles of the Republic, which was ever vigilant to avoid the concentration of power in the hands of a few. Also, the office of the Cazamorti was considered to be very demanding. Thus, the Councils preferred not to ask the same individuals to perform other onerous duties at the same time. The patricians that were elected to serve as Cazamorti had plebeian assistants who served as guards at the entrance gates to the city – *Ad Pillas, Ad Plocias, Ad Sanctum Lucam,* and *Ad Catenam,* and others who served outside the city.[53] These commoners were elected by the Minor Council and served under the *Cazamorti* from Dubrovnik who gave the assistants direct orders. The archival sources mention them as Cazamorti but it is clear from their names that they were, in fact, only assistants.[54]

From 1390 to 1426, the Cazamorti were elected by the Minor Council. The election procedure utilized by the Major Council, where the majority of the public officials were elected at the beginning of the year, is well known.[55] However, the election procedure of the Minor Council remains unknown. The councillors might have chosen the candidates by drawing lots and then voting or, they could have named the officials. In any case, it was always called an election.[56] If three officials were needed for a public function, the election procedure of the Major Council required nine candidates to be nominated. Positive and negative votes were written next to each candidate's name and the ones elected were marked. We can thus follow the exact election process for each candidate and for each office. No such information is available for the elections by the Minor Council. Three names are usually grouped together, one under the other, followed by a brace around those names and the words "are elected" – *electi sunt* or *facti sunt* –appear next to it. For the Cazamorti elected by the Minor Council, it was always specified that they were elected "by the authority given to the Minor Council by the Major Council."[57] It seems that the Major Council had to grant such authority for every election. On 1 January 1419, the elections for the Cazamorti were not held because the Major Council had not empowered the Minor Council to hold those elections. The elections were delayed until the next day when consent was given.[58] In 1426, the Major Council decided that it would elect the Cazamorti as quoted in the regulation above.[59] However, in the following years, they were again elected by the Minor Council.[60] We do not know the reason. It could be that the Major Council transferred some of its duties to the Minor Council.

The procedure prescribed for the elections of the Cazamorti on 15 January 1426 proves the importance of their office. In the fifteenth and sixteenth centuries, patricians were elected to serve as Cazamorti in their forties or fifties, usually in the middle of their careers.[61] From the names of those elected, we gather that they belonged to the five or six most illustrious patrician families.[62] The archival book *Speculum Maioris Consilii* (Mirror of the Major Council) registers all public functions of the Republic since 1440, including the names of the health officials.[63]

THE CAZAMORTI IN THE HIERARCHY OF OFFICES

David Rheubottom suggests that senior patricians tended to occupy more prestigious offices. To measure the hierarchical ordering of offices, he used the average number of years from admission into the Major Council until the first appointment to an office. His sample consists of patricians who entered the Major Council between 1455 and 1490. Rheubottom found that election to first office usually came between three and ten years after entering the Major Council. He stated that, on average, it took 27.2 years to be elected to the office of Cazamorti. For the sake of comparison, for that group of men, it took 30.1 years to become a senator, 31.2 years to become a member of the Minor Council, and 33.1 years to become a rector. The most respected offices were those that Rheubottom called the "inner circle" of political power: the judges of the civil and criminal courts, members of the Senate, members of the Minor Council, the rector, the count of Ston, and the overseers of public officials.

Rheubottom also studied the availability of senior offices to various cohorts of the Major Council from 1455 to 1490. A member of the Major Council could be elected to one of these posts after approximately thirty years of service. The positions of the Cazamorti or of the *Advocati del proprio* (attorneys of the Civil Court) most often served as steppingstones for those inner circle positions. The experienced senior patricians usually held those offices one year prior to election into the inner circle.[64] Other common routes to the top were through the posts of officials responsible for the grain supply, municipal attorney, or customs officials. Such posts accounted for over 80 percent of the posts outside the inner circle held by senior patricians. Rheubottom was able to demonstrate that while there were many inner circle positions – around forty a year – there were relatively few offices that served as preparation for the top ranks of those patricians who had between twenty and twenty-five years of service.

This paucity of available functions created a serious bottleneck in the higher echelons. From 1455 to 1459, when there were quite a few senior men in the Major Council and only nine patricians were elected to inner circle posts for the first time, this congestion increased. With many senior patricians available who could not all be elected to inner circle positions, this group was most likely to be holding the posts of Cazamorti or one of the other positions that were held prior to entering into the inner circle. Rheubottom's demonstration of the competition for senior functions at the top is further proof of the importance that the Ragusans attributed to the function of the Cazamorti and the high esteem in which this office was held, a post that a Major Council member could occupy only after twenty-five to twenty-nine years of service.[65]

BANISHMENT FROM DUBROVNIK

On 18 January 1431, the Minor Council adopted a regulation that ordered the Cazamorti to not, in case of plague in a Dubrovnik family, which, as they mention, God in his mercy should forbid, expel or isolate anyone without first informing the rector of Dubrovnik and the Minor Council.[66] The act of banishment was the most severe punishment and it is clear that only the rector and the Minor Council could make such a decision.[67]

DIVERSIS ON THE CAZAMORTI AND THE
1437 PLAGUE EPIDEMIC

Diversis was one of the very lucky people who, in 1437, became sick with plague and survived. In his book the Description of the illustrious city of Dubrovnik, he describes the climate and the geographical position of the city. He notes that "this city manages to stay healthy, untouched by plague outbreaks, sometimes for sixteen and even twenty years." He attributes it to "the healthy

air and the abundance of drinking water" and elsewhere to "the smart government of the city that elects Officials Against the Plague and adopts plague control measures."[68]

In the section on permanent offices of the Republic, Diversis devotes a
whole chapter of his book to the Cazamorti: "For this office five noblemen of
the best repute and among the most cautious when facing death are elected to
examine and keep a vigilant eye on those who come ... from plague-infected
areas."[69] Diversis has nothing but praise for the Cazamorti and stresses that it
is because of the successful health measures that the city was spared several
plague outbreaks. He describes how the infected are not allowed to enter the
city but are confined to the islets of Bobara (St Barbara) and Mrkan (St Mark)
or the town of Cavtat. Diversis reveals that the Cazamorti are empowered to
lengthen the stay of the infected in isolation but are not allowed to make it
shorter. The Cazamorti also supervised the local counts, who had to report the
cases of plague on the territory under their jurisdiction. Two ships cruised constantly and made sure that no ship docked on the territory of the Republic without permission. Diversis commends the Ragusans for sending the children, who
are more likely to succumb to the disease, to safer locations outside the city
during epidemics. If a patient died at home, the person who took care of him
and those who buried him had to go into quarantine at Danče, just outside the
city walls.

Diversis compliments the Ragusans on their health protection measures
and notes that this was not the case in the cities of Greece, Illyria, and Italy. He
also mentions the temporary officials such as the commander in chief of the
flotilla or the election of a certain number of patricians who have to stay
behind to govern the city in case of plague. He also describes "the beneficial
measures that they adopt when plague becomes rampant and almost everyone
has fled the city." He applauds the courage of the elected patricians who, risking their lives, have to stay in the city at all cost. Special regulations for
governing during the plague were adopted by the Senate.[70] In 1437, when
plague was rampant from 2 April to 24 June, "ten patricians stayed to govern
the city, nine of whom died of the disease within fifteen days." The only survivor was Marin Šimunov Rastić (Resti), an eighty-three-year-old patrician,
who tirelessly governed alone until the others returned.[71] Diversis did not forget to report that the old patrician repeatedly asked for reinforcements when
the epidemic had subsided but that the citizens still refused to return to the
city. The archival sources confirm that Rastić was awarded five hundred
hyperperi for his effort.[72] In this way, adds the chronicler, "with beneficial help

and salutary measures they saved themselves, the city, the sweetness of freedom and they protected the city from plague." Diversis does not mention that the fine for a patrician refusing to serve, which was five hundred hyperperi, the equivalent of 250 Venetian ducats, was exorbitant, while the fine for those who dared to leave the territory of the Republic was one thousand hyperperi. He concludes that "the care for saving the city, its security and its protection" became even better after the plague outbreak and that the "Ragusans formulated new laws and new measures that had to be respected in such cases." Diversis explains that the plague epidemic stopped on 24 June 1437, the feast day of St John the Baptist. Since then, to give thanks for the return of health to the city, every year on that day, the Ragusans held a procession in the presence of the rector and the Minor Council. Diversis's vivid descriptions of the Plague Control Office are corroborated by archival sources.[73]

On 21 May 1437, for a period of four months, the patricians who stayed in the city to govern during the plague hired a doctor of medicine, Jacobus de Prothonotariis from Messina, with a salary of 200 hyperperi. In case the Councils refused to confirm his employment when they returned to the city, the patricians had decided to pay the physician from their own funds. The doctor survived the plague but he did not linger in Dubrovnik.[74]

DUTIES OF THE CAZAMORTI

On 17 March 1439, the Major Council adopted an extensive regulation known as the *Ordines observandi tempore mortalitatis* (Rules to obey in case of an epidemic). It says that in case of an epidemic outbreak, should two or three people die of that epidemic in the city, the Cazamorti are obliged to report it to the Minor Council, under the threat of a fine of fifty hyperperi each. After that, the physicians should declare the nature of the disease. If they diagnose it as plague, the Minor Council should, immediately or the next day, inform the Senate under the threat of a penalty of one hundred hyperperi for each member of the Minor Council. The Senate should then promptly equip an armed galleon and elect its captain. His salary should not be limited in any way but decided by the Senate as it sees fit. That galleon should be armed with great haste in order to ply the seas off Dubrovnik and defend the city and its district. Also, a special guard should be formed on land.[75]

The regulation about the officials who have to stay in Dubrovnik during the grape harvest, *Ordo eorum officialium qui habent stare Ragusium tempore vindemiarum*, adopted by the Major Council on 28 March 1444, stipulates that at least one of the Cazamorti has to stay in the city.[76]

The basic mission of the Cazamorti was to implement the plague control regulations that the Councils adopted on a regular basis in order to achieve a complex system of plague defence. During every new plague epidemic, new protection measures were added, ushering in change over time. Thus, each new plague outbreak represented a watershed year. The responsibilities of the Cazamorti increased manifold as new duties were added to an already long list of tasks they had to perform. Their work became more complex, demanding greater coordination with the authorities and the subordinates that they were assigned. They supervised the entrance of the ships into the city harbour as well as the arrival of overland caravans; during epidemic outbreaks, they decided who should be sent into isolation and organized the whole protection effort; to maintain public order, they had to punish delinquents. In the beginning, they gave orders only to the lowest level of employees, including the barber, the guard, and the gravediggers, so-called *kopci* (male) and *kopice* (female).[77] Later on, they supervised those who worked in quarantine: the priest and the plague doctor. When necessary, the Cazamorti employed local assistants. It is clear from these examples that they performed complex tasks and, over time, developed wide-ranging executive and judicial powers (see Chapters 7, 8, and 9). If we take all these elements into account, it is not at all surprising that the Senate eventually decided to give the Cazamorti a salary.

On 12 February 1457, the Senate adopted a regulation in which the Cazamorti are called *officiales cazamorti salariati in civitate*. This is a significant change of their status and represents an important milestone in the development of the Health Office. They are no longer working *per angariam*, for free, as mentioned in the 1426 regulation, but as *salariati*, officials with a salary.[78] The fact that from then on the Cazamorti were paid for their work not only corroborated the importance of their function but also confirmed the high esteem in which they had been held during the sixty-seven years of the existence of their office. It is also a sign that their duties were considered uncommonly burdensome, with few candidates eager to perform them. However, there is no indication in the archival sources of the amounts that they were paid.[79] Would the fact that they were from now on salaried employees of the state possibly mean that the patricians somehow suffered some erasure of their noble status? Working with commoners was not new for the patricians; in their business ventures, they often associated with commoner merchants, often from the elite group of citizens, the members of the confraternity of St Anthony. Other patricians, such as the judges of the Criminal Court, were also paid a salary. The rector was also paid a salary. After 1457, the health officials continued to be elected from the six most prestigious patrician families in Dubrovnik. That did not change. Were the health officials worried about their loss of status? There is evidence that they always took it in consideration. Commoners were not allowed to make decisions concerning patricians. Thus, whenever a commoner could have authority over a patrician, the decision was changed in order to put a patrician in charge and preserve the patrician status (see Chapter 8).

The office of the Cazamorti was of crucial importance for the survival of the Republic. During the yearly elections, their term of office was arranged to overlap in such a way that two new officials started six months after the term of those who were elected earlier. Thus, the most experienced among them had the opportunity to initiate the newly elected colleagues in all the sensitive details of their demanding office and ensure its continuity.[80] Until 1457, the Minor Council gave specific instructions to the Cazamorti. After that date, this role was taken over by the Senate. In the sixteenth century, the Cazamorti were called the health officials. They were elected in the Major Council but when more officials had to be added during the year, they were elected in the Senate.

PLAGUE CONTROL MEASURES, 1457–1482

As plague raged with increased intensity during the deadly epidemic of 1457, the plague control measures were reaffirmed and further elaborated. According to the regulation of 12 February 1457 adopted by the Senate, three overseers were elected who had to find several candidates to serve for a monthly salary: one priest with the salary of ten hyperperi, a guard with a salary of five hyperperi, one barber (amount of salary unknown), and two commoners with a salary of six hyperperi. The two commoners, *doy de povolo*, had to patrol the city twice a day in search of the sick. They also had to patrol the suburbs as often as they were asked to do so. If they found a sick person, they had to immediately inform the overseers, who in turn would send physicians to diagnose the disease. If the patient was not in danger of dying, they transferred him to the islet of St Peter, near Cavtat.[81] However, if he was gravely sick, the overseers could decide whether to have him transported or leave him at home. In any case, they had to make sure that he had everything necessary for his treatment and survival; a priest had to hear his confession and give him communion and other sacraments. The family members of the sick person were also sent to the islet of St Peter, where they were accommodated in one of the houses set up for that purpose and provided with all the necessities. If a member of the family sent to St Peter became sick, he was immediately isolated and sent to another place where everything necessary for his survival had to be procured. The priest and the guard had to stay in St Peter permanently. To get an exact picture of the infection rate, the commoners patrolling the city had to write the name of the infected, the date, and the address of the house in a book. On the back of the same book, they had to mark the date and the names and the number of family members that were sent to St Peter. To keep abreast of the health situation, information from this book was read in the Senate on a predetermined day of the month. The barber had to be at the disposal of those at St Peter and of those in the city who were infected. He was answerable to the overseers. If a patrician or a reputable citizen became sick, it was necessary to inform the rector and the senators who would then decide on the measures to undertake. If anyone lent a deaf ear or was walking around with visible plague buboes, the senators could decide to punish that person as they saw fit.[82]

Owing to the nature of their calling, the priests working with the infected had to stay in quarantine. Given the danger to which they were exposed, their duties were tantamount to the death sentence. Although he received pay for his services, the barber, who was sent instead of a physician to treat the infected in the quarantine, could not expect a better outcome. The barber used to administer drugs, mostly *theriac*, perform phlebotomies, or incise mature buboes. If the sick person was a patrician, only the Senate had the authority to decide his fate. At his expense, he could be left in his home under guard or he could be transported outside the city, usually to his country home. To avoid any abuse of power, when deciding about the cases of patricians who were closely connected as blood relations and business partners, the decision was put to a vote in the Senate.

On 17 June 1457, the Senate decided to reduce the quorum to twenty-five members. Such a decision was also part of the 1438 special plague regulàtion.[83] On 5 July 1457, it was decided that the Senate would meet outside the city on the island of Daksa, in Ombla or in Gruž.[84] In December 1457, the Senate decided to build a Church of Our Lady and a cemetery at Danče, a neighbourhood of Dubrovnik just outside the city walls. The sculptures that adorn the portal carved by local artists and showing Our Lady with Christ flanked by two angels, much too big in proportion with the central figures, underline the Gothic style of the entrance (see Figures 4.1 and 4.2). The church was built to prevent

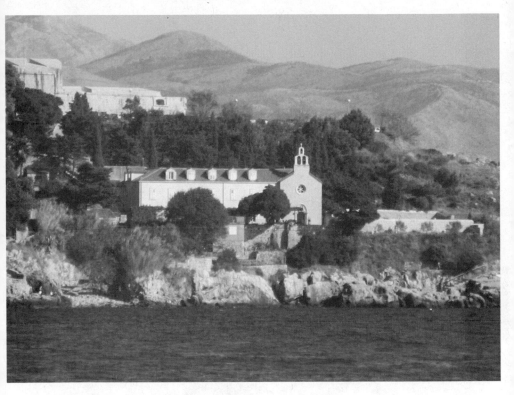

Figure 4.1 Church of Our Lady at Dance

the poor who would die of plague at Dance from dying "like sheep" and to "provide them with a sacred Christian place of burial."[85]

On 26 March 1466, the Senate adopted a new regulation that paid particular attention to cleaning and disinfection of infected homes.[86] Of particular interest is the second paragraph of this regulation, which was not adopted. It was a proposal for the Cazamorti to freely decide which belongings of the infected should be burned, keeping in mind that the total value should not be higher than ten hyperperi. This proposal did not pass because most Senators considered that burning the property valued at ten hyperperi was too big a loss for certain citizens. Clothes were to be washed at the expense of the commune. In the next paragraph, this amount was reduced to five hyperperi.[87] It has to be mentioned that the amount of ten hyperperi represented four months of a labourer's income.[88] Workers employed in textile manufacturing could not bear such a loss. Although senators were aware of the dangers of new plague outbreaks, they refused to put added pressure on socially disadvantaged citizens and chose a compromise. Law had to be tempered with humanity and charity, even if it meant further risk of disease.

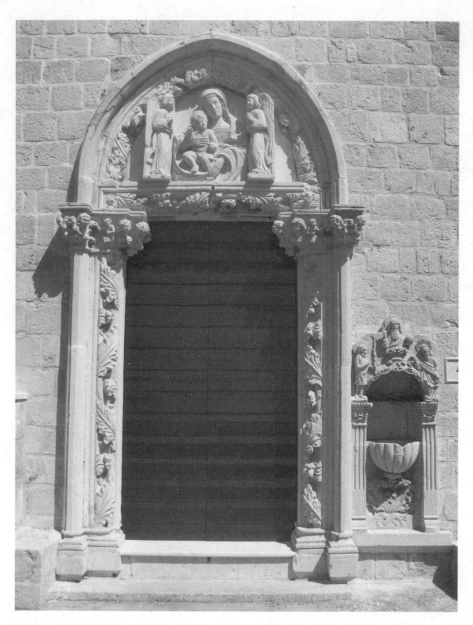

Figure 4.2 Church of Our Lady at Dánče, portal

In the last paragraph of this regulation, the senators instructed the Cazamorti to send the infected and the suspects to St Peter and not to Lokrum, the island that is situated very close to the city of Dubrovnik. Those who were already in Lokrum were to be moved to St Peter. The reasons for closing down the Lokrum quarantine were, in essence, political. At that time, the Ottomans were close to the borders of the Republic. If unprotected Lokrum, so close to the city, were to fall into the hands of the Ottomans or the Venetians, Dubrovnik itself would be threatened. To avoid such a scenario, the senators decided to send the infected elsewhere to concentrate on the appropriate defence of Lokrum.[89]

On 20 May 1466, the Major Council decided to build special housing for the accommodation of the isolated at Danče. Furthermore, a plague doctor was hired to improve medical assistance. A number of gravediggers, laundresses, and guards were employed. The latter were to make sure the infected and the suspects as well as the persons working in quarantine did not have any contact with the healthy.[90]

On 16 October 1469, the Major Council adopted a regulation that emphasized the importance of the office of the Cazamorti. It states that senators are allowed to perform some duties usually assigned to the members of the Major Council, duties such as those of treasurers, trustees, and Cazamorti, the term of office being *tam ad vitam quam ad tempus* – for life or for a period of time, according to the duration of each office.[91] This decision of the Major Council was probably motivated by the fear that there could be a shortage of qualified candidates for these essential services due to the recurrent plague epidemics.

In the fifteenth century, the plague years had a major impact on the size of the Major Council. Rheubottom has established that the cohort born in 1437 was unusually small with only twenty members. This was reflected in the small number of new members of the Major Council around 1455. In the plague year 1466, eleven members of the inner circle died; in 1482, forty-two members of the Major Council died; twelve of those were members of the inner circle. We know that the Cazamorti were elected among the senior members of the Major Council. These mortality numbers probably also reflect the rate of mortality among the Cazamorti. In times of high mortality, there was a numerical compensation. For example, in the aftermath of the 1466 plague, the size of the inner circle was sharply increased. In this way, losses could be replaced and numbers maintained.[92]

On 26 March 1482, the Senate, faced with a growing threat of another epidemic, adopted a wide-ranging regulation for the protection against the plague, called *Provedimenta contra pestilentiam*.[93] Due to the high mortality of one of the deadliest plague epidemics ever to hit the Republic, discipline was lax, so lax that even the Cazamorti avoided spending any time in the infected city. Most residents abandoned the city and sought refuge in the countryside. Thus, four of the nine paragraphs of this regulation deal with the obligations of the Cazamorti and threaten them with a fine of twenty-five hyperperi for each violation. The regulation stipulates that in the future, not two, but all three Cazamorti have to be permanently present in the city. They were to meet every morning, and on the basis of the most recent data, decide how best to protect the Republic. They had to name special guards who were to supervise gravediggers and make sure that the gravediggers had no contact with the healthy and that they did not cause a fire. This regulation, like many later ones in the sixteenth century, reflects a major mistrust of the gravediggers (see Chapter 7). Furthermore, the Cazamorti were asked to submit a list of infected homes to the Senate, which had the authority to decide the fate of the infected goods.

In 1482, the Senate ordered two deep holes to be dug outside the city as well as a deep collective grave at Danče to receive all those who died in the Danče quarantine. Probably because there was no more room for the suspects of infection at Danče, it was decided to move them to the islets of Mrkan and Bobara.[94] After thirty or forty days, they were allowed to go anywhere they pleased, except back to their infected homes.

During this time, people were dying from other diseases as well. Malaria was constantly present in Ston, north of Dubrovnik, as were dysentery, typhus, and other infectious diseases.[95] Sufferers were not allowed to come into contact with the healthy. These diseases had to be reported to the authorities, just like plague, so that their true nature could be determined. The rector and the Minor Council, always afraid that the Ottomans could use the chaos caused by a plague epidemic to invade their territory, had to keep guards and spies on the borders of the Republic. An invasion never took place because the Ragusans invested vast amounts of money into strengthening their massive defence walls and considerable energy into honing their diplomatic skills.

Three months later, on 27 June 1482, the Senate adopted other regulations concerning more rapid disinfecting of homes, better control of the gravediggers, and listing of the property of the deceased.[96] More attention than ever was paid to disinfecting homes and clothes. The authorities assigned special sums of money for additional employees: four commoners to supervise the cleaning of infected items, twenty women to launder clothes, four to six women to clean and disinfect homes, and two boats with a crew to transport infected goods from the city. With special care, infected clothes and other items were taken to

Dance to be washed. The Cazamorti had to make sure that all homes were cleaned and disinfected with vinegar, those of the poor at the expense of the commune and others at the expense of their owners.

MISTRUST OF THE PLAGUE SURVIVORS

Particular attention should be paid to the first paragraph of the regulation adopted on 27 June 1482, by which the Senate decided to employ the women who survived the plague, the *resanatae* – the recovered – to wash the infected items since they could handle them without endangering their lives.[97] It was a rational move in the right direction that contributed to the advance of plague control measures. Since the *resanati* were at least temporarily immune to the plague, some of them used to break into abandoned houses and steal. If proven guilty, they were given exemplary sentences. On the one hand, the authorities badly needed their services and, on the other, they did not trust them. This ambivalent attitude towards the plague survivors continued in the sixteenth century and became evident during the 1526–27 disastrous plague upsurge (see Chapter 7).

The death rate started decreasing only at the end of 1482. As mentioned in the regulation of 14 October 1482, the infected were sent into quarantine at Dance. This regulation consists of nine paragraphs, three of which deal with gravediggers. Under the threat of being hanged, gravediggers were forbidden to pass from the section for the sick to the section of the healthy suspects within the isolation compound. Likewise, if a cloth item was found on the path where they had passed while carrying the dead on the way to the funeral or returning from it, they were liable to be hanged. It was determined that the gravediggers, who were among the poorest of the *resanati*, would often spread the disease by throwing infected items along the way where other people could pick them up.[98] It is obvious that the gravediggers, either out of ignorance or because of pecuniary interests, did not observe the quarantine regulations. Expensive clothing of the wealthy deceased represented too much of a temptation for becoming rich overnight. Whenever supervision relaxed a little, things were hidden and presents from the relatives of the deceased remained undeclared. Authorities put in motion energetic measures to get rid of these dangerous practices.

In December 1482, two gravediggers, Mihoč from Rijeka Dubrovačka and Živan Pupak, were caught stealing at Dance. According to the regulation of 14 October 1482, they were sentenced to death by hanging. The fate of these two unfortunate gravediggers, who were "hanged by the neck in order to separate the soul from the body," was decided with twenty-one votes in favour of hanging and eighteen against.[99] It is possible that at a time when hundreds were dying, the authorities, aware of their own shortcomings, felt frustrated and helpless. Unable to stop the epidemic, they may have been looking for a scapegoat. In a society with a definite class bias, such punishment was reserved for the individuals from the lowest social class who were not protected either by their social rank or an institution such as a confraternity. It goes without saying that the social constellation in Dubrovnik was such that not a single patrician was ever hanged for violating plague control regulations.

This was the first time anyone in Dubrovnik had been sentenced to death for contravening plague control measures. Such a harsh sentence represented a serious escalation of repressive measures unheard of in previous plague outbreaks. It is interesting that in both 1482, and later in 1527, individuals were sentenced to death for stealing infected items. Because it was believed that disease was caused by some agent that taints the environment or objects, the health officials persistently traced the route of each infected item. Their insistence on the origin of infected items was related to the fear that such goods could cause a recurrence of the plague epidemic.

One could ask whether, at this point in time, the health officials were truly interested in plague management or whether the escalation of repressive measures was a pretext for the expansion of judicial powers. Broadened judicial powers, even if they were not the original objective of plague control measures, were certainly a by-product of combating plague. Increased state control occurred also in other plague-stricken cities around Europe (e.g., Venice, Geneva, Florence). The early development of sanitary measures in Dubrovnik (see Chapter 1) and the establishment of pharmacies and hospitals available to the whole population (see Chapter 3), even before the appearance of plague, testify to the genuine interest of the patricians for the citizens' welfare. The regular hiring of physicians and surgeons since the 1280s is further proof of the patricians' desire to offer the best possible health care in their Republic. As fear of plague recurrence grew, of necessity, every successive cycle of adopted measures became more repressive. From the documents of the Ragusan councils, we learn that measures promulgated during an epidemic were enforced during a limited time – only for the duration of that epidemic. Every epidemic had its official beginning and its end, registered in the archival documents. After the end date, the special measures adopted during that plague epidemic were lifted. In Chapter 6, we discuss the special measures taken for the 1526–27 and 1533 plague outbreaks and the dates when they were lifted. In fact, from 1482 until 1526, there were no major plague outbreaks in Dubrovnik. Therefore, very few plague regulations were adopted during that period and the measures previously endorsed were not applied. This proves that the increased judicial powers granted to the health officials were valid only for a limited duration. From the evolution of plague defence in Dubrovnik, it becomes evident that the patricians were wholeheartedly interested in fighting plague. Because they were not able to stop plague even with the strictest measures applied, they felt frustrated. The increased repression was probably the result of their fear and impotence. The health officials must have felt threatened as their state, as well as their whole way of life, was in jeopardy. They had to fight plague but they could not completely isolate Dubrovnik. Had they done so, all trade would have stopped and the economy would have suffered. Therefore, they tried to find a compromise – they implemented the plague control measures and continued to trade. The economy, the state, the citizens of Dubrovnik, all had to be rescued, and the responsibility for bringing this about rested squarely on the shoulders of that small group of patricians. Since the Republic was their responsibility, from the patricians' point of view, a threat to them was a threat to the safety of the whole state.

As a group, the patricians continued to apply repressive policies adopted by the Councils, but as individuals, they must have had their misgivings. This is evident from their reluctance to serve as health officials. The fact that the death penalty for the gravediggers was adopted with a majority of only three votes in favour also suggests that there were some personal doubts about strict repression.

During a plague outbreak, the Ragusans were usually in constant fear of attack from their outside enemies, the Ottomans and the Venetians. For this reason, during every plague epidemic, the Ragusans habitually first organized the defence of their territory: two fast ships were ordered to ply the seas from the southernmost to the northernmost point of the Republic; additional guards were posted on the city walls and more soldiers were added at the entrance gates.

In the fifteenth and sixteenth centuries, the Ragusan society was characterized by stable relations between patricians and commoners. The patricians allowed commoners to trade and become even richer than the patricians themselves (see Chapter 1, p. 28). The wealthy commoners, especially the members of the confraternity of St Anthony, shared the interest for the common good of the Republic with the patricians and believed in the same civic ideals of freedom, prosperity, stability, and social tolerance. They were more interested in imitating the patrician lifestyle than in taking over power. Citizens of the lower social classes had better protection, a higher standard of living, and certainly superior health care in Dubrovnik than anywhere else in the region.

The Major Council, the Minor Council, and the Senate each functioned within its own area of responsibility. This was still the "golden age" of Dubrovnik. There is no evidence that the patricians felt threatened by any group within the society because they provided a stable environment for all. Fissures in the solidarity of the patrician class were not yet apparent. A major division of the Ragusan patricians into two opposed factions occurred in the seventeenth century. The Senate took over most of the decision making, while the role of the Major and Minor Councils was diminished. The Republic slowly became an oligarchy and the city experienced a serious decline after the 1667 earthquake.[100]

The patricians definitely resisted change. Ragusan society was based on conservatism, pragmatism, continuity, and order. The Ottomans certainly represented a major headache for the Ragusans but, then again, as usual, the Ragusans adopted a pragmatic attitude and undertook all the measures within their power to get acquainted with the Ottomans and their culture. The relations that the Ragusans maintained with the Ottomans made it possible for them to remain masters of their own house and defend the Republic until 1808. By that time, with the influx of new players – namely, France, England, and Russia – in the Mediterranean, who the Ottomans were no longer able to influence, the international context had completely changed.

DUBROVNIK AS A FORERUNNER OF PLAGUE CONTROL MEASURES

The first extant source in the State Archives of Dubrovnik referring to the Plague Control Officials dates from 1390, but it is clear from the text that these officials were elected even before that date because they were given the same authority as those who had been elected before them. It is possible that they were elected ever since the quarantine legislation was implemented in 1377. It would have been a logical next step in the development of plague control measures. The regulation dated 5 January 1397 defines the elections of plague control officials and lists their duties. Although they were regularly elected since 1390 or even earlier, it is in 1397 that they joined the list of permanent officials of the state, to be elected every year at the beginning of January. We thus find them elected in January 1398 and 1399 and the years that follow. The archival documents reveal that the Ragusan Republic had established the earliest recorded Plague Control Office, or Health Office, as it was later called.[101] This development represents an important landmark in the history of plague control measures and the history of public health policy. Above all, the plague control measures were firmly rooted in the social, environmental, economic, and political structures of Dubrovnik, a wealthy and ambitious city with a centralized government that maintained full control of the state apparatus and gave full support to the actions of the health officials. The search for common good was part of the Ragusan Christian ideals and their aristocratic republican identity. Thus, their approach to plague was based on their political ideals that included keeping their state free of epidemics.

The health officials did not have any medical training, but they were experienced administrators of noble rank, usually elected to this duty after more than twenty-five years of service in the Major Council. They were men who knew that they had to find a way to tackle any problem facing their homeland. They were entrusted with judicial and executive powers in matters concerning plague control regulations. The Councils gave the health officials wide-ranging duties and extensive authority in their field of activity but, according to the Ragusan custom, they refrained from giving away legislative powers. The status of the health officials was strengthened by the 1426 regulation that prescribed their election by the Major Council. The process of the establishment of the Health Office had reached its final phase with the 1457 regulation when the Senate decided to give the health officials a salary. In the same period, they started supervising a whole range of lower-class personnel working for the Health Office.

During the deadly 1482 plague flare-up, strict new plague control regulations were adopted that dealt with the obligations of the Cazamorti, the gravediggers, and the plague survivors, and new, more threatening repressive measures were enacted. The 1482 regulations demonstrate a special preoccupation with contaminated goods as a source of infection and led to the death sentence of two gravediggers caught stealing infected goods from Danče.

The Ragusan health officials were convinced of the communicable nature of plague, its transmission from person to person, and through suspicious goods. They maintained their pragmatic stance, and despite all the medical and

Table 4.2
Founding of the Health Office in Dubrovnik and in Italy

CITY	TEMPORARY OFFICE	PERMANENT OFFICE
Dubrovnik	1390	1397
Milan	1424	1448
Pavia	1450	1485
Venice	1462	1486
Siena	1462	1486
Florence	1496	1527
Lucca	1481	–
Cremona	1480	–

religious theories prevalent at the time, they put the isolation of the sick at the core of all their protection measures. With their approach based on administrative experience and observation, they were able to organize practical plague protection measures.

According to the chronology regarding northern Italian cities, established by Ann G. Carmichael, it becomes evident that the Ragusan Health Office became permanent many years before similar offices in Milan, Pavia, Venice, Siena, and Florence (see Table 4.2).[102]

PLAGUE CONTROL MEASURES IN NORTHERN ITALIAN CITIES

In 1374, Milan and Mantua were the first cities to declare a temporary travel ban on persons arriving from plague-infected areas. In 1400, Milan was the first city to use a river, the Adda, as a natural sanitary barrier. In the jubilee year, when great numbers of pilgrims travelled to Rome from France and Germany, the Milanese authorities, to keep them well outside of populated centres, had assigned the pilgrims obligatory routes on the other side of the river Adda and had created a sanitary cordon. At the moment of the plague outbreak, two plague hospitals were opened and a system of control of suspected cases was put into effect. A leading city official was named to assure the execution of detailed plague orders. Plague hospitals were later moved out of town and patients kept separate from one another. Teams of doctors, barbers, apothecaries, and nurses of both genders cared for those patients. The Milanese ad hoc measures against the plague are of immense significance because they became the precursors of the health measures later adopted by the Italian maritime states.[103]

The fifteenth century was marked by a series of mild plague outbreaks with a lower mortality than in the fourteenth century. They were often localized in the poor districts of the city. By the 1450s, many northern Italian city administrators were persuaded that there was a connection between the poor and the plague. At the same time, they came to the conclusion that plague is a communicable disease. Therefore, they thought that the lazarettos were the best solution for dealing with this problem. Most Italian cities, starting with Venice, established plague hospitals before the Health Office. Because plague came to be considered as the disease of the poor, cities felt an increased urgency to open the lazarettos and round up the destitute, the refugees, and the migrants. These groups were targeted, among other reasons, because it was impossible to ascertain from where they had arrived, that is, from a healthy or from an infected place. It has been argued that the plague legislation of these cities aimed to gain greater control of the population, especially the poor. By controlling the poor, they hoped that they would get rid of the plague.[104]

On 11 May 1400, the Venetian Senate took its first known measure against plague when boatloads of Ragusans fleeing the plague were refused entry. Richard Palmer, the authority on plague control development in northern Italy, notes that it was a retaliatory measure because Dubrovnik had refused entry to Venetian ships when Venice had been infected.[105] However, this measure became policy only in 1423 when Venice took another decisive step against the plague with the establishment of the Lazareto Vecchio. The populous city on the lagoon, the most important trading partner of the Levant, and therefore the most exposed to plague infections, the city that could not protect itself with city walls or gates, established the plague hospital before the Health Office. On 28 August 1423, the Senate ordered a hospital of at least twenty rooms to be built in a peripheral zone of Venice. The sum of one thousand to two thousand ducats was put aside for this project. The hospital was to accept the infected Venetians, those who became infected at sea and the foreigners who became sick while travelling to Venice. The lazaretto was intended, above all, for persons without residence, including refugees, migrants, and beggars, in order to prevent them from circulating in the city and spreading disease. Still, the consent of the patients was necessary for admission to the lazaretto. This suggests that the state was not yet ready to enforce unpopular measures. The authorities provided financing through the Ufficio del Sal (Salt office), while the religious orders cared for the infected and the dead. It was the first time that the state took over the fight against the plague. Until then, it was the Church and the monasteries that fulfilled this role. In 1438, the procurators of St Mark took over the administration of the finances of the lazaretto and decided to make much larger investments to increase its estate. Over time, the lazaretto was enlarged to receive all the plague sufferers of any social status, with or without known residence.[106] Since the 1420s, the Venetian Senate started banning people arriving from plague-infected areas from entering Venice. In 1471, another hospital was built – the Lazaretto Nuovo – where the plague survivors and the persons suspected of infection could stay while they recovered and were disinfected. The two lazarettos thus became the basis for the control of plague in Venice.[107] It has to be pointed out that Venice was one of the biggest cities in Europe at that time. Therefore, the organization of plague control measures in the city of that size, for such a large number of people, was a particularly challenging task from every point of view: organizational and financial. Jane Stevens Crawshaw emphasizes that the lazarettos were crucial institutions for facilitating trade and that it was important for Venice to project a position of strength in the face of epidemic disease. The task was daunting but Venice was wealthy and ambitious to protect its citizens and its trade. The sheer fact that Venice was able to maintain the lazarettos for many centuries is a remarkable achievement. The lazarettos represent an attempt to care for the plague patients and ensure their reintegration into society. Before the end of the fifteenth century, they were adopted in other Italian cities such as Ferrara, Florence, Milan, Mantua, Genoa, Siena, Parma, Udine, and Recanati, before they were embraced by cities all over Europe.[108]

According to Palmer, the development of the Venetian Health Office met with a number of hurdles. It was first proposed in 1459 that three nobles of good repute be elected by the Senate to preserve the city from plague.[109] Although this decision was adopted, it was not put into effect. A year later, a similar proposition was adopted by the Senate but the officials were not elected. Then in June 1461, three nobles were elected as health officials but on a temporary basis. Throughout the sixteenth century, the Health Office suffered from a serious shortage of funds. Employees were sometimes not paid for years. Although it took almost three more decades, until 1486, for the Health Office to attain permanent standing, it played a crucial role during the major plague epidemics, especially in 1575–77.[110] The Venetian Health Officials were called *Provveditori alla Sanità* and sometimes, out of respect, they were referred to as our most distinguished nobles – *primi nobili nostri*. They always had legislative, judicial, and executive powers.[111]

Renowned historian Carlo M. Cipolla claims that there is no doubt that Italy was far ahead of other European countries in the field of public health. He reports that the first temporary health boards in France were established only at the end of the sixteenth century (Lyon in 1580). The first quarantine for ships and the first permanent health office in England were established in 1543. European countries north of the Alps were slow to adopt the plague protection measures and paid a heavy toll.[112] Plague outbreaks in those countries were more frequent and more violent.[113] Samuel Kline Cohn, who has studied the plague tractates of sixteenth-century Italy, laments the fact that to date, no one has plotted the pace or geography of the formation of permanent health boards in Italy. According to him, the period from 1575 to 1578 may have proven to be an important stimulus, with, for instance, the formation of health boards in Palermo and Florence.[114]

In Chapter 5, the control of arrivals in Dubrovnik, as practised by the health officials in the first thirty years of the sixteenth century, in times of health and during the catastrophic 1526–27 plague outbreak, will be analyzed. In Chapter 6 and those that follow, we will be able to observe how the experience gained during the fifteenth century influenced the implementation of plague control measures in 1526–27, during the last major plague outbreak in Dubrovnik.

a six-month imprisonment, on 7 July 1501, Peroto Torela, a Catalonian, who had arrived from Apulia in Italy, had to declare under oath that he would not bring to Dubrovnik anyone other than his family, his servants, and a nephew.[15] Particular attention was paid to ships moored in the port of Dubrovnik. On 20 August 1501, two ship owners, Bartulić Tomašević and Pavlić Marinović, both originally from the island of Lopud, returned from Sicily with a crew of about ten sailors each. All of them together and each one of them individually, under the threat of a fine of one hundred ducats and a six-month imprisonment, and whichever other punishment the health officials might impose, had to give a sworn statement that the crew had spent the last two months in places free of plague and had not been in touch with people from infected areas.[16] Likewise, on 3 December 1501, Ivan Antićević, owner of a galleon, originally from Lopud, had returned from Ancona with Antonio Pasquini, a merchant from Florence, and a crew of fifteen sailors. All of them individually, under the threat of usual penalties, had to pledge under oath that they had spent the last two months in plague-free places. In the record, the professions of the sailors are marked next to their names: *nauchier* (helmsman), *scrivan* (scribe), *chalafat* (waterproofs the ship), *marangon* (carpenter), and *bombardier* (artilleryman).[17] This record demonstrates the detailed attention health officials paid to the identification of each individual who arrived on the Ragusan territory.

Plague was not present in Dubrovnik in 1502, but judging by the number of arrival records, the health officials did not diminish their vigilance (see Figure 5.2). However, merchants could rather easily avoid the usual penalties and the destruction of their goods by burning if they simply omitted mentioning that they had arrived from infected places. Merchants could also count on the fact that the messages took almost two weeks to reach Dubrovnik.[18] Circumventing the truth did not help Marin Petrov Radaljević and his servant Bogeta from Ombla, who had returned on 4 May, and Radonja Radovanović, who had returned on 19 May, all three from Skopje in Macedonia. On 1 June, the health officials had sent a letter to two Ragusan patricians, who were still in Skopje, inquiring about the presence of plague. Their letter was delivered on 12 June in the afternoon and answered very respectfully on 13 June by Vladislav Junijev Sorkočević (Sorgo) and Luka Nikolin Bunić (Bona).[19] They confirmed that plague had spread to Skopje in January and was still rampant in an area with a diameter of two to three miles around the city. They added that many people had died in March and that plague was widespread in Kratovo, Polog, and Božovče Polje in October. The health officials received the letter on 23 June and did not the arrivals of travellers, the Ragusans wanted to achieve an increased control of the access to their territory. They registered each individual's name and profession, point of departure, his final destination, and the purpose of his trip to Dubrovnik. The health officials prohibited domestic and foreign travellers from visiting Dubrovnik if they had been at a plague-infected port up to two months prior to arriving in the city.[10] It is not difficult to imagine how such plague control measures obstructed the mediaeval traffic of people and goods, which moved slowly even under normal circumstances. In spite of all the delays and financial losses caused by these measures, they were still useful because they contributed to the interruption of the chain of infection.

In the manuscript, the testimonies of the witnesses begin on 2 January 1500. The persons who were suspected of having arrived from plague-infected areas were sent into quarantine on the islet of Supetar (St Peter) close to Cavtat.[11] The health officials learned that Đuro, the parish priest from Župa, who had returned from Rome where fifteen hundred years of Christianity had been celebrated, and who was confined to his house, celebrated Mass in the church of St Peter in Župa near Kupari, eight kilometres southeast of Dubrovnik. Under the threat of a penalty, they interrogated Božidar Grubišić, who declared under oath that the priest had in fact said Mass on the day of St Peter the apostle but that the members of the congregation had not approached him during Mass.[12] On 8 August 1500, the health officials interrogated the priest Lukša Radovanović, who was suspected of having received a cap and a pair of socks from Paul, the priest, who had just returned from Rome. Lukša, the priest, swore on his life that he had never received those items.[13] From this episode we gather that the health officials not only carefully monitored the persons suspected of transmitting plague, but they also questioned them about the origin of their possessions made of wool, cotton, linen, or silk, which were likely to be infected. The Senate was also concerned with the pilgrims returning from Rome and, on 26 September 1500, decided that the health officials could leave them in front of the city walls at the Pile gate, close to the sea, for eight days and later admit them into the city proper if none of them were suspected of being sick.[14]

Dubrovnik was a city that attracted craftsmen, artists, physicians, surgeons, notaries, chancellors, and many other specialized individuals from various countries. They were usually issued a permit of residence for their family members and their servants. Under the threat of a penalty of one hundred ducats and a six-month imprisonment, on 7 July 1501, Peroto Torela, a Catalonian, who had arrived from Apulia in Italy, had to declare under oath that he would not bring to Dubrovnik anyone other than his family, his servants, and a nephew.[15] Particular attention was paid to ships moored in the port of Dubrovnik. On 20 August 1501, two ship owners, Bartulić Tomašević and Pavlić Marinović, both originally from the island of Lopud, returned from Sicily with a crew of about ten sailors each. All of them together and each one of them individually, under the threat of a fine of one hundred ducats and a six-month imprisonment, and whichever other punishment the health officials might impose, had to give a sworn statement that the crew had spent the last two months in places free of plague and had not been in touch with people from infected areas.[16] Likewise, on 3 December 1501, Ivan Antićievič, owner of a galleon, originally from Lopud, had returned from Ancona with Antonio Pasquini, a merchant from Florence, and a crew of fifteen sailors. All of them individually, under the threat of usual penalties, had to pledge under oath that they had spent the last two months in plague-free places. In the record, the professions of the sailors are marked next to their names: *nauchier* (helmsman), *scrivan* (scribe), *chalafat* (waterproofs the ship), *marangon* (carpenter), and *bombardier* (artilleryman).[17] This record demonstrates the detailed attention health officials paid to the identification of each individual who arrived on the Ragusan territory.

Plague was not present in Dubrovnik in 1502, but judging by the number of arrival records, the health officials did not diminish their vigilance (see Figure 5.2). However, merchants could rather easily avoid the usual penalties and the destruction of their goods by burning if they simply omitted mentioning that they had arrived from infected places. Merchants could also count on the fact that the messages took almost two weeks to reach Dubrovnik.[18] Circumventing the truth did not help Marin Petrov Radaljević and his servant Bogeta from Ombla, who had returned on 4 May, and Radonja Radovanović, who had returned on 19 May, all three from Skopje in Macedonia. On 1 June, the health officials had sent a letter to two Ragusan patricians, who were still in Skopje, inquiring about the presence of plague. Their letter was delivered on 12 June in the afternoon and answered very respectfully on 13 June by Vladislav Junijev Sorkočević (Sorgo) and Luka Nikolin Bunić (Bona).[19] They confirmed that plague had spread to Skopje in January and was still rampant in an area with a diameter of two to three miles around the city. They added that many people had died in March and that plague was widespread in Kratovo, Polog, and Božovče Polje in October. The health officials received the letter on 23 June and did not waste time. On the same day, the three returnees from Skopje, because of their false statement upon arrival to Dubrovnik, were sentenced to six months of imprisonment in the Rector's Palace and a monetary fine of one hundred ducats each.[20] It is interesting to note that two health officials voted against the sentence. The reason could be that almost two months had already elapsed and no one had fallen sick. It is also questionable whether the travellers who returned from Skopje had known about the presence of plague in that area.

At a time when plague was not rife in Dubrovnik, such a sentence was undoubtedly a threatening example to all the other individuals who might have tried to circumvent the plague control measures. On 27 November 1486, the health officials had acted in a similar way, which demonstrates the continuity and consistency of their decisions over time. In that year, the health officials, belonging to five of the most renowned patrician families of Gundulić (Gondola), Lukarević (Luchari), Ranjina (Ragnina), Gučetić (Goze), and Menčetić (Menze), sentenced the crew of the ship of the deceased Vasilije Vitković to a fine of one hundred ducats each. They had returned from Recanati in Italy and falsely declared that they had arrived from plague-free places. Since their return, some of them and thirteen other persons in Dubrovnik, and nine other persons in Trstenik on the Pelješac Peninsula where they had stopped, had died of plague. Under oath, the health officials had questioned the patrician witnesses Ivan Markov Gučetić (Goze) and Marin Šimun Nikolin Gučetić (Goze), who had also returned from Recanati.[21] They declared that plague was rampant in Recanati and that religious processions had been held for the protection of the city. In their sentence, the health officials mentioned the need to stop a "bigger fire from being ignited" and referred to the well-known regulation, *De ordinibus contra eos qui veniunt de locis pestiferis* (Against those who arrive from pestiferous regions) from 5 January 1397.[22] The 1502 case is different from the 1486 case in that no one died of plague, but the danger of false declarations always created utmost concern.

The chroniclers offer a wealth of information for the year 1503. Serafino Razzi warns that in 1503 the plague flare-up had spread from Barletta to the island of Koločep, from Alexandria to the island of Šipan, and from Chioggia to Konavle, but that with God's help and efficient guards it did not penetrate into the city.[23] According to the Anonymous chronicler, in 1503, there was a great scarcity of grain due to the war between the French and the Spanish for the conquest of Barletta, Manfredonia, and Naples. That war was probably the reason for the higher number of arrivals in Dubrovnik noted in 1503. The

Ragusan authorities had bought sufficient grain in Sicily so that they could come to the rescue of their neighbours on both sides of the Adriatic but the expanded maritime traffic increased the likelihood of plague. The Anonymous chronicler and Razzi both confirm that plague had spread from Barletta in Apulia, and that because of it, the Ragusan authorities had prohibited all sick people arriving by land and sea from entering the city.[24]

At the beginning of April 1503, plague was rampant on the Pelješac Peninsula. Therefore, on 24 April 1503, the authorities gave the health officials wide-ranging powers to burn all articles in the houses where someone had died of plague in Žuljana, on the Pelješac Peninsula, as long as they had previously made a list and had estimated the value of those items.[25] Soon after that, the Senate gave permission to the health officials to spend from the state treasury as much money as necessary to stop the plague from escalating in Konavle. Likewise, they were permitted to burn suspicious items and distribute grain, oil, and salt to the infirm and the isolated persons suspected of being infected. Persons found responsible for spreading plague could be punished by the health officials. Since the plague attack was not dying down, the authority of the health officials continued to grow. Thus, if the inhabitants of Konavle did not obey the regulations, the health officials were allowed to burn their houses and even the inhabitants themselves within the houses.[26] There is no evidence that this threat was ever implemented. On the other hand, to those who obeyed and stayed in their homes, the state distributed food.

In May, since the plague had started to subside in Konavle, the Senate permitted traffic between houses and places that were not infected. The Senate asked the health officials to prohibit the import from the hinterland of wool, blankets, and other items that they considered suspect during the month of September 1503. If such items were found, they could be burned.[27] The health officials also questioned the origin of the wool brought to Dubrovnik and they examined the storage space of the patrician Šiško Franov Đurđević (Georgi). On 15 July 1503, under the threat of a fine of one hundred ducats and a six-month imprisonment, he had to promise not to buy any more new wool.[28] The concern about wool continued. On 11 May 1504, the health officials decreed that all the rough wool blankets – schiavine – bought from the Vlachs had to be previously washed in the sea or a fine of twenty-five hyperperi would have to be paid.[29]

The penalties for seafaring persons became increasingly more threatening. The most likely reason for the increased threat was the occurrence of the Franco-Spanish War in southern Italy that brought with it an increased risk of plague. On 13 June 1503, the rector and the Minor Council asked Andrija Splentić to sail to Apulia and to take with him a man from Naples. In Bari, Splentić became infected with plague. The rector and the Minor Council did not permit him to return to Dubrovnik. Neither could he cast anchor on any coast, or could he disembark on firm land for two months, under the threat of usual penalties, to which they added the burning of his caravel – *brusarli la charavela*. This decision was revoked the same day, probably due to the fact that Splentić had undertaken that trip at the request of the authorities.[30]

On 18 June 1503, Petar Živković, Đuro Živanović, Petar Damjanović, and Cvjetko Nikolić, residents of Župa, Kupari, and Čibača, arrived from Trieste and were threatened with the death penalty by hanging – *pena dele forche* – if it was discovered that they had visited a plague-infected place during the last two months.[31] Constant threats contributed to the deteriorating relations between the health officials and the citizens. In more remote places, the assistants of the health officials were physically attacked. Thus, on 10 July 1503, Pavko Vučičić from Šipan was threatened with a one-month imprisonment if he ever again attacked or insulted an assistant of the health officials.[32] Such incidents happened more often as citizens became frustrated with the plague control measures that limited their daily activities and prevented them from making a living. Still, the threats continued. On 31 July 1503, the health officials asked Luka, the messenger, to announce in all the usual public places in Dubrovnik that from then on, no one was allowed to travel into the hinterland without the permission of the health officials. According to the decision of the health officials, this decree was accompanied with the threat of being branded with a hot iron, exposed on the column of shame, and tortured.[33]

The health officials always paid close attention to persons attending pilgrimages and fairs. On 3 August 1503, they questioned Grgur Ratković, a hat maker, Ilija Dobrijević, Radoje Radovčić, and Vukosav Radonjić, all of whom had returned from a fair in Bakar, fifteen kilometres east of Rijeka in the northern Adriatic. They had to vouch that they had not visited a plague-infected destination in the last two months, under the threat of usual penalties. The same applied to a man from Kotor who had arrived with them. The four of them had to state under oath that this man had not visited Kotor in the last two months, which meant that plague was widespread in Kotor.[34] Therefore, the Ragusan authorities had interrupted all communication with this city until the danger subsided.

On 30 August 1503, the health officials were asked by the Minor Council to put into confinement Pietro Antonio de Castiglione, who had arrived from

Venice. He was to be lodged in the house of Nikola Vitov Džamanjić (Zamagna) at Ploče with a guard at the door who would be paid by Castiglione himself.[35] It was also decided that the merchants who were getting ready to attend a fair in Recanati would not be sent into quarantine on the islet of Supetar (St Peter). The Minor Council was quite lenient and permitted them, while they waited for their ships to take them to Italy, to stay in the area between the inner and the outer city wall, under guard at their own expense.[36] On 9 September 1503, Stjepko Damjanović, owner of the caravel, with ten members of the crew, arrived in Dubrovnik from Trapani in Sicily. He had to swear, under the threat of the usual penalties, that they had not stopped in an infected port.[37] On 25 October 1503, the Minor Council decided that Rafael Federikov Gučetić (Goze), member of the Minor Council, should help the health officials to assess the value of the goods that belonged to the people from Cavtat, which were to be burned.[38] This is another example that demonstrates that whenever serious decisions involving the property of the citizens were concerned, the health officials had to consult the Minor Council or the Senate.

Penalty threats were increased again in 1504. In some cases, shaming by exposure on the *berlina*, the column of shame, was added. On 10 January 1504, Jakša Antićievič, galleon owner, had arrived from Ancona, a city suspected of plague infection. Under the threat of a fine of one hundred ducats for each one of them and being exposed at the *berlina*, all the persons in his ship, including the owner, other merchants, passengers, and crew who had arrived with him, were prevented from disembarking from his ship. The health officials posted guards in front of his ship, which was anchored in the harbour.[39] There is no mention of the how long all of them were confined to the ship. The threats of shaming, which were until then reserved for peasants only, were also applied to seafaring persons. In this particular case, patricians were not present on the ship. It is well known that, in order to protect the dignity and authority of the patricians, and also out of class solidarity, the authorities did not impose physical sanctions on the patricians.

In 1504, the health officials concentrated on preventing contact with the individuals from the hinterland where pockets of plague infection still remained. Particularly the inhabitants of Ombla and Župa, close to the road leading to Bosnia, were warned not to accept anyone from Trebinje in Herzegovina into their homes or boats. The inhabitants of the suburb of Ploče were forbidden to receive anyone in their homes without the permission of the health officials. Buying goods at Ploče, which were not inspected by the health officials, was forbidden, again because the road from Bosnia ended at Ploče.[40] Nikola Franov

Marković and Borko Dedojević, who had arrived from Srebrenica, were sent into quarantine on the islet of Supetar, under the threat of a fine of twenty-five hyperperi and a three-month prison sentence.[41] On 24 May 1504, the Minor Council had set aside a sum of thirty hyperperi for the health officials to feed the infected people who were sent to the lazaretto on the island of Šipan.[42] On 15 June 1504, the Minor Council decided that no one should have access to the suspected items that the Cazamorti had stored at the fish market, which were unloaded from the infected ship of Jakov Martinov Jakoević from Šipan who had returned from Alexandria.[43]

From 1505 to 1510, there are fewer records of arrivals. Also, the texts of the records become shorter and offer much less information – usually just the names of those arriving, their place of origin ,and the oath that they had to take. The main reason for fewer records was the absence of plague epidemics in those years. The same lack of information can be observed in the works of the chroniclers Razzi, Ragnina, the Anonymous, and Sanudo. On 27 January 1505, the health officials, who always paid particular attention to places where crowds of people gathered, questioned eight travellers who had returned from a fair in Trani, Italy.[44] There is also an intriguing record from 17 July 1505. The health officials ordered Gabriel Balcaero, a Catalan merchant, to stay in his house without ever going out, under the threat of the usual penalties, because he was suffering from leprosy.[45] This is the only case in the *Libro deli Signori Chaz-amorbi* where this disease, which was rampant in Europe in the twelfth and thirteenth centuries – that is, before the appearance of plague – is mentioned. The measures against leprosy remained recorded in the archival sources and in the memory of the future generations. They became a useful precedent for the implementation of isolation during plague upswings that followed.

The health officials also supervised the payment of confinement fees. Marin Nikolin Gundulić and Nikola Radaković were quarantined in a private house and had to pay the owners a confinement fee. Marin promised to pay fifteen *grossi* to each of the men from Lastovo and he promptly paid his share. However, Nikola refused to pay and had to be coaxed by the health officials to pay the fifteen *grossi* before he was allowed to leave.[46] On 13 June 1506, Lovre Nikolin Ranjina (Ragnina), the Ragusan ambassador to the Vatican, returned from Rome and, like all the other travellers, had to take an oath that he had not arrived from an infected city.[47]

In 1511, the number of arrival records is low and then, suddenly, it doubles in 1512. Then, in 1513, the number declines and remains low until 1522. In the archival sources for this period, there is no mention of plague outbreaks, which

incurable fever can designate any communicable disease, including plague. This could explain a considerable number of arrival records for 1517.[59]

In 1522, there are only two arrival entries in the *Libro deli Signori Chazamorbi*. The Ragusans knew that the Ottoman Empire did not apply any plague control measures and often asked a person to testify under oath what he knew about the travels of another individual. On 15 April 1522, Đurađ Ivanović confirmed under oath that Cvjetko Lužanin, who had returned from Istanbul the day before, had not been in any infected places in the previous two months. Under oath, Đurađ declared that Cvjetko had stayed in Maleševci near Sofia, where he had received a letter from Marin Rastić (Resti). He also stated that Cvjetko's visit to Prijepolje had to do with one of his horses. On 20 April 1522, under the threat of paying a fine of two hundred ducats and staying in prison for six months, Orsat Fran Džamanjić (Zamagna) declared that he had arrived from Naples via Apulia, and that he had not stayed in a plague-infected area.[60]

On 11 July 1523, Ivan Tomin, the guard of the port of Dubrovnik, transmitted the order of the health officials to Pasko. Marinov Marsić, the owner of a galleon from the island of Šipan, who had arrived from Messina and whose ship was anchored near the island of Lokrum. He was ordered, under the threat of a fine of one hundred ducats and a six-month prison sentence, to go, without stopping anywhere, straight into quarantine at Polače on the island of Mljet with all his crew.[61]

On 9 August 1523, Vlaho Bernardov Kabužić (Caboga), the guard of the port of Dubrovnik, relayed to Marko Radojević and Ivan (?), both grip owners, the order of the health officials to go, with their crews, to the islet of Supetar and stay there until told otherwise, under the threat of a fine of one hundred ducats and a six-month prison sentence for each one of them, and for each transgression, if they disobeyed.[62]

In the 1520s, the Ottoman territorial expansion in Europe reached its peak. The Sultan Suleiman (1520–66), who had succeeded Selim I, occupied Belgrade in 1521 and went on to defeat the Hungarians at Mohacs in 1526.[63] These momentous events placed Dubrovnik in a very delicate political position. Although they sympathized with their Christian brethren, the Ragusans had to tread very carefully when dealing with the Ottomans. After 1526, when the Croatian and Hungarian alliance came to an end and the kingdom was dismembered, the Ragusans were left without their royal protector and became increasingly dependent on the Ottomans. The 1520s brought major political changes to the region, and the relations with the Ottomans became unsettled. The Ragusans repeatedly tried to improve and solidify their relations with the

Sultan and the Porte but there were several unpleasant incidents with the Herze-govinian Ottoman officials. In 1522–23, the Herzegovinian *sancakbey* (district governor) constantly endangered the Dalmatian coast with his military cam-paigns until he finally occupied Skradin near Šibenik.[64] When he started forti-fying Skradin, he asked the Ragusans to supply him with fifteen ships, builders, and, most importantly, building materials.

The Ragusans tried to avoid this obligation in several ways. They informed the sancakbey about the dangers to which their ships would be exposed from the Venetians and the pirates in the northern Adriatic. They also tried to pay off the sancakbey by offering gifts and money if he released them from this duty. They stalled and they negotiated. It was also a time when the French and the Spanish fought for supremacy in the Mediterranean. While the Spanish were winning that battle, the French tried to improve their relations with the Ot-tomans. During that time, Dubrovnik worked very hard to maintain good rela-tions with all of them – the Ottomans, the French, and the Spanish.[65] In 1523, the Ottomans tried again to raise the Ragusan customs duty to 5 percent. New negotiations and gifts for the sultan worth 5, 560 ducats were necessary to re-solve the issue.[66] Then, Mehmed beg Alibegović, a new Herzegovinian san-cakbey, was sent to Mostar. He immediately started questioning the Ragusan rights to the region of Konavle and demanded the overall revision of the whole issue. In 1525, he also organized a conspiracy to take over the Ragusan Ston. These events caused great uneasiness and concern in Dubrovnik and were only resolved with the death of this uncompromising individual.[67]

Although plague was not rampant in 1524, the number of arrivals registered by the health officials was on the rise. This indicates that the health officials expanded their supervision of the arrivals in the case of a variety of risks – political, commercial, or health-related. It is not by coincidence that the major-ity of the arrivals noted in 1524 were from regions under Ottoman rule: Bosnia, Herzegovina, Montenegro, Serbia, Albania, Romania, and Greece. Accused of smuggling goods from the Ottoman-ruled territory through Ston, and not pay-ing the customs duty they owed, the Ragusans obviously wanted to document as precisely as possible the movements of their merchants in the Ottoman-controlled regions. Merchants were not the only ones on the roads; physicians, too, were often travelling to reach their patients. On 25 March 1524, Fiorio (Cvjetko), the barber, who had arrived from Sarajevo where he accompanied the physician from Genoa who had treated the Herzegovinian sancakbey, under the threat of usual fines, took an oath and testified that in the previous two months he had not been in a place where plague was rampant.[68]

On 26 May 1524, Luka Radov, the town crier, confirmed that following the order of the health officials, he had announced everywhere in the city and informed every family that no one should by day or by night, under the threat of fines to be decided by the health officials, accept in his home a stranger, male or female, a Ragusan or a foreigner who came from outside of the Ragusan territory. No one should disobey this order without notifying the health officials.[69] The health officials were obviously aware of some danger that made them wary. The customary fines were all of a sudden increased by a notch and were accompanied by physical punishment and torture. Such threats were usually made only in crisis situations during the plague epidemics. Was this the reflection of the unnerving developments around Dubrovnik?

On the same day, Cvjetko Vlatković from Šipan, helmsman of Pavao Cvjetkov, who had arrived from Naples, vouched under the threat of the usual fines and ten jerks of the rope that he had not stayed in places where plague was rampant.[70] On 13 July 1524, Đuro Miloradović and Vitos Ratković, who had arrived from Dandovichi, took a similar oath on pain of the usual fines, three jerks of the rope and of breaking their noses – *squassi 3 de corda e spacarli lo naxo*.[71] On 10 August 1524, Toma Stjepanović, who had arrived from Istanbul, found himself constrained by the usual fine and five jerks of the rope on top of that.[72] On 12 August 1524, Ivan Beran from Zaton, who had arrived from the island of Vis, was also threatened by the usual fine and an additional five jerks of the rope.[73] On 7 November 1524, Nikola Pavlović from Slano, who had arrived from Barletta, and Mihoč Pavlović from Slano, who had arrived from Dalmatia and from the island of Rab, took an oath on pain of the usual fine and the punishment by torture – *pena de tortura*.[74] On 12 November 1524, Vlatko Vukotić, who had arrived from Borac, swore that he had not been in any pestiferous places, under the threat of being branded with four hot irons and four jerks of the rope – *ad pena de 4 bole et 4 trati de corda*.[75] On 16 November 1524, Cvjetko Banjanin, who had arrived from Vraneši, accepted under oath the punishment of four jerks of the rope and being branded on the face with five hot irons – *4 trati de corda e de 5 boli sul vixo* – if he were not telling the truth. On the same day, Petar Rusković, who had arrived from Herzegovina took an oath on pain of every physical punishment.[76]

The "jerking of the rope," a version of the *strappado*, was a terribly cruel punishment. The torture consisted of hoisting the subject by a rope fastened to his wrists behind his back and letting him fall to the full length of the rope by the sheer weight of his body. This procedure, extraordinarily painful for the joints, was usually repeated three times. It was considered a more severe punishment than a two-year prison sentence. But, as stated by Nella Lonza, Croatian researcher of the judicial system of the Ragusan Republic, it was usually not life-threatening. Therefore, it could be applied without fear of severe consequences. In Dubrovnik, it was customary to make sure that the tortured person did not suffer permanent damage to his health. Also, medical care was given to help him recover. The jerking of the rope was executed in public. In sixteenth-century Dubrovnik, the beam and the set of pulleys were installed near the small Onofrio fountain, in the central public space of the city, close to the St Blaise Church and the Rector's Palace.[77] Such forms of physical punishment were common in other European countries at that time. For example, during the 1523–26 plague outbreak in Empoli, Tuscany, many citizens who had contravened the plague control measures were punished by the jerking of the rope.[78]

Branding left a permanent scar on the face of the sentenced. Lonza explains that, marginalized by a mark of disgrace, the sentenced were transformed into a visible warning to other citizens and were forced to live on the edge of society. The branding also warned the judges in case of repeated violations. Ilija Mitić, a jurist, adds that branding was used before imposing a temporary or permanent banishment from the Ragusan Republic.[79]

When the area around Trebinje in Herzegovina was infected with plague in 1524, plague appeared on the border of the Republic.[80] On 12 June 1524, the health officials ordered Luka Vučičijević from Trsteno to bring his farm animals, including oxen, pigs, and goats, to Dubrovnik for inspection. They obviously suspected that the farm animals could also transmit the plague. This is the only record in the whole manuscript that mentions animals.[81]

In 1525, most of the arrivals registered were from the Ottoman-occupied territory – the Ragusan hinterland, Albania, and Greece. They were followed by the arrivals from Italy and Croatia. The same situation prevailed in 1526.

From 11 until 28 January 1527, only six arrivals in the city were noted. From 28 January to 16 June 1527, there is a total gap in the arrivals records in the manuscript. That pause is due to the most disastrous plague epidemic to ever hit Dubrovnik, during which the government abandoned the city for the suburb of Gruž (see Chapter 6). After the return of the Councils on 17 June, the health officials and their scribes resumed the recording of the arrivals on the same page where they had stopped in January. We know, therefore, that there are not any missing pages. On 18 June a whole new team of health officials was elected and new scribes, guards, a plague doctor, a barber, and gravediggers were designated – all of them supervised by the health officials.

After 17 June 1527, the records of travellers' arrivals in Dubrovnik became more frequent than ever, and the threats of fines were sometimes substantially increased. The highest number of records in the whole thirty-year period covered by the manuscript was registered in 1527. Until then, the health officials required the travellers to take an oath declaring that they had not visited an infected area within the last two months. After 17 June 1527, that period of time was often extended to within six months with increased threats of fines and punishment, including the death penalty.[82]

The striking characteristic of the arrivals in 1527 is that most of them are from within the Ragusan Republic. Out of 144 departure points, 99 locations are very close to Dubrovnik, only 23 are from Italy, and the rest are from the hinterland. It is obvious that in 1527 Dubrovnik was bypassed by most international traffic. The travellers were local people who had arrived from Lopud and Šipan (11 from each), Slano and Župa, Ombla, Ston, Koločep, Cavtat, and other places or islands close to the city. Numerous records do not refer to arrivals at all. They include the sworn declarations of individuals testifying that they had not been sick in the last two months or that no one was sick in their household or that they had not been in touch with infected persons. In fact, the first record on 17 June 1527 reveals that under the threat of a fine of one hundred ducats and a six-month prison sentence, Matko Maksić declared under oath that in the last six months he had not been in contact with anyone who was infected and that no one had been sick in his house during that period.[83] On 19 June 1527, under the threat of a fine of fifty ducats, Julije Cvjetkov Turčinović swore, at the risk of losing his life and all his possessions, that no one had become sick in his house since 15 April.[84] On 20 September 1527, Petar Suglatino affirmed under oath that in the last two months he had not been in contact with infected or recovered persons and that he would not be from then on.[85]

At the risk of losing their lives, most individuals were asked to swear an oath that they had not been in contact with the infected. On 5 August 1527, Bernard Binčulić (Binzola) certified under oath, at the risk of losing his life, that his servant girl, recovered from plague, had not touched any infected goods and had not been in contact with any infected persons.[86] On 14 August 1527, under the threat of the usual fines, Marin Krstov Gradić (Gradi) declared under oath, that since the death of his servant girl two months ago, he had not been sick.[87] On 24 August, Petar Nikolin Prodanello took an oath, at the risk of losing his life, that in the last two months he had not been in touch with any sick or recovered persons and that the infected individuals had not been in his house.[88] On 18 November 1527, under the threat of a fine of one hundred ducats and a six-month prison sentence, Fran Orsatov Džamanjić (Giamagno) testified under oath that he had neither been nor worked in the house of his brother Sarakin since Tuesday a week earlier.[89]

The following cases demonstrate that the health officials paid particular attention to the control of the circulation of infected goods. On 26 August 1527, the health officials wrote to all the local counts and captains asking them to announce everywhere on the territory under their jurisdiction that whoever had goods at the Customs Office should come and pick them up within eight days. If they did not obey, the goods would be sent, at the expense of the owner, to a place where infected goods were cleaned.[90] On the same day, Marko Jakovljev Lukarević (Luchari), who worked for the health officials, was sent to Zaton to close several patrician houses and to make sure that none of them left their houses or courtyards. The patricians were threatened with a fine of one hundred hyperperi if they disobeyed.[91] On 13 September, under the threat of a fine left to their discretion, the health officials announced to the monasteries of St Thomas, St Simon, St Andrew, St Mary of Castello, and St Mark that if they possessed infected goods, those items should be cleaned. They all swore on their conscience that they did not have any and that their infected goods had already been sent to the designated place for cleaning of infected items.[92]

On 26 August 1527, Marin Primov Milatović, Luka Mihojević from Ston and Katarina, the servant of Mihić Sinišin were prohibited by the health officials from leaving their homes, courtyards, or vineyards and were only allowed to go under guard to buy the necessities of life, under the threat of a fine left to the discretion of the health officials.[93] On 2 September 1527, Luka, the town crier, announced to all those who were sent by the health officials to Kantafig, the western suburb of Gruž, that they were not to leave Kantafig, with or without guard, except under guard to get water from the canal.[94]

On 12 September 1527, Luka, the town crier, announced on behalf of the health officials, in front of three churches in the east and in the west of the city that if anyone harboured in their houses persons who were sick or were not feeling well, these persons should be reported to the health officials. Should they not report these cases, they would all be hanged.[95] The harshness of the threat in this case, demonstrates the extent of fear of unreported plague cases.

On 16 September 1527, Radonja Miobradović, the town crier, threatened the wife of Anton Kriještalo that she should not go out of her house under the threat of six jerks of the rope and being branded with a hot iron. The town crier also threatened all the women living in that house or courtyard that they would be lashed if they left their homes.[96] This example shows that the penalties reserved for women were always harsh.

In the thirty-year period from 1500 to 1530, the highest number of arrivals, 189, was recorded in 1527. In that year, the health officials registered many individuals arriving from places within the Republic. The ratio of arrivals from within the territory of the Republic indicates that plague was rampant not only in the city but also in smaller communities. On the other hand, arrivals by sea were extremely limited in 1527, as Dubrovnik remained a destination systematically avoided by merchants and goods alike. In 1528, only 50 arrivals were noted; in 1529 only 28; in 1530 not more than 16.[97] The sudden drop in the registered arrivals after 1527 corresponds to the disappearance of plague from Dubrovnik.

At the beginning of 1528, the control of travellers' arrivals was reduced and the threat of fines for those arriving from infected ports was scaled back from six to two months. On 7 July 1528, under the threat of three jerks of the rope, Vlahuša Antunović and his companions from Ombla, who had arrived from Venice, vouched that they had not been in a place suspected of infection in the previous two months. On the same day, the health officials ordered the whole party to return from the island of Mljet. The ship owner Vlahuša was given five jerks of the rope and his mariners, one each. They were told to return to Mljet without stopping anywhere and ordered to report to the guard of the health officials in Mljet. They were prohibited from leaving the island without the permission of the health officials.[98] In this case, the health officials obviously suspected that the sailors had anchored in an infected place and imposed strict sanctions. In 1528, the longest entries do not refer to arrivals but to trials that the health officials led against those who had contravened the plague control measures.

On 15 February 1530, by the order of the health officials, the chancellor Marino communicated to the patricians Jeronim Lukin Bunić (Bona) and Šiško Jurjev Gučetić (Goze) that, under the threat of a fine of one hundred ducats and a six-month prison sentence, they should not go outside the walls of the house or outside the gate of its garden where they were confined at Ploče. Similarly, their guardian Fran Stanetin Stanov was threatened with the fine of one hundred hyperperi and a three-month prison sentence, if he should see them going out from the confinement without notifying the health officials.[99]

From 1500 until 1530, 1,551 arrivals from 224 different places of departure mainly in present-day Italy, Croatia, Bosnia-Herzegovina, Albania, Kosovo, Serbia, Greece, Turkey, and other countries were registered in the *A recto* part of the manuscript (See Figure 5.1).[100] Most of the travellers arrived from Barletta (92), Venice (75), Senj (69), Albania, the exact place of departure not

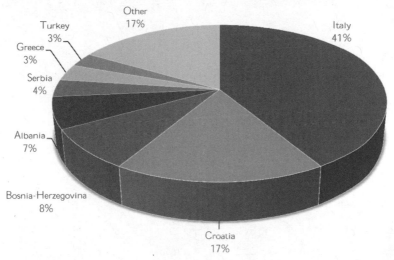

Figure 5.1 Travellers' Arrivals in Dubrovnik according to the Country of Departure, 1500–1530

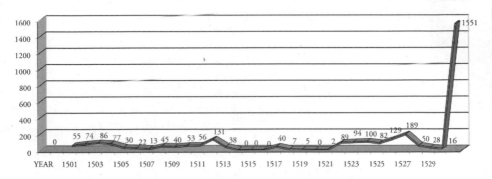

Figure 5.2 Travellers' Arrivals in Dubrovnik Registered by the Health Officials, 1500–1530

specified (58), Ancona (54), Manfredonia (38), Apulia (35), Sarajevo, also known as Vrhbosna in the past (34), Sofia (33), Patras (32), Otranto (31), Ortona, Skopje (29), Sicily (27), Bari and Novi Pazar (24), Alexandria, Lanciano and Lopud (20) (see Table 5.1).[101] The highest frequency of recorded arrivals occurred in the years 1502–03, 1511–13, and 1525–27. The two peaks at the time of plague epidemics in 1502–03 and 1526–27 illustrate the fact that the health officials entered the arrivals more conscientiously when the danger of plague infection was higher and adopted a more relaxed attitude when that danger subsided or was absent (see Figure 5.2). The *Libro deli Signori Chazamorbi* mentions a great variety of places of departure of persons travelling to

Table 5.1
The Place of Departure of Travellers Arriving in Dubrovnik, 1500–1530

Abruzo de la Marcha	2	Colfo de Ranpan (?)	1
Adrianople	13	Comoran (?)	1
Albania	58	Corfu	10
Alexandria	20	Corinth	1
Ancona	54	Coruña	1
Apulia	35	Cotrone	1
Argento, Albania	1	Cres	1
Banjani	4	Crete	4
Bakar	6	Čibača	1
Bakarac	2	Dalmatia	13
Bar (Antivari)	8	Dandovići	1
Bari	24	Donji Vlasi	2
Barleta	92	Dürres (Dyrrachium), Albania	10
Beyrouth	3	Drobnjaci	1
Bisceglie (Beseglo)	1	Drago Mjesto	1
Biela, Albania	2	Dubravica	1
Biesti	11	Fano	1
Bitola	1	Fermo de la Marcha	2
Blagaj	1	Ferrara	1
Bojana	2	Flanders (Fiandra)	3
Bologna	1	Foča	5
Borac	2	Fojnica (Chvojnica)	6
Bosnia	12	Fortore	2
Brgat	1	Francavilla al Mare	1
Brindisi	3	Gacka	1
Brodarevo	1	Gallipoli, Italy	2
Brsečine	1	Genoa	3
Bulgaria	1	Gianto	5
Calabria	5	Goražde	5
Calexo (?) (Calais?)	1	Grude	1
Catania	5	Hercegnovi (Castel Nuovo)	6
Cavtat	11	Herzegovina	1
Cephalonia	1	Hum	1
Cernica	6	Hungary	5
Cetina	1	Hvar	13
Chania	2	Istanbul	19
Chierenza de Levante	3	Istria	1
(Clarencia, Greece)		Janjina	1
Chios (Scio)	5	Javnich (?)	1
Chuziarna (?)	1	Jeleč	1
Civitanova de le Marche	1	Jelove Planine	1

Jeseri (?)	1	Orašac	5
Koločep (Calamota)	5	Ortona	29
Konavle	1	Otranto	31
Konjic	4	Pastrovići	1
Koper	3	Patras	32
Korčula (Curzola)	14	Pelješac	7
Koroni (Coron), Greece	1	Pesaro	17
Kotor (Cattaro)	1	Piergo, Albania	12
Krajina	1	Piva	1
Kreševo	1	Plovdiv (Philippopolis)	2
Kruševac	6	Poljice	2
Kupari	1	Ponente	5
Lanciano	20	Popovo Polje	3
Lastovo (Lagosta)	9	Poreč	4
Lepanto	5	Požega	2
Lezhë (Lexina), Albania	18	Prača	2
Lim	1	Preveza	1
Livno (Chlievno)	4	Priština	1
Lopud (Isola de Mezo)	20	Prizren	1
Ljubomir	2	Provadia	1
Ljubovinje	2	Prozor	1
Makarska	1	Rab	3
Manfredonia	38	Ravenna	3
Marche	12	Recanati	6
Messina	10	Rodon, Albania	1
Mlini	2	Reggio di Calabria	1
Mljet (Meleda)	1	Reggonta, Albania	1
Mola	2	Rijeka	6
Molfetta	6	Rimini	1
Monopoli	3	Rodi di Puglia	12
Montenegro	1	Rodos	1
Morača	1	Romania	5
Moravica	1	Rome	3
Morea	1	Rovinj	1
Morlachia	6	Rudine	1
Mostar	6	Rudnik	7
Naples	15	Sandžak	2
Nikopol	4	Sant'Angelo del Monte	2
Nikšić	1	Saplaninie (?)	7
Niš	4	Sarajevo (Vrhbosna)	34
Novi Pazar	24	Sardinia	3
Novo Brdo (Novamonte)	2	Scala de Sora (?)	1
Olovo	3	Scala Isaverde (?)	1
Ombla	7	Senigallia	3

Table 5.1
The Place of Departure of Travellers Arriving in Dubrovnik, 1500–1530

Senj	69	Vlorë (Valona), Albania	12
Serbia	2	Vasto	5
Shkodër (Scutari), Albania	2	Venice	75
Sicily	27	Vidin	6
Skopje	29	Vis	10
Slanich de Arbania	6	Volos	2
Slano	8	Vraneš	3
Smederevo (Samandria)	16	Vrbica	2
Sofia	33	Vrege (Vriega), Albania	2
Sulmona (Sol Monte)	2	Vrsinje	1
Split	4	Zadar	14
Srebrenica	8	Zakynthos	1
Srijem	1	Zaton (Malpho)	6
St. Maria	1	Zvornik	14
Ston (Stagno)	4	Župa (Breno)	5
Sv. Juraj near Senj	1	Total	1,551
Syracuse, Sicily	4	Question mark indicates unidentifiable	
Syria	3	place names.	
Šibenik	5		
Šipan (Giupana)	14		
Šumet (Gionchetto)	1		
Taranto	4		
Termoli	4		
Terni	1		
Thessaloniki	3		
Tomaševo	1		
Trani	10		
Trebinje	4		
Tremiti Islands	4		
Trepča	4		
Treviso	1		
Trieste	8		
Tripoli	2		
Tripolis, Syria	1		
Trnovo	5		
Trogir (Traguri)	3		
Trstenica	5		
Trsteno	2		
Turkey	11		
Ulcinj (Dolcigno)	1		
Uggiza, Albania	1		

Dubrovnik and can therefore be a useful source for economic historians who study the geographical distribution of the Ragusan maritime and caravan trade.[102] The places from which the travellers departed indicate that the Ragusan maritime activities were widespread and covered the whole Mediterranean and beyond. In fact, Ragusan ships rarely stopped in Dubrovnik as they constantly plied the seas and transported goods between foreign ports.

To conclude, we have to say that all the activities of the health officials demonstrate that they believed in the communicable nature of plague. It must be emphasized that, during the latter part of the fifteenth century, administrators of northern Italian cities had come to the same conclusion. That was unusual for the time because the belief in the communicable nature of the plague was contrary to all the medical theories of plague as well as the teachings of the Church. The isolation of the infected and of subjects suspected of infection constituted the core of all the health officials' actions. Their attitude can even be discerned in the vocabulary used. Although its mechanism was not understood, the word *infection(e)* was used thirty-eight times in the *Libro deli Signori Chazamorbi* manuscript.[103] The terms *miasma* or *corrupt air*, often used by physicians, were never mentioned – neither in the manuscript, nor in the decisions of the Ragusan Councils.

In the first quarter of the sixteenth century, the Health Office was an experienced and well-organized governmental plague control agency that gathered information about the spreading of plague epidemics and controlled the access to the Ragusan territory. The health officials had a difficult task of reconciling a successful international trade with the fight against plague outbreaks that trade could bring. Since they belonged to the same patrician social class as many merchants, the health officials showed flexibility in their approach and struggled to strike a balance between these two opposing goals. Past experience and direct observation were the most valuable tools of their pragmatic approach. A lot of organizational talent as well as considerable financial means were necessary to achieve that goal in an epoch that was centuries away from the discovery of the aetiology and pathology of plague.

However, at the end of 1526, when the catastrophic plague epidemic erupted in the city, everything changed in Dubrovnik. In a desperate battle for survival, the Health Office did not hesitate to use fines, trials, imprisonment, torture, and other measures of repression, as we will see in subsequent chapters of this volume.

6

The Disastrous Plague Epidemic of 1526–27

Donato Muzi, a physician from Venice, was in his first year of service in Dubrovnik when he was called to examine a young female patrician who had high fever. He lingered at her bedside and suddenly noticed right in front of his eyes two buboes typical of plague developing on her body. He fled quickly, persuaded that his patient was doomed. Honouring his professional duty, before returning home, Muzi informed the Ragusan authorities about his diagnosis of plague. Soon he noticed the same symptoms on himself. He had high fever, a headache, and buboes in the femoral area of his right leg and under the armpit. Since he was a firm believer in bloodletting in every fever, he wanted to perform a phlebotomy on his right arm, but not one of his colleagues dared to approach him.[1] Muzi discloses that the whole city of Dubrovnik and especially his two servants were witnesses to what had happened to him.

The young patrician girl had died in the meantime and the news that it was plague had spread quickly. Finally, someone gave Muzi a lancet and, using his left hand, the young and fearless doctor let almost 600 millilitres of blood from his vein on the right arm. Muzi was persuaded that this procedure had saved his life. Mirko Dražen Grmek emphasizes that Muzi's clinical description of the first victim of plague remains precious because it is the only one from the 1526–27 disastrous plague epidemic in Dubrovnik. It supplements the rather vague information supplied by the chroniclers. Furthermore, the rapidity of plague transmission from the patient to the young doctor reveals that in this case the *Yersinia pestis* infection was transmitted by the human flea *Pulex irritans*.[2]

In spite of strict control of travellers, mariners, and goods at the points of entry, the most disastrous plague outbreak to ever strike the Ragusan Republic after 1348 claimed its first victims on 6 December 1526. The chroniclers Razzi and Ranjina report that the plague was brought into the city of Dubrovnik by the Ragusan tailor Andrija Gunčević, who had returned from Ancona.[3] Since Ragusans believed that he had caused the death of many citizens by nonchalantly disregarding the plague control measures, he was sentenced to death in a public and cruel fashion that was common at that time.[4] The unfortunate tailor was tied to a cart and dragged through the city while being pinched with hot irons until he expired. He did not contract plague himself but his mother and his daughter-in-law became sick. He was accused of bringing infected goods into the city.

However, according to a Sicilian chronicler, the plague attack of the 1520s started after a ship from the Levant had docked in Syracuse. For the next ten years, it was carried from region to region by the constant movement of troops, as the French and the Spanish fought over the control of Italy while all of the Mediterranean was threatened by the rise of the Ottoman navy. Rome was infected in June 1522, Florence in August. During the 1526–28 plague breakout in Florence, people were dying at the rate of five hundred a day.[5] Because maritime trade was vigorous on both sides of the Adriatic, and infection prevalent in the ports, it was almost impossible to completely avoid getting infected.

In November 1526, plague was rampant in the city of Šibenik, further north on the Dalmatian coast.[6] According to the Venetian historian Marin Sanudo, in Split, the city in Central Dalmatia, the plague epidemic claimed six thousand to eight thousand lives.[7] From there, it spread to Brač, the island closest to the city of Split. The Croatian geographer Andre Jutronić reports that, according to the data gathered by the Venetian syndics, the population of Brač was reduced from 4,500 to 2,700 people.[8]

After the first few plague victims had died, the bustling city of Dubrovnik, usually noisy and overflowing with dockworkers loading and unloading goods from all sorts of ships – brigantines, carracks, grips, galleons, or caravels – as well as from overland caravans, suddenly fell eerily silent. Tradesmen from the hinterland and ship captains started avoiding Dubrovnik and directed their goods to other destinations. Manufacturing ground to a halt. The economic decline caused by plague led to enormous financial losses: the textile, leather, fur, and wool manufacturing all but stopped; ship building and goldsmithery could not prosper; maritime and overland trade were reduced to a minimum.

To avoid famine, bakeries hurriedly churned out large quantities of bread. Wealthier commoners with their families and those patricians who were allowed to leave the city sought shelter in their suburban residences or on the islands, while the poor, with nowhere to flee, awaited their uncertain fate in their humble dwellings within the walled city.

Under such grave circumstances, those governing the Republic – the chosen members of the Senate, the Minor and the Major Councils, and, above all, the health officials – had to stay on duty and put their lives at risk. By the nature of their functions, they had to be familiar with the circumstances of previous plague outbreaks, special regulations, and plague control measures that had been enacted in the past. Plague tended to recur in virulent form every five, ten, or twenty-five years, just long enough for the public memory of the previous plague to need some deliberate refreshing. This would open the way for changes and enhancements of plague control.[9]

The Ragusan Republic undertook the first plague control measures in 1377 with the implementation of quarantine, continued in 1390 with the founding of the first recorded Health Office, and by the 1526–27 outbreak, a tradition of plague control regulations had been part of government policy for 149 years.[10] However, a fresh outbreak of plague put the city's health culture to severe tests. Pressed by the terrifying circumstances of fear, misery, and death, the Ragusan Councils very rapidly adopted a whole series of measures to protect the homeland. The Senate acted promptly. Already on 6 December 1526, the day that the first victim had died of plague, the Senate ordered the health officials to start exercising the powers that had been bestowed on them in 1524 in order to preserve the health of the people.[11] Dubrovnik gave full support to the health officials and the Republic footed the bill without wavering.[12]

The health officials had to find housing for the infected families in special places designated for that purpose.[13] They also had to punish severely those who did not obey the plague control regulations. As well, they were entrusted with special powers that allowed them to burn the belongings of plague victims. Their authority covered not only the city of Dubrovnik but the whole territory of the Republic.[14] The infected, and those suspected of being infected, were soon sent into quarantine on the island of Mljet, on the islet of Supetar near Cavtat, or to Danče, just outside the city walls.[15]

Two days later, on 8 December 1526, the Senate designated ten guards, between the ages of twenty and fifty, to be permanently available to assist the health officials.[16] Also, three officials were designated to remove the beggars and those with festering wounds from the city, to organize their food supply, and arrange for their religious assistance.[17] The deep-seated fear that the Almighty could be punishing people for their sins by sending plague prompted the Ragusans to build a chapel dedicated to St Roch, the principal patron saint against plague and the main intercessor who could placate "God's wrath" and ask for God's mercy.[18] Some Senators suggested that the health officials should close the churches for a few days to avoid large gatherings that could contribute to the spreading of the epidemic. It was also proposed that women, children, and those unable to work should remain in their homes, but the Senate rejected these suggestions.[19]

At the end of the month, on 31 December 1526, *magister I*van Mednić, *medicus chirurgus*, a native of Kotor, applied for the position of the city plague doctor. Pressed by the urgency of the epidemic, on the same day, the Senate approved the applicant's contract and all the monetary demands that he had made.[20] The aforementioned plague control measures demonstrate that the authorities acted without delay. To protect the citizens of the Republic from the plague epidemic, which was claiming human lives in unprecedented numbers, they utilized all the measures at their disposal.

The absenteeism of the members of all three governing Councils was always a sore point. Under the dramatic new circumstances, it was feared that absenteeism would increase.[21] Therefore, on New Year's Day 1527, the Minor Council ordered all the members of the Senate to be present at a predetermined time. The decision was made that the absentees would be punished with monetary fines, according to regulations, except for those who were sick or absent from the Republic. All private appeals were abolished and solely matters of public interest were to be dealt with by the governing Councils.[22]

Barely three days later, on 3 January 1527, the Senate adopted various plague control measures for the protection of the state against plague – *pro mediis contra pestem que cepit sternire in civitate*.[23] These measures were adopted by thirty-six votes in favour and only one against. The Senate ordered the homes of all those who had died of plague to be burned with all their belongings except for fine silk and textiles intended for trade. The decision about which items were to be burned was to be made jointly by the Minor Council and the health officials. Just as in the past, to avoid conflicts between the two jurisdictions, the Senate decided that the Minor Council would have the last word in case of disagreement.[24] Under the threat of a monetary fine of one hundred hyperperi for the head of the household, it was decided that women and children younger than fourteen years of age would be prohibited from leaving their homes.

The heads of households and their servants, women selling bread, women keeping taverns and selling wine, and butchers were the only persons allowed to go out. Preventing children from unnecessary gathering in the city was a justifiable measure. They might have been much more vulnerable to plague infection than adults.[25] It is obvious some reasonable decisions, likely to alleviate the consequences of the epidemic, were made. The authorities took great care to avoid famine in the city. Since the economy was paralyzed, the government and wealthier individuals distributed financial aid and foodstuffs to the most destitute citizens. They also made sure that the women who were baking bread were regularly supplied with grain.[26]

The Minor Council judged that infected items in private homes were not being burned fast enough. Impatient, and dissatisfied with the health officials, the Minor Council threatened them with a monetary fine of one hundred ducats and ordered them to burn, that same night, the home of Leonard Đurašević, the prison guard at Danče, who had died of plague. Under the same threat, the health officials, with the help of their assistants, had to burn all the items contained in the homes on Zvijezdić Street and in all the other infected homes in the Republic. The commercial items intended for sale were the only exception. The health officials could not have them burned without first consulting the Minor Council.[27] In no uncertain terms, the Senate asked the health officials to execute all the orders without discussion or hesitation. The Senate ordered them to choose two individuals from among themselves who would supervise the burning of infected homes. If the health officials refused to obey, the Minor Council would choose for them.

From then on, the health officials chose those individuals among themselves.[28] Of all the unpleasant duties that they had to perform, the burning of the homes of their fellow citizens was a task they tried to avoid at all costs. Was the burning of homes and household items a sensible plague control measure?[29] The enormous fires burning during the night must have terrified both the living and the dying. However, instead of curtailing plague, the flames may have allowed the rats and their fleas to spread even further. Although the measures were taken in community's best interest, we have to conclude that such a measure may not have attained the desired goal. Both the government and the health officials obviously acted in a realm full of unknowns. With such a hit and miss strategy, some of the efforts proved to be efficient while others were counterproductive or simply not useful.

The health officials worked under exceptionally difficult circumstances. Physically and mentally exhausted, they probably feared for their own lives and those of their loved ones, like every other citizen. In the adverse circumstances of the times, they coped as best they could. To make them obey, the government had to threaten the health officials with laws, regulations, and exceedingly high monetary fines. Even though the services of the health officials were indispensable, the Minor Council did not hesitate to discipline them. On 12 January 1527, under the threat of a monetary fine of one hundred hyperperi for each transgression, it ordered all the health officials to remain in the city, day and night without exception.[30]

The Ragusan patricians often had to perform duties that they did not enjoy and that took them away from their private business, families, and other pursuits. Although they never wavered as a group, as individuals they must have had their misgivings about many offices but especially about the duties of the health officials. They probably felt endangered by the epidemic, on the one hand, and threatened by other social groups, on the other. Their hesitation is evident from their unwillingness to serve in this capacity. It is not difficult to imagine that they felt the same urge as other citizens to escape to their urban villas or to the islands. Moreover, they were aware that the repressive measures of the state that they governed could also be used against them. The plague obviously created tensions that the patricians found difficult to resolve. As individuals, they may not have supported the repressive measures that were increased during every new plague epidemic. This is evident from the way they voted. The most repressive measures usually received the minimal majority. They did not embrace the duties of the health officials with enthusiasm, but they were aware that their social status obliged them to accept them, however grudgingly. Dubrovnik was a society where the survival of the group took precedence over individual rights. The patricians found protection in their social rank more often than in their individual rights. Why did they not rebel? Because they were acutely aware of the fact that, in comparison with other regions of Dalmatia, the Ragusan model of government offered them a superior standard of living.

We have no record of the feelings of the Ragusan health officials in 1527. However, a hundred years later, during the plague epidemic in Prato, a small town thirty kilometres northwest of Florence, one health official expressed his feelings in a note on the first page of the *Libro della Sanità* by Cristofano Ceffini. This note, written in a handwriting different from the author of the book, reads, "one learns at the cost of human life what happens when one receives from God the scourge of an epidemic without having any light or experience wherewith to guide one's conduct in so exacting a task." Carlo M. Cipolla shows that the correspondence of the health officials of Prato conveys a sense of intolerable fatigue, constant worry, loneliness, and self-questioning: "Conflicts, abuses and infringements of regulations, petty quarrels, and a never-ending series of problems and difficulties – every day the health officials had to face such things, while indefatigable vigilance was required as the bells of the churches kept announcing new deaths."[31]

Strict security measures were observed in 1527. Patricians and commoners were asked to keep guard at the city entrance gates under the unceasing supervision of the health officials. If any of them were still outside the city, they had to return the same day.[32] The Senate released from prison the persons who were serving sentences for less serious transgressions, while those who had been sentenced by the Criminal Court were banished from the Republic. Ragnina, a Ragusan chronicler, reports that the plague epidemic lasted twenty months. During that time, the state treasury spent forty thousand ducats for charitable purposes, for the arming of two hundred soldiers who kept guard in the city, and for four hundred armed soldiers at Brgat Hill, eight kilometres northeast of the city.[33]

The capacity of the burial places dug within the city was soon exceeded. Thus, the Senate ordered the health officials to bury the dead in church crypts and monasteries, burial grounds of the religious confraternities, and communities outside the city.[34] It was also necessary to speed up the production of lime and to make sure that those who had quick lime also had sufficient quantities of wood for burning. Lime had to be made within eight days and had to be sold at the usual price because it was used to disinfect dead bodies.[35] On 28 January 1527, the government ordered the sale of grain and oil to be moved outside the city, which indicates that, even at such an early date, the idea of temporarily leaving the city was contemplated.[36] Financial aid and foodstuffs were distributed to the craftsmen and textile workers, especially the weavers, most of them women, who were out of work.[37]

Since the epidemic did not subside even during the coldest winter month, on 31 January 1527, the Senate ordered a whole new range of plague control measures. In winter, bubonic plague was accompanied with the extremely virulent form of pneumonic plague that had a tendency to spread excessively fast and claim its victims almost immediately. The patricians had to bring fifty men from the islands and fifty from the coast to organize squads of commoners and peasants to keep order. They were to guard the city fortifications of Minčeta, Revelin, and Lovrijenac. The Minor Council had to make sure that, together with the rector and six members of the Minor Council, at least twenty-five senators were present in the city every week. Three judges and ten senators were asked to stay in the city to process court cases. Five members of the Major Council also had to stay to assist the Minor Council. If four officials usually performed a function, two of them had to remain in the city. From then on, just three health officials, not all of them as before, had to stay in the city.[38]

This regulation finally brought a more just distribution of both the heavy responsibilities and the onerous tasks performed by the health officials, but it did not reduce their fines. Each absence of the health officials was still punishable by a fine of one hundred hyperperi while the fines for all the other functions were just twenty-five hyperperi. Such treatment is a testimony of the importance of their office. However, it is also a demonstration of tactless methods brought about by a certain degree of state repression. In years when plague was not rampant, the Health Office consisted of five individuals who were elected for a year with overlapping terms.

How many health officials lost their lives in 1527 while serving the Republic? We can search for the answer in the *Speculum Maioris Consilii* (Mirror of the Major Council), which lists the names of all the public officials in the Ragusan Republic since 1440. In 1526, two health officials were elected on 12 January, two more on 28 January, and the last two on 6 April, for a total of six. They were Jeronim Stjepanov Gradić (Grade), Miho Antunov Sorkočević (Sorgo), Marin Đurov Gučetić (Goze), Andrija Antunov Benešić (Benessa), Luka Markov Bunić (Bona), and Nikola Dragojev Gučetić (Goze). If all had survived, their duty would have ended on the same date, a year from their election. What happened is that the elections of health officials became more frequent in 1527. Due to ill health of the serving health officials, two more health officials were added on 8 December 1526 for January, two on 14 January, one on 30 January, and one on 21 February 1527. Four assistants were added on 8 March 1527. Five health officials were elected on 18 June, three on 27 September, and one on 25 November 1527, for a total of nineteen in the year of the worst plague epidemic.[39]

In 1527, the following patricians were elected as health officials: Stjepan Nikolinov Gundulić (Gondola), Stjepan Pavlov Lukarević (Luccari), Miho Marinov Bučinčić (Bocignolo), Luka Nikolin Bunić (Bona), Nikola Marinov Gundulić (Gondola), Serafin Orsatov Džamanjić (Zamagna), Jeronim Pavlov Gradić (Gradi), Orsat Martolov Rastić (Resti), Marin Stjepanov Džamanjić (Zamagna or Giamagno), Frano Pandolfov Benešić (Benessa), Pavao Marinov Gradić (Gradi), Ivan Marinov Pucić (Poza), Stjepan Marinov Bundić (Bonda), Dimitar Matov Ranjina (Ragnina), Paskoje Trojanov Crijević (Zrieva), and Nikola Džorin Palmotić (Palmota).[40] It is significant that on 18 June 1527, upon their return to the city, the senators elected five new health officials, almost as many as were usually necessary for the whole year. We have to conclude that

Decisions of a purely practical nature follow. First of all, the Senators had
to elect six to eight patricians in their thirties, who would, with pay, govern the
city if the councils had to withdraw to Gruž, the suburban port of Dubrovnik.
One of those patricians elected would have to take over the role of the rector.
Simultaneously, the Senate had to organize the defence of the Republic against
enemies attacking by land or sea. In those uncertain times, following the battle
at Mohács in Hungary, the Ottomans could easily have decided to occupy the
Ragusan Republic. And Venice, a competitor in diplomacy and trade, was also
a potential threat. Moreover, the Saracens, the North African pirates, who made
frequent plundering excursions to the Adriatic islands, were never far away. It
seems, however, that, no matter how vulnerable and how easy a prey the
Republic might have become, the threat of plague infection acted as a deterrent
in those crucial months of 1527. On the other hand, the city walls, several
metres deep, successfully protected the city, a reality that even the Ottomans
could not ignore. Therefore, to further improve their defence, the Ragusan
authorities added two hundred more soldiers to be posted along the fortifications and the city entrance gates. One galleon and two brigantines with eight
oars each were to be armed and sent to patrol constantly between Molunat,
forty kilometres southeast of Dubrovnik, and Zaton, the bay eight kilometres
northwest of the city. The sailors, defending the Republic from the sea, could
choose to spend their free days either at home or on their ships.

The merchants and other commoners, between the ages of eighteen and
sixty, had to keep guard. Each group was made up of twenty members of nobility and fifteen commoners. In case of avoidance of these duties, hefty monetary fines could be applied, which, in those times of scarcity, few could afford
to pay. Those serving prison sentences for minor offences could buy their freedom by volunteering for guard duty. In addition, the authorities had to provide
the necessary food supplies for those who had to remain in the city. Four bak-
ers and six women had to stay behind to make and to sell bread. They were
given five hundred *staria* of ground flour. For the needs of the government, ten
thousand ducats from the state treasury of the Republic had to be transferred to
the Dominican Monastery of the Holy Cross in Gruž.[48]

On 7 February 1527, after they had declared that they could not and dared
not practise medicine because of plague, the physician Bartholomeus Barisonus
and the surgeon Hieronymus Pavanellus asked for an unpaid leave of absence
of three months. The government was happy to oblige and thus reduce the expenses of the state. The physicians always avoided serving in plague stricken
cities. At that time, the physicians considered plague a major calamity that was

not within their jurisdiction.[49] Ever since the first appearance of plague in the fourteenth century, physicians usually abandoned the infected cities. On the one hand, they were acutely aware of the danger a plague outbreak represented and, on the other hand, they were also conscious that their knowledge and skills were inadequate to deal with this disease. Since they were quite well-off, they could afford to take an unpaid leave of absence. Moreover, because they were highly educated, their qualifications were considered too precious to let them die of plague. This being said, there were at least two medical practitioners who died of plague while serving in Dubrovnik. The surgeon Johannes della Dolce Calderia from Naples arrived in Dubrovnik from Lecce in 1455. On 18 May 1457, the Senate gave him the permission to leave the city but he stayed and died of plague on 5 October 1457. The physician Gabriel de Galvano served in Dubrovnik since 1476. He left a testament that states that on 18 April 1482 he had died of plague.[50]

Donato Muzi was also a salaried physician since 2 June 1526. When he asked for a one-month leave of absence on 23 February 1527, the Senate acquiesced to his demand. During his absence, Muzi was given his full salary, probably because of his contribution to diagnosing plague in the city and because he himself had survived plague. In April, he was allowed to go with his family wherever he pleased so he left again, returned on 27 August, and was hired again. He stayed in Dubrovnik until 1536.[51]

Just as they hired surgeons and physicians, Ragusans contracted state pharmacists at least since the 1300s, the earliest period for which the archival documents are available.[52] Three pharmacists are mentioned in the Ragusan legal documents of the 1526–27 plague period. Since 1520, Gaspar de Antonio from Rimini worked in Dubrovnik. At the beginning of 1527, he died of plague, as did his wife Nikoleta and his daughters. On 14 February 1527, his son Antonio Gaspari inherited his father's pharmacy, but a month later he died of plague and so did his brother Julian. With their deaths, the whole family of apothecaries was wiped out. In their wills, the two brothers, the last of the family to die, left all their property to Miho and Nikola Zlatarić. The third pharmacist, Battista di Giovanni from Brescia, who was active in Dubrovnik for fifteen years, is mentioned in a 1526 legal document as *aromatarius*, a herbalist. By May 1541, he had also died.[53]

In order to provide spiritual assistance to those in need, the Senate asked the vicar of the Ragusan Archbishop to assign four deans of the Cathedral of St Mary to stay in the city. Furthermore, to ensure the preservation of the sacred relics, they were hidden in the cathedral and sealed by a wall.[54] In fact, owing to the unceasing care of the Ragusans, the sacred relics were later transferred to the new cathedral, built after the earthquake of 1667, and have been preserved until the present time. On 25 February 1527, the Major Council decided to lower its quorum requirement. Instead of 150 members, just one hundred were required to be present when major decisions were made; only eighty members were required when other matters were discussed. The quorum of the Senate was reduced to thirty-one members and its powers were limited. For example, it was not allowed to name ambassadors, the treasurers of St Mary, or the officials whose term of office was for life.[55]

Since the plague epidemic continued to rage unabated, on 12 March 1527, the government finally decided to abandon the walled city and move to Gruž. Seven patricians were elected to stay behind to govern the city with Nikola Franov Tudišić (Tudisi) as rector.[56] It was previously decided that these gentlemen would be rewarded with four hundred to seven hundred hyperperi. In the port of Gruž, the government met at the Dominican monastery of the Holy Cross.[57] At their first meeting, on 24 March 1527, not more than twenty-two senators showed up – insufficient even for a reduced quorum. The dramatic consequences of the epidemic became obvious to all.

Deprived of their regular surgeons and physicians who had left the city at the time of the greatest need for their services, the authorities usually hired plague doctors. As if he had sensed that his colleagues were going to retreat, on 31 December 1526, Ivan Mednić from Kotor – Johannes Mednich de Catharo – offered his services as a plague doctor – *medicus pestis*. His application, written in Italian, is preserved in the State Archives of Dubrovnik. His contract, written in Latin, was adopted by the Senate on the same day.[58] In his application, Mednić emphasizes that his father Pavao was born in Dubrovnik, and that thus he himself originates from this illustrious city to which he would like to return together with his five sons.[59] He writes that it is his duty to practise as a plague doctor not because of monetary gain but because he wants to care for the citizens of Dubrovnik with love and compassion, without regard to the danger to his own life.[60] Mednić promises to perform phlebotomies, incise buboes, and faithfully care for the infected and those suspected of infection. He is ready to prescribe medicines, and to this effect he attaches a list of his recipes.[61] He adds that other Ragusan physicians may verify his recipes.[62] For his services, he expects two hundred gold ducats paid in three equal instalments during the year. If necessary, and if the Senate expressed its interest, he is ready to serve beyond this first year. On top of his salary, he asks the Senate to allocate him three ducats per month for life for his five sons. The state was supposed to pay for the unguents, plasters, and other medicines.

The Senate confirmed the contract and accepted the conditions of *magister* Mednić. Written in the formal legal style, the contract does not show any major corrections in the text, which lead us to believe that difficult negotiations between the two parties, which were frequent in such situations, did not take place. From the tone of Mednić's application, one gets the impression that he wanted so badly to be accepted in Dubrovnik that he would have settled for more modest conditions. The authorities in Dubrovnik, for their part, were under considerable pressure to fill this crucial position. Therefore, the only difference between the application and the contract can be found in the clause concerning his sons. We have examined the contracts of physicians and surgeons during two centuries, from 1348 to 1529, and have not found any clause concerning children. What made the senators accept this clause in Mednić's case? Did they want to make sure that he would stay in Dubrovnik after the expiry of his contract? Did they consider that in the future they will be able to offer Mednić less, or were they in such a difficult situation that they simply had to accept his conditions? The fact is that the Senate allocated three ducats per month for his sons but added that this amount is given under the condition that Mednić stay in the employment of Dubrovnik after the expiry of this one-year contract. If Mednić did not honour his obligations, adds the Senate, he would lose his salary, and the clause concerning his sons would be null and void. Should Mednić die during the validity of his contract, he would not receive his salary for the remaining period. His sons would still receive three ducats per month for life as long as they stayed in Dubrovnik for good and served the Republic as needed. The Senate was quite aware that their plague doctor could succumb to plague and did not want to pay a considerable amount of gold after his death. This condition is not surprising given that it was common in northern Italian cities.[63] The clause about Mednić's five sons is highly unusual. Does it demonstrate that there might have been a human streak in the Ragusan approach, or is it proof of the fact that the Ragusan Senate was in a very difficult bargaining position?

We know that the Ragusan patricians entertained close relations with the leading families in Kotor, only eighty-seven kilometres south of Dubrovnik. They could thus easily get information about Mednić's surgical education and practice, his reputation, and his standing in the city. They knew that Mednić had been trained by a qualified surgeon in Venice and that he had worked in Kotor as a community surgeon. This was not the first time that the Ragusans employed a surgeon from Kotor. In 1483–84, they had hired Michael from Kotor – Michael de Catharo.[64] The plague doctor's situation was not only dangerous; it was also unpleasant because he had to stay in isolation forty days after the epidemic had died down. The plague doctor was not allowed to come in contact with other people, and he was not allowed to treat the patients who suffered from other diseases.

In Venice, on 7 February 1527, the Ragusan patrician Vlaho Sorkočević (Sorgo) recruited Jacobus Rizo as plague doctor. He was hired for a six-month period with a salary of 160 ducats. Rizo was also given free lodging for him and his servant. The government was obliged to supply him with medications to treat the infected. He was to care for the plague sufferers and receive free food as long as he stayed, together with his servant, in isolation.[65] However, Rizo's behaviour proved questionable. The information in the archival sources is sketchy, but it seems that he committed several acts of theft and outright robbery. Evidently, before hiring a candidate, the government, pressed by the urgency of the plague, had little time to verify the professional and moral credentials of this individual. The unethical plague doctor was thus in the position to profit from the grave circumstances in the city.

The Minor Council empowered the health officials to investigate and punish him as they saw fit. Since the health officials found that Rizo had committed a serious crime, the Senate had to be consulted.[66] However, the archival texts give us only a partial insight into Rizo's case. When the authorities completed the investigation on 10 September 1527, Rizo readily agreed to give up any further demands and he quietly disappeared from Dubrovnik.

Up to that point in time, salaried foreign physicians had been employed in Dubrovnik for at least three centuries. Rizo's candidature is the only one that turned out to be utterly unsatisfactory. The other plague doctor, Ivan Mednić from Kotor, who was working in Dubrovnik during the same period, is described in the archival sources as a man who always responded when it was necessary to diagnose plague or the cause of death. Mednić administered drugs as necessary and fulfilled all the conditions of his contract.[67] The government was obviously satisfied with his services because, upon the expiration of his contract, it hired him for another year, albeit under different conditions.

In spite of the minimal distance from the city, governing Dubrovnik from Gruž proved to be difficult. The councils did not meet because they could not maintain even the reduced quorum that had been prescribed on 25 February 1527. The main reason for that situation was high mortality among the councillors. There were also difficulties with the food supply. Some patricians, their self-discipline and their morale at an all time low, had fled the city. On the island of Šipan, there were incidents involving several patricians who took advantage of the temporary weakness of the central government. Six noblemen were punished with a fine of twenty-five hyperperi. Common thieves and those breaking into abandoned homes were punished by hanging. It is documented that Ivaniš was hanged at Danče for thieving and breaking the wall of the Revelin fortress in Dubrovnik.[68]

In the second half of April, the mortality from plague was slowly diminishing and the authorities, although few in number, tried to keep order in the Republic. They sent several patricians into *kaznačine*, the rural territorial units, to supervise the work of the health officials' assistants, who had been chosen among the most reputable commoners. The patricians were empowered to punish the violators of the health regulations as well as the designated gravediggers, the *kopci*, who were hired to bury the dead at the expense of the commune.[69] On 12 April 1527, it was decided to allow healthy persons who were quarantined on the island of Mljet to return home while poor homeless people were sent to live in some wooden barracks in Kantafig, the western section of Gruž.[70]

The Councils were also in charge of the valuables belonging to those who had died of plague in various quarantine compounds. These items were held in a wooden house on the island of Lokrum. Some people suspected of plague, who were also staying on Lokrum, were later taken to the suburb of Pile and then, on 28 April 1527, back to the city where they were assigned various duties according to their social status. Men were employed to transport items while the women were asked to bake bread and disinfect homes.[71] Burial within the city of those who had died outside the city was forbidden and efforts were made to keep the city clean and disinfected.[72]

On 8 June 1527, the Senate adopted a new regulation regarding the reduction of the quorum of the Minor Council. The Senate also decided that the infected persons who had returned to the city could be ordered to stay in their homes and would not be allowed to come in contact with healthy people. However, if they so wished, they were permitted to stay in their villas outside the city and could spend their quarantine time there.[73] To resume a more orderly functioning, the government was doing everything in its power to entice the patricians to return to the city.

After a three-month absence, on 16 June 1527, the feast of the Holy Trinity, the government returned to the city. Of the seven patricians who had been designated to remain in the city to run the government during the exodus, only one, Nikola Franov Tudišić (Tudisi), survived. He was there to open the gates of the city when the others returned. Holy mass was celebrated. The aid of the Holy Spirit and of St Blaise was invoked. The extraordinary measures adopted in February remained in force until 16 November 1527. From that date on, in order to be legally competent to make decisions, the assemblies of all the Councils had to observe the usual quorum. In the end, government authorities, even with the reduced numbers of patricians available to serve, and especially owing to the service of the health officials, managed to save the Ragusan Republic from defeat by the invisible enemy. They also succeeded in keeping at bay the potential political enemies who threatened with plunder and territorial conquest.

All Ragusan chroniclers mention approximately the same mortality rates for Dubrovnik. The Anonymous chronicler states that plague struck on 6 December 1526 and insists that the disease was the result of the "wrath of God" – *Non fu mortalità, ma ira di Dio* – which lasted a full year and claimed the lives of 75 noblemen, 84 noblewomen, and 20,000 commoners, including the famous poet Šiško Menčetić. The chroniclers Nikola Ragnina and Serafino Razzi report that 19 Dominicans and 25 Franciscan friars perished in the monasteries; 160 nuns died in 5 convents. However, in the 3 convents that were permanently locked, all the nuns had survived. This confirmed the efficiency of isolation as a plague control measure. The chroniclers also concur that about 20,000 commoners and 164 patricians perished in the Dubrovnik plague onslaught of 1526–27.[74] In 1498, the Ragusan Republic had reached the highest demographic boom in its history – there were almost 90,000 inhabitants. There were 2,000 patricians, together with their families, for a total of almost 8,000 inhabitants of the city of Dubrovnik. In 1536, the population of the Republic had fallen to about 65,000. This has led Nenad Vekarić to conclude that the drastic population reduction of more than 20,000 citizens between 1498 and 1536 was the result of the plague epidemic of 1526–27. The latest estimates of demographic data indicate that one-fourth of the population died during that period.[75]

In 1528, there were still some pockets of plague infection on the territory of the Republic, especially in Ston. On 14 January, the Senate authorized the health officials to spend fifty hyperperi to assist the infected poor who were confined in Ston and sent them some grain. The health officials were also told to use their own judgment on how best to fight the plague.[76] Ivan Mednić's first contract expired at the beginning of 1528 just as the plague epidemic subsided. On 11 January, he offered his services but no longer as a plague doctor, rather as a surgeon. Again, he offered to stay permanently in Dubrovnik knowing well that it depended on the goodwill of the authorities. He emphasized that he was ready to perform the skull trepanation, set broken or dislocated bones, incise abscesses, and treat other diseases that were the responsibility of a surgeon. If plague should rear its ugly head, God forbid, he was ready to treat the infected for any salary that the authorities would approve. He obviously considered that it was better to leave the crucial decision about the salary to the Senate. In the sixteenth century, the salaries of medical men were lower than before. The authorities were well informed about the availability of physicians and surgeons and not only did they offer lower salaries but they imposed additional duties. The medical men had to visit and treat the sick in prisons, give their opinion during court investigations, which often involved torture, and report woundings in street brawls as well as cases of prostitution and sodomy.

On 11 January 1528, the Senate approved Mednić's contract with a salary of one hundred ducats and a free residence.[77] Although they were satisfied with his services, the Senators allocated Mednić only half of his previous salary. They were aware that plague had receded and that soon their city would again be attractive for many other surgeons. There was also another reason for their thrift. During the 1527 epidemic, trade was significantly reduced but the expenses of the state for the defence of the Republic and the care of the sick had increased exponentially. If we add up Ivan Mednić's salary of one hundred ducats, thirty-six ducats for his sons, plus free lodging, which was worth another fifteen ducats, and add the income from individual patients, we have to conclude that he was quite successful in providing for his family. On 12 March 1529, a contract was signed between Mihoč Ivanović and Ivan Mednić in which he promised to treat the patient's syphilitic abscesses for eight ducats – a truly royal fee for just one patient.[78]

Finally, one could ask why, despite all Ragusans efforts and a lengthy experience with plague control measures, Dubrovnik could not avoid the calamitous 1527 plague epidemic. The most likely reason is that a grain shipment full of infected rats and their fleas had arrived from the Levant, a constant source of plague infection. Plague always originated on the Ottoman-controlled territory where the plague protection measures were not applied. It could have been brought to Dubrovnik directly on an infected ship or indirectly via an Italian port city. If a captain tried to hide the fact that his ship, its crew or its cargo, had arrived from a plague-infected port, such a false declaration, if it were not discovered by the health officials, was sufficient to endanger the city.

The plague attack of the 1520s may have started after a ship from the Levant had docked in Sicily. During the French-Spanish War for the control of Italy, constant movement of troops facilitated the spread of plague across the whole region. Another possible cause is the particular virulence of the plague bacillus, or its mutation. The fact that it was a major plague outbreak, which affected a number of cities on both sides of the Adriatic, among them Rome and Florence, would add credence to the theory of an increased virulence of the plague pathogen, in comparison with the fifteenth century when plague outbreaks were relatively mild and the mortality low. Another element to support this theory is the fact that the worst plague outbreaks in Dubrovnik, in 1348 and 1526, both started in December and raged during the winter months while most other plague flare-ups reached their peak in summer. Such an evolution of the epidemic would also favour the presence of the pneumonic form of the plague, which is more deadly than the bubonic form.

Moreover, at that time, the Ottomans expanded their navy and fought for political and commercial domination in the Mediterranean and the Adriatic, thus increasing the likelihood of plague infection. Dubrovnik and Venice, as well as other maritime cities, had built powerful trade navies with many more ships than before. Those ships constantly plied the seas in search of trade, especially with the Levant, whence the plague arrived. Lastly, it has to be pointed out, that in spite of all the plague control measures, epidemics could not be completely avoided as long as the cause of the disease and the mode of its transmission by rat and flea vectors remained unknown. This knowledge was acquired only at the end of the nineteenth century, during the third plague pandemic.

The last major plague outbreak in the city of Dubrovnik occurred in 1533. Nikola Ragnina reports that the plague was brought from the Ottoman territory, that it lasted three months (six according to the Anonymous chronicler). Seventeen male patricians, nineteen female patricians, and 2,600 commoners lost their lives. Two galleons and one *fusta*, a fast ship, were armed for the defence of the city.[79] Serafino Razzi reports that the plague outbreak started on 27 March and lasted until 4 July. After that there were smaller flare-ups for another twenty months. The rector and the Senate were asked not to leave the city for a while because it was considered that their trips could cause the epidemic to last longer. According to Razzi, the state had spent fifty thousand ducats to combat the epidemic, but Ragnina quotes the sum of only one thousand ducats. The Senate adopted the usual protection measures in times of plague, ensured the defence of the state, and issued specific orders to the health officials concerning the infected and their homes. The quorum in all the Councils was reduced.[80] On 4 April, three new assistants of the health officials were elected, and three more health officials were added on 23 December 1533.[81]

At the end of May, the Senate decided to build, at the expense of the state, the votive Church of the Annunciation situated close to the Ploče gate, next to the chapel of St Luke, in the hope that the "Almighty God with the intercession of the glorious virgin would liberate the city from plague."[82] On 10 July, the Senate threatened the health officials with a fine of one hundred ducats if they did not live up to their responsibilities – namely, stay in the city at all times, free the city from infected goods, post proper guards where necessary, and perform all their duties as stipulated. The health officials were asked to report to the Minor Council what they had undertaken. The rector and the Minor Council were also asked to make sure that those who did not obey were punished with the hundred-ducat fine.[83] On 2 October 1533, all the special plague measures were revoked because the city had recovered its "pristine health."[84] After 1533, the plague outbreaks were sporadic and occurred only in the countryside, not in the city itself. The health officials issued health passes for Ragusan ships and examined the equivalent documents held by foreign ships mooring in the port of Dubrovnik.[85] In the seventeenth and eighteenth centuries, plague was more prevalent in the Ottoman-controlled hinterland and kept the assistants of the health officials fully occupied on the continental border. Their duty was to prevent the smuggling of infected goods, especially on the route from the Ottoman-ruled Herzegovina through Ragusan Konavle to Venetian-ruled Boka Kotorska.[86]

After 1530, plague was no longer endemic in the Ragusan Republic. Sadly, the 1575–77 and 1630 epidemics affected all of Italy and caused an unprecedented loss of life. Although she does not provide any further explanations, Jane Stevens Crawshaw claims that there is no sign that the lazarettos were effective at reducing the impact of plague over the first two centuries of their history. Despite all the efforts of the Venetians, and enormous amounts of money invested in the lazarettos, the 1575–77 outbreak in Venice claimed more than 46,000 lives, or more than one-quarter of the total population, making it the highest loss ever recorded in Italy. Of that number, 19,175 deaths occurred within the lazarettos, which represents 41 percent of the total mortality or 75 percent of the subjects sent there.[87] In the beginning, the authorities, fearing the consequences for Venetian trade, tried to deny or at least to downplay the presence of plague. The physicians who argued that the disease was "true plague" received various threats.[88]

Dubrovnik was spared both of these major plague attacks. Was it a stroke of luck or foresight? Was Dubrovnik's good fortune due to the measures of the Health Office or was it bypassed by infected ships and suspicious goods? Did some other factors play a role? It is impossible to tell.

Having studied the plague tracts in sixteenth-century Italy, Samuel K. Cohn noticed a fresh way of thinking among Italian officials and physicians after their close observation of the disease. He also discerned a marked shift – away from treating individual patients towards public health, hygiene, and political action – to eradicate the disease. Cohn reports that in Italy, the 1575–78 plague was a turning point for such concerns.[89] During the 1575–78 epidemics, new officials were elected, decrees were issued for keeping the streets dirt-free, clearing public latrines, ensuring clean water, and maintaining harbours purged of waste. Fundamental economic programs were proposed for ridding the cities of dire poverty that came to be recognized as a true cause of plague. Addressing social problems with vigorous political measures led to a new optimism by plague writers that the plague could be eradicated once and for all.[90]

Due to the efforts of Giovanni Filippo Ingrassia, the Protomedico of the Kingdom of Sicily, only 3,100 people perished in the 1576 epidemic in Palermo, a city of at least 80,000 inhabitants. Ingrassia successfully implemented the city's first permanent health board, oversaw the building of its first lazaretto, along with two other plague hospitals and two new hospitals for the convalescents. He enforced the rules of operation with military efficiency. He also recommended social measures to help the poor: charity, low-cost loans, and the suspension of sales taxes for the poor, while the rich, including him, would have to pay more.[91] All this lends credence to the effectiveness of quarantine and other plague control measures.[92]

In the next chapter, the Ragusan health officials assume a new role and become trial judges in cases of the plague survivors, the *resanati*, who contravened the plague control measures in the wake of the 1527 plague epidemic.

7

Plague Survivors as Plague Workers

When the surviving councillors returned to Dubrovnik on 16 June 1527, the special plague control measures prescribed by the Senate were still in force. Armed squads of patricians and commoners still kept guard in the city. For each office, the Senate instituted a schedule of calls of duty by a draw. According to the number of members in each Council, each quorum was divided into four groups. Each group was on call for one week and, during that time, all the members of that group had to remain in the city, day and night. Considering the extraordinary conditions under which they had to work, with these measures, the Senators tried to protect themselves and their colleagues from excessive fatigue, ill health, and too many absences.[1] The replacement of four health officials in January and four of their assistants in March 1527 confirmed that there was an inevitable turnover caused by the epidemic.[2] In the manuscript *Libro deli Signori Chazamorbi*, numerous records testify to the fact that after the plague epidemic started dying down in the second half of 1527, the Health Office resumed its regular functions, employing more people than ever before. The chancellors and the scribes, whose names appear in the manuscript, dutifully recorded the investigations and the trials against the violators of plague control measures.[3] When a document had to be presented to a patrician, this duty was performed by chancellors. Thus, Chancellor Troyano Pasqual de Primi notified Lovre Nemanjić on 10 August 1527 that, under the threat of a fine of one hundred ducats, he was forbidden from leaving his home until further notice from the health officials. On 11 August 1527, Troyano advised Lovre, the vice count of Ombla, that under the threat of a fine of fifty *hyperperi*, he was required to send all the recovered and the sick to specific places designated for the purpose of disinfection. If they did not obey, Lovre would have to report them to the health officials.[4]

The plague control measures were only grudgingly obeyed because they were often perceived as impinging on the class status, material interests, and personal freedoms of the citizens. Cases where there was no direct conflict with the authorities have not reached us because it was not compulsory to record them. Serious violations of plague control measures that required an investigation and a trial were documented on a regular basis. As previously mentioned, each new epidemic upsurge brought with it more rigorous measures to fight it and even harsher sentences for those who contravened them. The 1527 plague onrush ushered a new level of severity and even cruelty in the treatment of the citizens. It represented, without a doubt, a new landmark in the implementation of more rigorous plague control measures. The health officials held these trials because they believed that careful inquiry into the circumstances of each case of plague within their jurisdiction was necessary to stop the spreading of the disease. Today, owing to those cases, we can reconstruct the circumstances of the lives of the *resanati*, the persons who had recovered from plague. We are able to trace to what extent they were able to adjust to a new set of social rules dictated by the government and to follow the fate of the transgressors who had abused the temporary absence of the authorities during the epidemic. In the *Libro deli Signori Chazamorbi*, the destinies of the offenders, as well as the disruption and damage that they had directly or indirectly brought upon their neighbours, are recorded in great detail. The result of all these special circumstances was a generalized insecurity.

In smaller communities outside the city, the duty of punishing the violators of plague control regulations was performed by the assistants of the health officials. If they were not available, other government officials took over. Their duty was to make the rounds in their area of jurisdiction and immediately report to the local counts or the health officials every new case of plague and the arrival of travellers from infected areas or areas suspected of being infected.[5] Aware of the fact that it was much easier to hide cases of plague in remote villages than in the city, the health officials incessantly tried to supervise the whole territory of the Republic.[6]

Securing sufficient grain supply and avoiding famine were constant obsessions of the Ragusans because they could not feed their population with the amount of food produced in their territory. The survival of the Republic demanded a special effort in procuring wheat. The records mention that on 24 February 1528 Angelo de Maria da Ravenna arrived from Sicily with a full load of grain and signed a written oath that he had not visited any infected areas in the last two months.[7]

The *resanati* (the recovered) and the healthy were forbidden from leaving their homes for an additional fifteen days after the expiration of the usual quarantine period. The poor among the plague survivors were assigned difficult tasks that paid very little. The health officials employed the women to wash infected items and disinfect homes.[8] Men were employed as gravediggers, the *kopci*, who had to prepare graves, bury the dead, or carry heavy loads from the port to the city. When there were no men available, sometimes even the women, the *kopice*, helped with the burying of the dead. Employing those who could no longer get infected to perform such tasks was a rational move that led to a significant improvement of plague control measures.[9] The plague survivors lived in their homes or in quarantine and were escorted to work under guard. Although their services were badly needed by the authorities for the purpose of restoring a degree of normalcy after the epidemic, and even though their work was miserably paid, the government and the citizens did not trust them.[10] Many pages of the *Libro deli Signori Chazamorbi, A tergo* are filled with investigations against them.

This chapter covers the trials of the plague survivors from 16 June 1527 to 16 June 1528 in which the health officials acted as trial judges. The number of folios that the trials for each year occupy in the manuscript is indicative of the progress of the epidemic. It is obvious that most trials took place in 1527, at the height of the infection.[11] The Ragusan Republic did not have any professional judges.[12] They were elected for a year from among the more experienced patricians, who were usually at least forty years old. The Civil Court was established in 1448 and the Criminal Court in 1459.[13]

The health officials who served as trial judges from 1527 to 1530 were usually forty-eight to sixty years old.[14] Judges were overloaded with obligations that occupied all of their time. Thus, they could not perform any other duties, public or private, during that year. Their salaries were symbolic but they could hope to attain the highest political honours.[15] Therefore, it was not difficult to fill these positions as the patricians who desired to become members of the Senate, or fill other inner circle positions, served as judges. The judges were assisted by university-trained chancellors of the court, who were able to provide guidance for the judges and ensure uniform implementation of the law.[16] In spite of the formal juridical style used, the trial proceedings confirm the successful collaboration of the health officials with the chancellors.

Scribes, notaries, and chancellors were professionals trained in Italian notary schools where they had also studied procedural law. In order to satisfy the juridical form, especially when court decisions involved serious offences, chancellors used special manuals, prepared in Italy and sold to other cities. Because they recorded the official state acts, chancellors constituted an important component of the state apparatus.[17] This was particularly important in the Ragusan Republic where the judges were not professionally trained. In the registers, there is no change in the structure or style of the records when judges changed, but each new chancellor can be easily discerned. It is obvious that judges let themselves be guided by chancellors who were much more experienced and had a better grasp of the law. The chancellors also supervised the judges and made sure that court decisions were made within two months; they assisted the health officials in their trials of plague control offences; they supervised the clerks of the Health Office and made sure that the decisions of the health officials were respected. In the *Libro deli Signori Chazamorbi*, the names of two chancellors are mentioned: Pasqual and Marino. In one spot the chancellor signed his full name: Troyano Pasqual de Primi.[18]

In the Middle Ages, notaries and chancellors were hired in Italy (see Appendix A). In the sixteenth century, local commoners started assisting the Italians and, from the seventeenth century on, the commoners took over their duties. The highest honour that a commoner could attain was to become the secretary of the rector. He kept this position for many years and was held in high esteem. To emphasize his social status, the Senate recommended him for membership of the confraternity of St Anthony (see Chapter 1). If he died, the rector wore black mourning clothes and stood by his casket, which was considered an exceptional honour.

The chancellors had wide-ranging duties. Among other obligations, they had to be present when a suspicious death was being investigated. Their fees in such cases were one-third higher than those of the physician or surgeon. Although they had a lot of responsibilities, their salaries were rather modest.[19] However, they could supplement their income with fees that private persons had to pay for each service. If they failed in their duties, the penalties were severe – rowing on a galley or expulsion from Dubrovnik, for example. This demonstrates the importance that the Republic attributed to their profession.[20]

The health officials did not have a law degree. When plague was not widespread in the Republic, just like the judges of the Criminal Court, they gradually acquired experience by executing their tasks. The Ragusan electoral procedure made sure that the candidates belonged to different patrician families in order to share equally the danger and also to avoid the oligarchic concentration of power.[21] For example, in 1530, as noted in the *Speculum Maioris Consilii*, the following patricians were elected as health officials: Vlaho Božov

Sorkočević (Sorgo), Frano Pandolfov Benešić (Benessa), Leonard Mihov Đurđević (Giorgi or Georgi), Miho Markov Bučinčić (Bocignolo), Luka Mihov Bunić (Bona), and Dominik Markov Ranjina (Ragnina).[22]

The intolerant attitude towards the poor among the plague survivors was fostered in part by the opinion prevalent in the cities of the Western Mediterranean that the destitute lived in poor hygienic conditions and were the source of infection. It was widely believed that they transmitted plague.[23] During the 1576 plague outbreak in Palermo, Givanni Filippo Ingrassia, the *protomedico* of the Kingdom of Sicily, asked for another convalescent hospital to be built because those who had recovered from the disease in the lazaretto were victims of social exclusion. A special place was needed to care for them in order to demonstrate their good health to their neighbours. The community needed to be encouraged to accept the plague survivors back into their homes.[24]

The regulation adopted in Dubrovnik in 1482 that forbade the plague survivors from circulating among the healthy, going to work without guard, or throwing away infected clothing in public places was still in force. The death penalty by hanging was imposed for such violations and confirmed again on 31 August 1527.[25] There were also other situations that caused the gravediggers to get in trouble. From the dying or their relatives, the gravediggers used to receive expensive gifts of jewellery, fine clothes, money, or other valuables, which, according to law, they were obliged to hand over to the health officials.[26] However, some of them saw it as a unique opportunity to make money and they did not report the gifts received or would sell the infected items.

In Venice, the body clearers were accompanied by a guard when walking through the streets and had to have bells attached to their legs to warn others of their presence. People in the street were afraid of them and associated them with predatory images of wolves, lions, or scavenging birds. The public perceived the gravediggers to be profiting from the plague outbreak, an act considered immoral. Body clearers were seen as indulging in revelry, drinking, and immoral sexual acts; they were often accused of theft and of deliberately spreading plague. Many of them were convicted criminals who were given the opportunity to have their sentences cleared by doing this kind of work, but this did not help their image.[27] Numerous criminal cases were brought against them. The Venetian notary Rocco Benedetti relates that on 3 November 1576, four of the gravediggers were sentenced to death and hanged in St Mark's Square in Venice.[28] These men were feared but they were also envied. The chronicler Alessandro Canobbio observes that most of those who had served the Health Office in Padua from the beginning of the 1575–77 outbreak survived until the

end of the plague epidemic.[29] However, there is no mention that the plague survivors were hired as body clearers, as was the case in Dubrovnik.

Giulia Calvi has studied about three hundred trials of the Health Office in
Florence and patiently reconstructs the stories of the common people as
recorded during the 1630 devastating plague flare-up. Calvi reveals that the
acts that the authorities interpreted as criminal turned out to have been strategies of survival and self-help for the poor: "The people of Florence broke the
quarantine in order to protect their interests – to continue working at their
trades, to find ways to feed their families, to tend the sick or retrieve their belongings from the meddling bureaucrats. Despite the great odds against them,
they were determined and resourceful, hardly an anonymous mass suffering in
silence from forces beyond their control."[30]

At least temporarily immune to plague, the resanati of Dubrovnik were in
an advantageous position compared to all the other social classes, which elicited
envy on the one hand and mistrust on the other. They could no longer contract
plague but they could transmit it by transporting and selling infected items.[31]
That is why local authorities of rural communities, the kaznaci, under the threat
of penalties to be announced, forbade any contact with plague survivors or the
infected.[32] The resanati used to break into abandoned houses and steal valuables, even livestock and wine. If proven guilty, they were given exemplary
sentences that included public branding, lashing, and hanging.

The surviving citizens, returning to their homes after the plague epidemic,
often discovered that they had been victims of theft. On 13 August 1527, Miho
de Staj wanted to help Mrs. Đivana to have her stolen items returned. Once
they had been returned, she refused to reveal the name of the perpetrator. Miho
de Staj noticed Radula Vladisaljeva, a woman from Konavle, handling infected
items and saw her in contact with healthy people while she sold salad at Pile.[33]
From such incidents, we learn, in passing, that life in the city assumed a degree
of normalcy, and that peasant women from the countryside used to bring fresh
vegetables to the market. Đivana Rakova, a woman from Kantafig, had also
been a victim of theft. However, her stolen items – four candle holders, one
box, and two pitchers – were returned.[34] Fearing the dissemination of plague,
next-door neighbours used to report transgressors to the health officials. A case
in point is Mada Krilina, a woman who, on 23 August 1527, reported Vlahuša
called Upećialo, a peasant, living on the property of the patrician Marin Nikolin
Menčetić (Menze). Mada Krilina accused Upećialo of not disinfecting the
items in his house after having survived the plague. She also accused him of

marrying another plague survivor and inviting many healthy people to their wedding, who, she feared, would all become sick.[35] Further developments in this case were not reported.

The case of Mihoč Božov Šimša was much more tragic. Interrogated by the health officials on 24 August 1527, Mihoč declared that he was living with Kata "Risanata," Kata "the Recovered," the servant of the patrician Đivo Paladinov Gundulić (Gondola), the woman who infected him with plague. Mihoč was treated by Ivan Mednić, the plague doctor. He admitted that a boy had stayed with him who had become infected with the plague, survived, and later disappeared. The health officials were of the opinion that Mihoč was guilty of grave violations of plague control measures and that, together with Kata "Risanata," he was responsible for the dissemination of plague. During an uncommonly short trial, he was sentenced to death and hanged the next morning at Danče.[36] It is debatable to what degree Mihoč was aware of his transgressions and whether a man of such a humble social standing could actually be knowledgeable about the transmission of plague infection. Mihoč Božov Šimša was given an exemplary sentence to frighten others into obedience. His case demonstrates that plague survivors were still somehow deemed capable of transmitting disease. They were not allowed to mingle with healthy people and, because of that, they were subjected to constant government control and harassment. Mistrust of this kind led to the harsh treatment of the survivors.

In principle, the resanati did not represent danger for people around them. Some hid their sickness at home without ever reporting it to the health officials. Others, aware of their acquired immunity, came in contact with the infected and their belongings without fear, and could in this way transmit the infection. The next case shows that even people in places far from the city knew how to protect themselves from infection. On 8 September 1527, the patrician Federik MCnčetić (Menze) accused Luka Ivanović from Plat, a community thirteen kilometres southeast of Dubrovnik, of secretly breaking into homes, stealing valuables, and then fleeing to Hercegnovi. Luka was caught and started giving back the stolen items. He claimed that he could not return two gold rings and two silver ones that he had stolen from Pavao Marković because he had given them to his sister Nikoleta for her wedding. Vukosav Paoković from Glavša reported that Luka tried to touch him and wanted to hit him. Vukosav then removed all his clothes so that Luka could not infect him. Naked, Vukosav left all his clothes right there on the spot where he had removed them.[37] Vukosav obviously knew that he could become infected by touching infected clothing or infected people. His action made sense, even though he could not have had any idea about the actual mechanism of plague transmission. By removing his clothes he prevented Luka's infected fleas from getting onto his garments.[38]

Then there is the unique case of two female plague survivors, Radosava Paskojeva from Župa and Stana, the servant of the patrician Nikola Prodanello, who entered the city on 6 October 1527 to sell fruit and vegetables at the Pile gate. They were not wearing any special warning sign. Paladin, the captain of Pile, asked them when they had contracted plague and found out that Stana had been sick at the time of the Carnival, six months prior to that date. Radosava, who had also recovered several months earlier, declared that the day before, when she came to the city to bring some pomegranates and vegetables to her friends, she had worn her scarf around her neck – *fazoletto sopra el collo*.[39] This is the only case documented by the health officials that indicates that plague survivors had to wear a warning sign on their clothing.[40] However, if Radosava and Stana had contracted plague several months prior to that date, even according to the most rigorous quarantine orders of the sixteenth century, by the date when they were stopped at Pile, they should have been considered healthy. It is possible that the rules in such cases were not well defined so that decisions could vary from case to case. This scenario might also be read as another case of harassment of the recovered. As usual, the social status of the accused played an important role in this process.

In contrast with the above situation, a remarkably explicit order of the Health Office forbade burial in public places in the city. The gravediggers Petar Dulčić and the town crier Radić Božićević, the *parlabuć*, admitted to burying two boys by the public road, *sulla via del commun*. On 4 July 1527, the health officials did not hesitate to sentence Petar Dulčić to four "jerks of the rope," standing at the *berlina* (the column of shame), and the burning of his beard and hair.[41] Radić Božićević escaped torture because of ill health but, in exchange, the health officials continued to withdraw from his deposit, every five days during the month of July, an amount that they had determined as a fine.[42] When inflicting pain, the ability of the sentenced person to withstand torture had to be taken into account. The city physician, who also cared for the health of the imprisoned, used to give his opinion in this matter in times when plague was not rampant.

From July 1527 to the end of the year, the investigations of breaking and entering, as well as thefts of valuables from abandoned homes where the occupants had died of plague, fill the pages of the *A tergo* part of the manuscript. Most of these cases took place in the small villages of Župa, a region southeast of Dubrovnik that was seriously afflicted by the plague. The gravediggers Matko Mlađenović and Pavao Lučić, both from Petrovo selo, were noticed in their boat on the Ombla River at night. They were seen entering the homes of the healthy and of those who had died of plague with the intention to steal. The local assistants of the health officials, answerable to the Health Office in Dubrovnik, complained that despite hefty fines, some violators remained defiant, as confirmed by several witnesses. During the investigation, which took place from 6 to 12 August 1527, both gravediggers were tortured by jerking the rope twice in order to elicit their confessions but they did not reveal anything – *fu tormentatto trati dua et non disse niente*.[43] Pavao Lučić acknowledged only that he took some garments to be disinfected with the permission of two women, Marija Lucina and Mada Cvjetkova. Both gravediggers, Matko Mlađenović and Pavao Lučić, were freed on 3 September 1527. The health officials probably concluded that incarceration during the trial and the torture that they had endured constituted sufficient punishment.

As these trials suggest, the jerking of the rope was used to elicit confessions and as a form of punishment. Used in several trials documented in the *Libro deli Signori Chazamorbi*, jerking of the rope is referred to as *tracti de corda* or *tratti di corda*.[44] So barbarous by present standards, this practice was in keeping with the customs of the time for those who defied authority. It was common throughout Europe until the eighteenth century. Indeed, confessions elicited by torture were considered the best evidence of all.[45] The accused had no attorney and could not appeal his or her sentence.[46] In Dubrovnik, the judgment depended on the majority of the trial judges finding the accused guilty or not guilty.

On 17 November 1527, Radosava, the wife of the street sweeper Petar Radičević, was accused of having kept some clothing items brought home by her husband. She admitted that she knew that, together with other plague survivors, her husband was often cleaning infected homes. Unanimously, the health officials sentenced her to public branding with a hot iron – *donna Radossava dover esser bulata con la bulla del commun* – one of the harshest types of punishment.[47] In the sixteenth century, a person was usually branded with two stamps on the face and one on the forehead. Due probably to some extenuating circumstances, Radosava was lucky to escape with only one mark on her face.

The trial of Mihoč from Župa, Antun Paskojević, and Deša Matićeva, all gravediggers, which lasted from 27 November 1527 to 28 September 1528, is the longest trial recorded in the *Libro deli Signori Chazamorbi*. The manuscript contains a detailed description of the investigation and frequent application of torture. Both men were first ordered by the health officials to stay confined to their homes in Pelegrin. They did not obey this order and, what is more, Mihoč also became involved with a woman plague survivor. On 28 November 1527, they were sentenced to lashing and three jerks of the rope. On 3 December 1527, at the fortress of Minčeta, the place chosen to administer justice, Mihoč, his hands tied with cord, was brought to face the health officials. He was first asked how many people he had buried, whether he had been paid for his work, and whether he had kept the infected items. The accused stated that, together with two other gravediggers, he had buried five hundred deceased persons but that he had been paid for only three hundred. Mihoč declared that he had buried the other two hundred for the love of God. Of the infected items, he had kept only one blanket and one old rough cover. He claimed that the other gravediggers, Antun Paskojević, Deša Matićeva, and Đivan Milovanović, had kept the rest of the garments and blankets, worth sixty ducats. Since Mihoč was only describing the violations of his companions and concealing his own, the health officials had him tortured again to make him admit his involvement.

The next day, probably quite exhausted and threatened with further torturing, Mihoč declared, "Gentlemen, I will tell the truth, do not torture me." He eventually admitted that all of them together had kept sixty dishes and 210 silver rings, all of these things divided into three equal parts. He claimed that he had buried these items under a rock in Pelegrin. Mihoč was then taken back to prison. Ten months later, on 18 September 1528, the five health officials – Luka Nikolin Bunić (Bona), Mate Franov Bobaljević (Babalio), Nikola Franov Sorkočević (Sorgo), and Bernard Marinov Binčulić (Binzola) – with Serafin Orsatov Džamanjić (Giamagno) presiding, all of them acting as trial judges, explained in their sentencing statement that Mihoč and his companions broke into homes and stole various clothes, money, and silver items. They hid those items and they did not disinfect them, thus causing the plague infection to spread. The health officials emphasized that the Senate had left them free to determine the sentence for Mihoč as they saw fit. On 4 October 1528, Mihoč was to be led on a donkey from the Pile gate all the way to Ploče – that is, through the whole city – and lashed in public. He was also to be exposed at the *berlina* for three whole hours as an example to those caught committing illegal deeds. After that, he was to be branded with three hot irons, two on his cheeks and one on his forehead, as a perpetual reminder of his offences and to frighten others – *ad perpetuam rei memoriam et terorem deli altri*.[48] To humiliate the sentenced, but also to act as a deterrent and a warning to others, the sentencing and the execution of the sentence were performed in public. The sentenced person was paraded through as many streets as possible as a mark of disgrace. On Sunday, in order to be seen by as many citizens as possible when the streets were crowded with people, he was obliged to ride a donkey facing backwards and hold the donkey's tail. The same type of punishment was prevalent in mediaeval and early modern Europe.[49]

The trial of the female gravedigger Deša Matićeva from Župa started on 8 July 1528. She was brought to the hall of the Major Council where she was asked when she had buried the plague victims. She declared that, in 1527, she had helped Mihoč from Župa and Antun Paskojević, from the Carnival time until the feast of St George. She had buried thirty-one persons. She admitted that she had kept mostly clothing items, citing a long list of names of their owners, some of whom were her relatives. She had also received two hundred silver coins and had given one hundred of those to Marin Rastić (Resti), captain of Brgat who sent them, in a sealed box, to the authorities in Dubrovnik. Regarding the old rough covers, she said that Antun and Mihoč had kept them and had put them away. When asked if she had buried any animals, she said that she had not.[50] Asked if she had in her possession other stolen items that were not disinfected, she answered that, other than those that she had mentioned above, she did not, and that the rest were in the possession of Margarita Petrova, consigned by the scribe Miho de Staj.[51] When interrogated about the amount of money she had shared with the other gravediggers, she declared that they had not shared anything, other than two hyperperi, because they had spent the rest on the burial of the poor who had nothing but their daily wages, which they would spend the same day – *poveri homeni che avevanno quello che ala giornata guadagnavan anche spendevan.*[52]

On 16 September 1528, after two and a half months, Đivan Milovanović from Župa, Deša's husband, promised under oath that he would bring Deša back whenever the health officials demanded to see her. The health officials threatened that if he did not, Deša's sentence would be passed on to him. Due to her weakness and on the recommendation of the physician, the health officials then decided to release Deša from prison. Several factors were decisive in setting Deša free. Her participation in the misdeeds was minor. She readily admitted to all the thefts. Because she had been a witness in the investigation against Mihoč, she was kept in prison until the end of that long trial. Poor health and the recommendation of the physician were also significant factors in her liberation.

To disinfect clothing Ragusans used to expose it to the fresh air in the space between the city walls, near the Pile gate. The investigation concerning the guards of infected clothing started on 5 June and ended seven days later on 12 June 1528. The following guards of infected clothing were investigated: Cvitko Radonjić from Konavle, Stjepan Vukosaljić, Marin Radičević, and Đuro Marketov, who was employed by the Health Office. Torture was administered in the interrogation of the first three accused. Cvitko Radonjić, brought from prison to the fortress of Minčeta and sworn in, revealed an intricate network of trafficking in clothing items and a variety of fabrics that belong to patricians and commoners. The accused were in touch with people outside the city to whom they sold the items, which they would throw from the city walls at night. Cvitko declared that Marin Radonjić knew the way to Belgrade, a route he had learned by having accompanied merchants on their travels, and that it was the guards' intention to take the stolen goods to Belgrade and Wallachia. Both destinations were far from the territory of the Ragusan Republic. Until then, the accused had prepared three bags of fine clothing and valuable fabrics including velvet, wool, and silk. Cvitko and his companions knew to whom these items belonged. The health officials, with Nikola Tripe Sorkočević (Sorgo) presiding, must have been shocked to learn that these persons, who were supposed to guard the city, dared to descend the city walls during the night, using a deep cleft next to the mills, to execute their well-prepared trafficking scheme. However, their plan was discovered in the early stages so that they only managed to sell smaller quantities of goods to individuals – some for cash, some on credit, and some for cheese and milk.[53]

The health officials were indignant to learn that the fourth accused, Đuro Marketov, was an employee of their office, which, as they put it, also "provided his means of subsistence."[54] With his misdeeds he had degraded the reputation and the honour of the institution for which he worked and he did so without any fear of God: *qual postponendo ogni timor de Dio e non havendo rispetto del officio nostro al qual serviva e del qual viveva*. Like the other three, he was brought from prison to the fortress of Minčeta, with his hands tied behind his back, and was sworn in. He promptly confessed his wrongdoing and was not tortured. He declared that he had sold, to a Gypsy by the name of Ivan, some damask, some silk and *raša* (*raxo*) for six *grossi* and some other fabrics for thirteen *grossi*.[55] It did not take long for the sentence to be pronounced. After a week, the first three accused were sentenced to death by hanging at Dánče. Đuro Marketov, the employee of the Health Office, was also sentenced to death by hanging in the space between the inner and outer Pile gates. He was to be hanged by the neck until his soul left the body, and his lifeless corpse was to remain hanging as a warning to others who would otherwise want to commit similar offences.[56] Meant to terrify, designed to serve as an example and, with any luck, as a deterrent, all four sentences were purposely executed in public.

Could such exemplary sentences act as a deterrent? With the severe punishment dealt to the gravediggers, who were, to tell the truth, vulnerable plague survivors, the health officials clearly intended to stamp out the offences that they deemed most dangerous for the citizens returning to the city. The plague epidemic ushered in a chaotic acceleration of life and death. Superimposed on that pervasive dread of infection, the threat of state repression for violations of plague control measures further accentuated the precariousness of life. The trials of plague survivors in the aftermath of the 1527 plague epidemic, as well as the trials of other groups of citizens that follow in the next chapters, certainly represent a new milestone in the implementation of ever harsher plague control measures. It appears that the higher the mortality in an epidemic, the more rigorous the measures implemented to fight it. The two seemed to go together.

William G. Naphy studied the trial records of the so-called "greasers," persons suspected of having intentionally spread plague, during the plague outbreaks in Geneva. In the 1530 plague epidemic, a conspiracy to cause the deaths of several rich people by spreading plague pus in their houses was discovered. It was led by a barber-surgeon who organized the whole operation and involved other plague workers, laundresses, and fumigators (*cureurs* and *cureuses*). Plague workers in Geneva were usually poor female foreigners. In the 1545 plague trials, many women were prosecuted but since they were perceived as tools of barber-surgeons, most of those acquitted were women. At the end of an exhausting four-year plague upsurge in 1571, there were 115 prosecutions for plague spreading and forty-four executions (twenty-six of those were women). As in Dubrovnik, most of the trials were held once plague had abated. During the plague outbreak, organizing time-consuming trials was not an option for the authorities because all their energies were sapped by the need to fight plague. In the 1571 cases, conspiracy ceased to be a prominent feature and barber-surgeons were no longer involved. Plague spreaders were perceived as individuals usually involved in witchcraft, spreading grease for financial benefit. They were not necessarily plague workers and the link with plague became secondary to the involvement with sorcery.[57]

In her study of the Florentine plague epidemic of 1630, Giulia Calvi found that most cases of assault and theft investigated by the Health Office were committed by the relatives and friends of plague victims who were trying to preserve their rights and property. To avoid the desecration and disgrace of mass burials, doctors, priests, bailiffs, and gravediggers were bribed and threatened, while the dead were secretly laid to rest.[58] Some of the same behaviour – concealing the disease, for example – was present in Dubrovnik a hundred years earlier. However, the violators of plague control measures were not relatives of plague victims who tried to protect the victims' rights. Rather, comparable to the ones in Florence, the judicial trials in Dubrovnik were the result of the difference in the economic and social status. Several questions come to mind. Did the educated groups of citizens and the illiterate common people have the same access to the information about the plague epidemic? To what extent could the common people understand and interpret the plague control measures? Could they apply them to their own situation? Were the gravediggers investigated in the above cases aware of their offences? Were they trying to outsmart the authorities or were they just trying to survive? In all probability, a bit of both might have been the case. The most significant difference between the health officials and the gravediggers seems to have been their social rank, which influenced their interpretation of the situation and coloured their views.

In his study of the 1630 plague epidemic in Monte Lupo, a small village situated thirty kilometres outside Florence, Carlo M. Cipolla found that "ignorance and penury were the main causes of non compliance with the rules, joined by egoism, avarice, and bullying to impede and negate the work of the health officials, and to encourage the lethal operation of the microbes." In Monte Lupo of 1630, as in Dubrovnik of 1526–28, the gravediggers still trafficked in the clothes of the dead, and the innkeepers ignored the plague control measures.[59] Calvi reports that, in the Ruciano Convalescent Home of 1630, owned by the Florentine hospital of Santa Maria Nuova, the employees organized a trafficking network to sell, in the city market, the bed sheets, blankets, and food that the state had provided for the plague sufferers. The public health magistrates found out that the mail carrier Jacopo had seduced two nurses and got them involved in a lucrative stealing venture. Transformed by the thieves, the hospital thus became a small factory where stolen linens were taken apart and made into aprons, socks, and a variety of garments. The goods were secretly spirited out of the hospital by a chain of accomplices that stretched from Ruciano to Florence. Calvi concludes that those who were normally excluded from more traditional forms of commerce were thus granted the right to take part in new forms of exchange. It was, according to her, "a sort of ritualized, somewhat predictable staging of the turning upside down of all things – of waste and license."[60]

In Dubrovnik, the plague survivors among the nobility were certainly not subjected to the harsh treatment reserved for the gravediggers. The surviving patricians were allowed to convalesce quietly in their homes and were definitely not treated as social outcasts. By contrast, the surviving gravediggers were members of the most disadvantaged social class and were without any protection from confraternities, hospices, or any other institution. After they survived the plague, and a probable stay in quarantine where they had lived in makeshift wooden huts in hygienic conditions that were worse than at home, and with only a meagre food supply, the authorities imposed an isolation period of fifteen more days for them and enforced a social segregation from the rest of the people, which continued long after that. Luka, known as Dulčić from Pile, for example, was followed as a resanatus even a year after he had survived the plague.[61] Living conditions in quarantine compounds were unpleasant, first, due to crowding, and second, due to the temporary nature of these shelters. Only the plague hospital at Danče and the lazaretto on the island of Mljet were actually permanent buildings that provided any comfort.

The inferior status of women is reflected in the destinies of the female plague survivors, enlisted as gravediggers. In general, with the exception of Deša Matićeva, who was exonerated after having spent almost a whole year in prison, the sentences these women received were harsher than those of the men of the same social rank. On the basis of the above cases, we can say that the authorities treated them in an unsympathetic manner.

The material analyzed in this chapter brings to light the exceptional abundance of precious information found throughout the *Libro deli Signori Chazamorbi* that allows the historian to reconstruct the daily lives of the common people during the plague epidemic. It also gives us the opportunity to recapture the emotions, attitudes, and behaviour of a social class that is not often mentioned in archival sources, which enhances our picture of the tapestry of life in early modern Dubrovnik.

In the next chapter, trials of patricians, ship owners, and local authorities who had contravened plague control measures are examined. The chapter makes evident that health officials had significant difficulties when it came to prosecuting and punishing members of their own social class.

8

The Health Officials and the Patricians

Suspected plague carriers and plague sufferers quite understandably feared being sent by force to a quarantine compound – an isolated and very uncomfortable place – where they would share their destiny with the dying and the rare lucky individuals who had survived plague. They all faced this prospect with apprehension, knowing that it would mean being separated from their loved ones and taken away from their homes where they could at least expect some security, protection, and care. As we discovered in the previous chapter, plague control measures were not applied equally to citizens of all social classes. Patricians, wealthy commoners, members of the confraternity of St Anthony or of St Lazarus, bankers, ship owners, merchants, abbots, and superiors of monasteries could expect better treatment than the members of the less-privileged classes, which included simple monks and nuns, poor priests and commoners, such as mariners, textile, leather and fur workers, artisans, servants, and peasants of the Ragusan Republic.

At the beginning of the sixteenth century, before plague became rampant, Ragusans returning from the hinterland, and suspected of arriving from plague-infected areas, were usually sent into quarantine on Supetar – the islet close to Cavtat, or to Kantafig, or Danče. Ship captains and their crews were sent to Lokrum or to Polače on the island of Mljet. In the second half of 1527, however, recalcitrant patricians created quite a few difficulties for their fellow noblemen, the health officials. This chapter covers the trials of the patricians, as well as some ship owners and two *kaznac* – the local authorities – who contravened the plague control regulations between 27 June 1527 and 23 May 1529.

On 21 June 1527, the patrician Antun Junijev Gundulić (Gondola) had been confined to his house because of plague but, in spite of this order, he walked around the city. He also sent his infected servant Simko Matković to Šumet, sick with the plague. The sentence imposed on Pompej Marinov Gundulić (Gondola) was rather lenient. He belonged to one of the six most influential patrician families, whose members were regularly elected to all governing bodies of the Republic.[8] This is another example that illustrates major differences between punishment for patricians and punishment for all other classes of citizens. The draconian regulation was made public only five weeks earlier, so one could have expected to see it applied in Pompej's case. Instead, this case demonstrates that the governing patricians were still allowed to be indulgent when members of their own social rank were concerned.

The health officials demonstrated consideration in profusion in the case of Miho Junijev Bunić (Bona), the patrician who was reported by Mihoč Stjepanov Garličić, the kaznac of Gruž, for refusing to pay the commoner Vlahota Antunović for being his guard during confinement.[9] The health officials circumvented the problem by designating a patrician in Gruž who would guard Miho's house as well as the houses of all other patricians suspected of plague infection. In this manner, the possibility of a commoner, the kaznac of Gruž, having authority over a patrician, was avoided. The patricians suspected of plague infection were prohibited from leaving their homes under the threat of a fine of one hundred ducats and three jerks of the rope.[10] For the first time, the patricians were threatened with corporal punishment. However, it probably remained just a threat because there is no record that it was ever implemented.

The trial of the patrician Renato Karlov Pucić (Poza) takes up five folios of the *Libro deli Signori Chazamorbi*.[11] On 2 January 1528, Marin Martolov Gučetić (Goze), the count of Ston, warned Renato to be careful not to come in contact with any person suspected of infection or already infected with plague when travelling to Gabela at the mouth of the Neretva River, accompanied by Božo Radovanov, his assistant and shoemaker by profession.[12] Renato gave his word of a patrician and promised to obey all the rules. Nikola Marinov Ranjina (Ragnina), also a patrician and sea salt merchant representing the Ragusan Republic in the Neretva Delta, was advised in writing of their arrival and of the warning given to Renato. Like many other patricians working on the border of the Republic, Nikola was a person trusted by the authorities. He was also in charge of implementing the plague control measures in the Neretva Delta.

Great vigilance was required because, there, at the mouth of the Neretva River, the Ragusans and the people from Ston used to come in contact with the Ottomans and their subjects with whom they maintained a brisk, lucrative trade. Still, attempts at smuggling were made on both sides. The Ragusan Republic shared one-third of the income from the salt trade with the Ottomans. The

Ragusans also used to sell fresh and dried fish, cotton, silk, and garments, while the inhabitants from the Ottoman-ruled area traded wool, leather, grain, meat, beeswax, and tallow.[13] The sea salt trade was hugely profitable for the Ragusans because the demand exceeded the supply: people raising livestock in the hinterland all needed salt. As previously discussed, the difficulty was created by the fact that practically no plague control measures were applied in the Ottoman-controlled areas. For this reason, all the Ragusan citizens, who had to travel to places like Gabela on the Neretva River on urgent business, knowing that these places were infected, had to exercise extra caution.

Božo Radovanov, Renato's assistant and shoemaker, who took Renato across the Neretva River in the boat, became sick and died of the plague five days later, which caused great concern both in Ston and in Dubrovnik. On the last day of Božo's life, the authorities in Ston closed down his house as well as other houses where he had spent some time. Božo was taken to the rocky islet of Škorpion, where five members of his family later died of the plague. Marin Martolov Gučetić (Goze), the count of Ston, with his assistants, following the specific orders of the health officials from Dubrovnik, then undertook a detailed investigation with a great number of witnesses in order to find the source of Božo's infection, where Renato and Božo had gone, what goods they had bought and from whom. In total, nine witnesses were interrogated. Renato Pucić declared that in Gabela they did not come in contact with persons suspected of plague infection since they had just gone to pick up some *aspri*, Turkish silver coins, some silver dishes and, a box with silver.[14] However, other witnesses revealed details that were truly significant for the investigation.

Nikola Marinov Ranjina (Ragnina), the sea salt merchant, notified the count of Ston by letter that Božo had gone into town at night to buy some shoe polish from Suliman Tabak, the Turk, who was known to live in an infected house in which three persons had died of the plague. Nikola also reported that Suliman had disappeared with his family at dawn and that he used to circulate all over Gabela. Nikola complained that he kept an eye on everything during the day but that he was unable to watch him at night. He mentioned that his sailors, who were the most loyal soldiers, did the same. In his letter to the count of Ston, Nikola strongly suggested that in the future more reliable persons should be sent to pick up Turkish money. Finally, he asked the count to send lime, roof tiles, and slabs as soon as possible; otherwise, he would not be able to save the sea salt pan (*slanica*) in which a great quantity of water had gathered for the first time in twenty years.[15] Nikola ended his letter with the phrase, *Christo de mal vi guardi* (may Christ protect you from evil).[16]

Frano Andrijin Benešić (Benessa), another patrician, in charge of guarding persons sent into isolation on the rocky islet of Škorpion, interrogated Božo's wife and son to learn the source of Božo's infection.[17] His son Vicko knew only that Božo had bought a cap from Nika Pavlova Jakuša, a woman who was cleaning infected items in the possession of the Sfondrati family from Dubrovnik, who had all died of plague. With the permission of the health officials, she later returned to Ston. Vicko said that they had washed that woollen cap before Božo started wearing it during his trip to Gabela. Vicko also said that, since he had started wearing that cap, Božo suffered from a headache. Vicko's testimony may seem insignificant but it could be the clue as to how his father had become infected. Considering its origin – the infected Sfondrati family from Dubrovnik – Božo's cap was probably infected with fleas. Thus, Božo may have been infected with the plague even before he left on his trip to Gabela. After that, the count of Ston, with his assistants, interrogated Vicko Marinov Brautović, the priest who had heard the confessions of Božo's wife, children, and mother-in-law.

The authorities wanted to find out whether Renato and Božo had brought from Gabela any other goods suspected of being infected. All replied that they did not know but that Renato had brought a silk *gipon* (a tunic) and a conger eel for his brother Pandolfo.[18] All declared that they suspected that Božo had become infected from that cap. Antun Marković stated that Božo had brought fifteen leather hides from the Neretva Delta after the 6 December St Nicholas feast. Next to be interrogated was Renato Pucić (Poza), who enumerated, day by day, all the places where he had gone and everything he had done. He stated that he had given the *gipon* to his brother Pandolfo, that he had never met Suliman because Suliman was not in Gabela at that time, but that he had sent Suliman a message proposing a meeting after the infection was eradicated. Luka Paoković, shoemaker, and Jerko Ivanović, tobacco merchant, both declared that they had seen twelve leather hides in the storage space of Đivo Hamzin. Both witnesses claimed that the leather hides were from Gabela because they were cut and tanned in the Turkish manner.

By the order of the count of Ston and his assistants, on 21 January 1528, Renato Karlov Pucić (Poza) and his brother Pandolfo were ordered to stay in isolation for one month. If they did not obey, they would each have to pay a fine of one hundred ducats and spend six months in prison. Both replied that they would go wherever they pleased and see whomever they wanted, refusing in advance to heed the count's order.[19] On 26 February 1528, Đivo Matijin, blacksmith, complained to the authorities that Renato Pucić (Poza) was coming every day to disturb the sea salt pan workers in Ston. Đivo reminded Renato that he was not allowed to circulate freely and the incident ended with them throwing stones at each other. This testimony was corroborated by three other witnesses: Petar Tomić, Lovro Marinov Menčetić (Menze), and Balaš, the Hungarian soldier who unsuccessfully tried to guard Renato.

On 20 March 1528, the health officials – Mate Franov Bobaljević (Babalio), Marin Stjepanov Džamanjić (Giamagno), Pavao Matin Gradić (Grade), and Nikola Franov Sorkočević (Sorgo), with Jeronim Lukin Bunić (Bona) presiding – having taken into account the offences of Renato Karlov Pucić (Poza) in Ston, sentenced him to one month in prison and a fine of one hundred hyperperi that he would have to pay before being released from prison. If he disobeyed, his prison sentence and his monetary fine would be doubled.[20] We can wonder why the authorities insisted on such a detailed investigation in the case of Renato Karlov Pucić (Poza) and Božo Radovanov. The explanation lies in the nature of the politically sensitive location where this incident happened: in an area between Ston, the border of the Ragusan Republic and the Ottoman-ruled region on the Neretva Delta. From the case of Renato Karlov Pucić (Poza), we gather that patricians often behaved arrogantly. In spite of it all, Renato successfully fulfilled the task that had been entrusted to him but, because of his quarrelsome temperament, he often clashed with people.

The priest Vicko Marinov Brautović heard the confessions of Božo's family members. Could he have committed a grave canon law offence by divulging the contents of their confessions?[21] It is possible that the term *confession* used in the archival text is not used literally and that it means that the priest asked the family members to explain what had happened, probably after a formal confession. However, that interrogation took place in quarantine at the moment when Božo's family members were already sick, an occasion when the priest usually administered holy sacraments. Thus, it remains unclear if the priest behaved correctly. He certainly showed a high degree of cooperation with the authorities. The count of Ston and his assistants also proved to be adroit interrogators in this incident. From the shoemakers they learned the crucial detail that before the end of 1527, Božo had bought leather hides of Turkish origin, probably to make shoes. There are, therefore, three possible sources of Božo's infection: the leather hides, his woollen cap, and his contact with the people of Gabela.

The investigation in this long trial showed that the health officials in Dubrovnik cooperated closely with the authorities in the Neretva Delta and Ston as well as with priests. In 1528, as we have seen above, the plague control measures were conscientiously implemented in Ston. Persons suspected of infection were kept at home under guard, the infected were sent to the rocky islet of Škorpion, and the houses of the infected were closed. All these actions demonstrate that the Ragusan Republic, in contrast with the Ottoman-ruled area on its border, implemented highly developed protection measures. In later centuries, when plague was present in Ottoman-ruled Bosnia and Herzegovina, the Ragusans organized a sanitary cordon. Their measures prescribed, among other things, the roads on which the merchants could travel, the places where they could trade, and the points where their goods had to be disinfected before trading. The Ragusans depended on the inhabitants of the Ottoman-ruled areas to respect these rules. To achieve their cooperation, they often wrote to the local Ottoman authorities and maintained a lively exchange of information with them.[22]

The owners of smaller ships and their captains, arriving from foreign ports, soon learned from painful experience that they could not escape the control of the health officials.[23] On 4 July 1528, they discovered that Bojan Matilović, a native of Ombla, owner of a brigantine, landed without the permission of the health officials in Mokošica, northwest of Dubrovnik, having arrived from Apulia, Italy. In Mokošica, Bojan unloaded and sold his wine. The witnesses reported that Bojan had also sailed to the isolation compound on the island of Mljet and after that he had landed without permission in Trsteno where Đuro Matilović, one of his sailors, had disembarked. Dragoje Marojević, the local kaznac, later saw Đuro Matilović, who had arrived from Trsteno to Mokošica by land.[24] The sentence was pronounced only ten months later, on 23 May 1529. Bojan and his sailors, who had been kept in quarantine for the duration of the trial period were lashed in public with their shoulders bared – *con le spalle nude* – and paraded through the city on a donkey. After that, they were taken to the *berlina*, the column of shame, and branded with three hot irons on the face. Bojan's brigantine was burned together with two smaller companion ships, the *navica* and the *pietronica* – *li sia brusato ditto suo Gripo con la naviza et pietroniza*. The homes of Đuro Matilović in Mokošica and of Antun Cvitković in Šumet near Komolac were also burned. On the same day, the health officials ordered Pavao Nikolin Lukarević (Luchari), a patrician, to personally go to Mokošica and Šumet to make sure that those houses were burned and that no trace of them remained.[25]

On 22 June 1528, Andrija Vlahotić, kaznac of Komolac, complained to the health officials that Marin and his father Vlahuša Bogunović had pronounced death threats against him because, according to them, Andrija, due to the testimony he had given at the trial, was responsible for the burning of the homes of Đuro Matilović and Antun Cvitković. Marin threw a stone at Andrija that hit his hand and another stone narrowly missed Andrija's wife.[26] These examples show that the kaznac occupied an unenviable position of split loyalty to the local inhabitants, on one hand, and to the health officials, on the other. The citizens, unable to voice their dissatisfaction to the distant health officials, made the local authorities bear the brunt of their fury.

The aforementioned sentences, other than the death sentence, were the harshest penalties ever pronounced by the health officials. The offenders were publicly shamed, lashed, branded, and disgraced for life. Finally, their houses were burned. Since Bojan did not possess a house, his ships were burned. The offenders were despoiled of their possessions and their existence was ruined.

Although the health officials were successful in developing an entire information-gathering network not only in the city but also in the countryside, the arrivals of sailors in smaller ships presented a challenge. At the end of 1528, it was observed that a certain number of ships arrived from ports suspected of plague and that their owners had carried out a well-prepared plan of landing in smaller communities without permission and without having declared to the local authorities their point of departure and the ports at which they had docked on their way. The trial against Rade from Slano, Radosav Lijepi Kos, his brother Petar, and Gromača, the son in-law of Nikša Krečić, started on 28 October 1528. Marino Dobrijelović from Poljice declared to the health officials on 21 May 1528 that, on his way back from Apulia, Radosav Lijepi Kos had wanted to land in Poljice but, since he was not permitted to do so, he had gone to see Rade from Slano, who lived on the island of Koločep. In Poljice, they were told that they should go to Dubrovnik to report their arrival but they did not want to do that because they were afraid of the consequences. The vice count of Koločep was asked to bring them all to face the health officials in Dubrovnik but they had fled by boat to Orašac, ten kilometres northwest of Dubrovnik, before he could round them up. In their absence, Rade from Slano and the other three accused were given a three-month prison sentence. If they did not obey, their houses would be burned as a permanent reminder and example to others.[27]

The last significant trial in the *Libro deli Signori Chazamorbi* was held from 4 to 7 May 1529 in the case of two kaznac, Mihan Radetić of Brsečine and Petar Jakšić of Trsteno.[28] Serafin Orsatov Džamanjić (Zamagna), the health official from Dubrovnik, came to Brsečine to hear the testimony of twelve witnesses after it had become known that Mihan, the ship owner from Brsečine, had died of plague. Mihan had returned from Bari and Mola in Apulia in his ship. When the members of his crew, Vlahuša Migljenović, Nikola Vučičijević, and Vicko Petrović, all from Brsečine, and Vlahuša Bogdanović from Trsteno, learned that Mihan had died, the crew took his ship and disappeared. After Mihan's death, the count of Slano ordered Mihan's widow and the relatives of the other crew members to be quarantined in Brsečine. Mihan's widow and the wives of the other crew members declared that Mihan had been sailing from Bari when a galley robbed him of thirty barrels of wine, leaving him with nothing to unload when he returned home. Mihan's widow described his sickness and his symptoms in detail. She mentioned that Mihan had returned with his crew on Saturday, 24 April, and that on the following Tuesday he had started to feel pain in his shoulders; the following Wednesday buboes had appeared in the groin area of his right leg – *a modo di carboni*, meaning that the buboes were becoming black. Mihan's widow declared that Mihan had been in pain and that he had died Sunday night. From this testimony, taking into account both the symptoms and the duration of the sickness, it is clear that Mihan suffered a case of typical bubonic plague. Mihan's is the most accurate description of the disease in this manuscript.

Nikoleta from Brsečine stated in her testimony that she had heard from Radoslav Radeljić, also from Brsečine, that in his ship Mihan had brought a few bags of linen. Nikoleta had also heard from her servant Milica that she had seen a woman from the island of Mljet coming out of Mihan's house carrying a load on her head in the manner in which linen is carried. Milica confirmed that on Friday she had seen a woman related to Đuro Glubišić come out of Mihan's house carrying a load on her head and a jug of milk. That woman then returned to Mljet with her husband and his brother. The following day, when Nikoleta returned to court, she complained to the health officials that the villagers in Brsečine had threatened her servant Milica because she had testified in Mihan's case.

Next to testify was kaznac Mihan Radetić of Brsečine, whose duty it was to inform the count of Slano and the health officials in Dubrovnik about the arrival, the sickness and the death of Mihan, the ship owner. When asked why he had not reported the arrival of the deceased Mihan, kaznac Radetić said that the sailors had claimed that they had arrived from healthy ports and that they were going to inform the health officials the following day and ask for permission to make another trip to Apulia. The toughest question that Radetić had to answer was why he had not reported Mihan's illness to the count of Slano or the health officials in Dubrovnik. To that, with a sense of foreboding, kaznac Radetić replied that he had not done it "because of his bad luck" – *che per mia mala ventura non lo fatto.*[29] When interrogated about the nature of Mihan's disease, kaznac Radetić tried to make the court believe that he did not know that it was plague. Asked why he had not reported Mihan's death, Radetić claimed that he had sent a boy with a message for the *vojvoda*, the military commander. Kaznac Radetić also declared that he had not seen Mihan and his crew unload any goods. Kaznac Radetić's testimony makes it clear that he had no intention of reporting Mihan's arrival, his illness, or his death.

Petar Jakšić, the kaznac of Trsteno, was also asked the same questions. He declared that the members of the crew had told him that they had permission from Dubrovnik to land. The sentence was pronounced on 7 May 1529. Both kaznaci were found guilty of not reporting the arrival of Mihan's ship, not stopping Mihan's crew from going to buy grain in Dubrovnik, and not reporting Mihan's illness or his death. Kaznac Radetić, who was primarily responsible for these offences, was sentenced to three jerks of the rope. Both kaznac Radetić and Jakšić were to be lashed while being paraded through the city for all the people to see – *al spectaculo de tutto il populo* – with a miter on their heads.[30] Following that, they were to be taken to the *berlina* where they would have to stay tied for two hours. After that, they were to be branded with three hot irons on the face and their houses would be burned.[31]

The offences committed in the above case were of the most serious kind. It is not surprising, therefore, to see that the sentences were heavy-handed. It is obvious from the testimony of kaznac Radetić that he had expected a severe sentence. However, for the authorities, the most disturbing aspect must have been the solidarity that had developed between the kaznac, the local authorities, and their villagers. In an attempt to protect the inhabitants of the community under their jurisdiction, the two kaznac completely disregarded the plague control measures. This sealed their destiny. In cooperation with the Senate, the health officials ruled quickly in order to set an example and terrify the citizens of the Republic as thoroughly as possible. Only a month earlier, on 11 April 1529, the Minor Council, in an attempt to put an end to secret landings in smaller ports, had adopted a regulation according to which the local authorities – the count, the captain, the fortress commander, and the vice count – could not permit a ship coming from foreign countries to land anywhere except in Dubrovnik. If they did not obey, the senators would punish them as they saw fit.[32]

In the second half of 1528, when plague occurred only sporadically, the health officials had the opportunity to improve their control over the mariners, especially those arriving from foreign ports. The Councils functioned with a full quorum and the number of health officials was increased from five to seven. Numerous trials, documented in the *Libro deli Signori Chazamorbi*, took place during this period and offer vivid proof of the ceaseless activities of the health officials. They were in charge of following the plague control transgressions, applying the existing plague control regulations, and, if necessary, proposing new ones such as the draconian one. A large number of witnesses testified in all the trials. There is no evidence that the draconian regulation, requiring only one witness, the accuser, was ever implemented. Likewise, despite the threat of the draconian regulation, the sanctions for the patricians did not include corporal punishment or the death sentence. They continued to be punished by monetary fines, quarantine, and prison sentences. The draconian regulation appears to have remained just a frightening threat to potential offenders.

The health officials regularly issued or refused permits for entering the city. They ordered people into quarantine and presided over trial procedures. Sentences had to be pronounced by the majority of votes. However, in all the trials documented in the *Libro deli Signori Chazamorbi*, the trial judges were unanimous in their sentences, usually expressed by the *formula tutti de una opinione* (all of the same opinion). At least three health officials had to be present as trial judges, but there could sometimes be as many as five.[33] In every team of judges, the most experienced health official usually presided. Probably to avoid overburdening the same patricians with judicial responsibilities, and to take into account the usual Ragusan concern about the concentration of power in the hands of a few individuals, after a month or two, the teams were rotated. In the new team, the trial judge from the previous team usually presided. In 1527, there were fourteen new trial judges; in 1528, only two; in 1529 there were just four.[34] Several health officials who were elected in 1527, served as trial judges in 1528 too. Serafin Orsatov Džamanjić (Zamagna), for example, served more often than any of his colleagues. He is listed as a trial judge in 1527, 1528, and 1529, but only sporadically, not during the whole year.

On 13 June 1528, when heads of twelve patrician families were ordered to stay confined in their homes and were not allowed to let their servants go out on errands, according to the rules concerning the patricians, members of the Minor Council joined the health officials in the sentencing. The presiding health official on that day was Pavao Marinov Gradić (Gradi), an experienced trial judge who had served since October 1527.[35] In 1528, he was fifty years old and had thirty years of experience in the Major Council. He served with Marin Stjepanov Džamanjić (Giamagno), who was forty-nine; Mato Franov Bobalje-vić (Babalio), who was forty-eight; and Nikola Franov Sorkočević (Sorgo), whose age is not known.[36] Some health officials did not serve as trial judges at all, which means that they were assigned other duties.[37] It is difficult to say whether this was a result of personal choice or coercion by the authorities. It is fairly likely, however, that the colleagues were aware of each other's interests and ambitions, which would have enabled them to figure out among themselves relatively quickly who was fit to serve as a trial judge. The activities explored in this chapter allow us to understand that, in 1528, the health situation was under control. Plague control measures were applied systematically, according to the established procedures.

Families that hid their plague patients and the merchants who concealed their infected goods represented a serious concern for the health officials, how-ever. These issues will be dealt with in the next chapter.

9

Concealing Symptoms of Plague, Importing Suspicious Goods, and Other Offences

The most common breaches of plague control measures were concealment of the symptoms of plague as they occurred amongst family or household members and failure to disclose the disease until death ensued. Although seemingly harmless, these offences resulted in the continued spreading of the disease. Such cases appeared from the very beginning of the 1527 epidemic. The health officials deserve credit for observing this phenomenon early and for trying to put a stop to it. Judging by the number of cases that were revealed and processed, it is clear that it was a matter of serious concern for the authorities. The trials relating to such offences, as recorded in the *Libro deli Signori Chazamorbi*, are examined in the first part of this chapter. The second part of this chapter explores the offences concerning the importing of infected goods, as well as offences committed by the nuns and priests.

CONCEALMENT OF PLAGUE CASES

The short duration of bubonic plague, only three to seven days, according to eyewitnesses, made it easier for the surviving family members to sound credible when they pleaded with the health officials that they had not recognized it as a case of plague. It is true that the initial symptoms, before the typical groin and armpit buboes appeared, looked very much like any other communicable disease. Complicating matters further was the fact that the pneumonic type of plague had an even shorter duration than bubonic plague, and its symptoms were even more difficult to recognize.[1]

On 23 June 1527, the patrician Ilija Đivov Bunić (Bona) reported the death of Marko, the tavern keeper. He noticed that Marko was not at work.[2] Lucija,

Marko's wife, told the patrician that Marko had gone to Poljice, forty kilometres south of Dubrovnik, when in fact he had died at home the preceding day.
Lucija pleaded that, as soon as she had noticed that Marko had a bit of fever,
she had reported the illness to Vicko, the guard of the health officials. Asked if
she had noticed any signs of plague, Lucija answered that she had not. She
claimed that her husband had felt some pain in his legs but that he had experienced such pains before.[3] In the *Libro deli Signori Chazamorbi* there is nothing more about this case. It seems that the investigation was not pursued for
lack of evidence. Most plague sufferers of the lower social classes were treated
with far less consideration. As we have seen in the previous chapter, the family of Božo Radovanov, the shoemaker from Ston, was sent to the rocky islet
of Škorpion right away. This was the usual procedure in the countryside as is
evident from the following case.

On 4 July 1527, Nuncijat Nikolin Luka, the captain of Trstenica on the Pelješac Peninsula, forbade a sick man from landing in Trstenica and ordered him
to return to Dubrovnik. The patient died on the boat while he sailed back to
Dubrovnik. The health officials called the barber and the physicians, who determined that plague was not the cause of that man's death. The health officials
accused Nuncijat of putting other passengers on the boat in danger and ruled
that he should have sent the man to a rocky islet. Nuncijat was ordered to pay
the cost of the inhumation of that man, in the amount of eight *hyperperi* and
seven *grossi*.[4]

Young Pasko, son of Marko Iljić and servant of Nikola Dragojev Gučetić
(Goze), patrician and member of the Senate, became sick on 11 July 1527.
Lady Jela, the senator's wife, noticed a wound on Pasko's hand. He told her that
he had burned himself with the candle. On the same day, all three left
Dubrovnik for Trsteno. Petar Jakšić and Damjan Marsić, *kaznac* of Trsteno,
both inquired about the wound on Pasko's hand. He replied that he had burned
himself – "kaznače, užegli smo se." Kaznac Damjan ordered Pasko to be kept
under guard. He died of the plague four days later. On his deathbed, Pasko con-
fided in his brother that four days earlier he had noticed a bubo (*bugnon*) on his
hand but he had not dared to tell the truth for fear of being sent to the isolation
compound at Danče.[5] Pasko's masters may have known that he was suffering
from the plague, but out of consideration for the young man they took him to
Trsteno, away from the city, and pretended that they did not recognize the disease. In posting a guard to isolate the patient, the kaznac in Trsteno acted according to the regulations.

On 16 August 1527, Andrija Banović from Ombla noticed that his female servant had become sick with plague. Immediately, he took her outside to the steep seashore. When she died three days later, he reported her case to the health officials.[6] On 18 September 1527, the health officials learned that, without informing them, Staneta Franov Stano had kept his maidservant in his house for several days after she had become sick. Staneta and his family members had been in touch with many healthy people who had gone to the vineyards to pick grapes. That made the matter even more serious. The captain of Brgat punished them by posting a guard in front of their house. Staneta stated in his testimony that he had gone to Dubrovnik with that servant and that she had become sick on the way back. He had taken her aside at once, had left her in the vineyard and had covered her with a sailor's blanket. After her death, he had asked the gravediggers Mihoč Ivanović and Antun Paskojević to bury her in secret. They preferred to first inform the captain of Brgat, who gave his permission for the woman to be buried next to the Church of St George. Both gravediggers were asked by the health officials to estimate the time of the woman's death.[7]

If members of the immediate family became sick, they usually died at home, and the survivors would inform the health officials only after their death in order to get permission for burial. Lucija, the wife of the leather tanner Maras, died in Dubrovnik on 31 October 1527. The health officials called Ivan Mednić, the plague doctor, to diagnose the cause of death. He confirmed that he had found evidence of plague on Lucija's body. The health officials learned that Maras left his home, both before and after his wife's death, and that he had been in contact with healthy people. Asked if he had known that his wife had plague, Maras stated that five days before she died, his wife had only complained that her back hurt because she had been very tired from making bread and that he had believed her. He said that he had gone out only to buy food, and, after her death, he had gone to inform the doctor and the health officials. This is the end of the investigation; Maras, it seems, managed to escape without any punishment.[8]

On 27 November 1527, Marin Alojzijev Rastić (Resti) informed the health officials by letter that Paskoje Kuzinović from Župa had reported his son's death of the plague and that he had asked for gravediggers to bury his son. The captain of Brgat also mentioned that Andrija Radovanović from Čibača, a community four kilometres southeast of Dubrovnik, had asked for gravediggers to bury his father. Andrija apologized for not reporting the case because he had not known that it was plague.[9]

CONCEALMENT OF SUSPICIOUS GOODS

Even before the disastrous plague epidemic of 1527, the authorities had paid particular attention to the import of goods suspected of being infected and they had questioned, under oath, each merchant or ship captain about the origin of their goods. On 16 March 1524, the patrician Vicko Nikolin Vučević (Volzo) brought to Dubrovnik some leather hides that he claimed to be from Turkey. He told the health officials that those hides had stayed in Ledenice, close to Kotor, for fifteen days and that they had been imported with the permission of the health officials.[10] However, others revealed that he had bought those hides from a salesman close to the city walls of Dubrovnik and that they had been brought from areas suspected of infection. Vicko was sentenced to spend one month in the prison of the Rector's Palace.[11] On 11 December 1527, Marino Vlahov had to declare under oath and under the threat of usual fines that the wool that he had brought was not infected and that those who have handled it have always been healthy.[12]

Even after the plague epidemic of 1527 was eradicated, the health officials doubled their supervision of the goods that were likely to be contaminated. They paid particular attention to wool manufacturing – *arte de lana*. Recorded in the *Libro deli Signori Chazamorbi* are thirteen wool manufacturing workshops in Dubrovnik. Six of those were owned by patricians: Šimun Antunov Bunić (Bona), Fran Pankratov Benešić (Benessa), Petar Nikolin Prokulović (Proculo), Dragoje Martolov Menčetić Crijević (Menze Zrieva), Federik Savinov Menčetić (Menze), and Orsat Junijev Đurđević (Giorgi); one was owned by Francesco Gotesco Fiorentino, a citizen of Florence; and six were owned by commoners: Marin Pavlov Radaljić, Petar Markov Radaljić, Martin Petrov Bisaljić, Božo *lanaro* (the wool manufacturer), Stjepan Šimunov de Alegreto, and Petar *texier* (the weaver).[13]

The growth of textile workshops dates from 1416 when Pietro Pantella and his half-brother Paolo from Piacenza, Italy, came to Dubrovnik. Unfortunately, Paolo died in 1417, but with the support of the Ragusan authorities, in 1419, Pietro developed textile manufacturing on a large scale.[14] The aim was to fulfill the demand for textiles in the hinterland and to free the Ragusan market from its dependence on foreign merchants, mainly Italian, who were importing woven materials not only from Italy but also from France and Flanders. Catalan merchants, who started importing Spanish wool of high quality, met a sharp increase in the need for wool in Dubrovnik.[15] Diversis reports in 1440 that four thousand pieces of woollen fabric were woven in Dubrovnik every year and that all classes of society benefited from this economic activity.[16] Many poor day labourers were employed in making yarn, carding, spinning wool, weaving, combing, dyeing, and trimming fabrics.[17] The limitations imposed on the import of raw materials would threaten their source of income and their existence. On 14 January 1528, the health officials issued an order that stipulated that, without their explicit permission and under the threat of a monetary fine of three hundred ducats and a three-month prison sentence, all owners of textile workshops were prohibited from stamping leather hides and woven fabrics, handing over wool for spinning, or contracting work for these activities. Marin Rugić, the scribe of the *Camera artis lanae* (Chamber of wool craft) was ordered, under the threat of losing his job, not to permit, without the explicit order of the health officials, the cotton fabrics to be stamped.[18] Thus, all wool and textile manufacturing in Dubrovnik was stopped for a while.

The consequences for the men and women employed in wool, leather, and cotton manufacturing were so serious that they were in danger of going hungry. In such cases, the Ragusan authorities reacted immediately and organized a free food distribution. Dubrovnik deserves credit for its initiative and, more importantly, for its social solidarity in such circumstances. Some of the day labourers were migrants from the hinterland where famine often reigned in years of poor harvest or constant warfare, and where no social measures existed to protect them. The Ragusan Republic was, therefore, a very attractive destination for immigrants. Despite the frequent plague epidemics, the population of the Republic was regularly replenished by newcomers, most often of Catholic faith, from the hinterland nearby where the economic and health conditions were much worse. The Ragusan authorities always made sure that the number of immigrants remained commensurate with the financial capabilities of the Republic.[19]

In 1528, the health officials were well aware of the fact that they were not dealing with an epidemic of disastrous proportions as in 1527, but with a phenomenon limited to sporadic cases in places where centres of infection still remained. In the opinion of the health officials, the sources of that infection were infected persons, persons suspected of infection, and the recovered. Goods that could easily carry the disease such as cotton, wool, fur, silk, and leather represented other potential sources of infection. These goods came from homes of individuals who were sick with plague or were imported from countries where plague was rampant. We will discuss offences concerning the importing of suspicious goods shortly.

On 13 June 1528, the health officials adopted two very strict regulations in order to deal with negligence offences such as failing to declare infected goods or concealing cases of plague or death of plague. With the approval of the Minor Council, it was ordered that heads of twelve illustrious patrician families, whether male or female, with their names spelled out, young girls, boys and young men, under the threat of a monetary fine of one hundred ducats and a six-month prison sentence, were forbidden from leaving their homes, until told otherwise. Since this regulation infringed on the freedom of circulation of members of well-known patrician families, it is understandable that the health officials sought the support of the Minor Council.[20] As was customary when important orders had to be communicated to the citizens, the health officials made it known, through the public crier, that every healthy or recovered person who still kept at home items that were not disinfected or aired would be punished by hanging – *pena delle forche* – and that if they were not declared to the health officials within three days, those items would be burned.

Those who could not satisfy this requirement because of lack of financial means were asked, under the threat of the above punishment, to report those items to the Health Office, which would make sure that the items were washed and aired at the expense of the commune. The recovered – the *resanati* – were also warned, under the threat of the above punishment, not to give or loan to anyone cotton, silk, or woollen items from their homes without the specific permission of the health officials. In the second part of this regulation, the Senate ordered all men and women under the age of twenty to stay in their homes the day after the announcement. The Senate also ordered, under the threat of a monetary fine of twenty-five hyperperi, all houses to remain locked and only one servant would be allowed to go out. This fine was to be paid by the house owner, whether male or female. Men older than twenty years were allowed to circulate freely.

The Senate decided that all heads of family, male or female, of any social rank or standing, would be punished with a monetary fine of one hundred ducats and a six-month prison sentence if they failed to report to the health officials the sickness from any disease of their family members, and that they would be hanged if, by such concealment, they caused the infection and the death of another person.[21] As well, the Senate warned that no person should dare sell or buy an item made of wool, cotton, or anything similar. The Senate had these decrees publicly announced by the messenger Luka Obad, *rivier*, in the presence of the chancellor.[22] These ordinances, like many others, make it obvious that the health officials adopted their regulations with the assent, advice, and accord of higher authorities – namely, the Minor Council and the Senate.

General insecurity caused by the possibility of new infections and the fear of strict regulations started to change the quality of neighbourly relations. Furtive eyes were present everywhere while gossip and hearsay followed the endless movement of goods.[23] In the atmosphere of the maximal control of citizens, on 21 June 1528, the priest Frano Sabatin reported Anuhla Nikolina, the woman who was his neighbour on Bratutova Street, north of Prijeki path. He declared that from his balcony he could see Anuhla give a package of wool to Mara Pavlova, her niece who had recovered from plague. He added that the day before, Anuhla's daughter, who lived with her, had become sick with plague. He gave the names of three female neighbours who knew about these events in Anuhla's home. On the same day, the health officials interrogated the women Lucija Vlahotina, Mara Lucina, Đivana Antunova, and Anuhla herself. Mara Pavlova testified the day after. The first three neighbours gave the same testimony as the priest Frano Sabatin and added that Anuhla's son Đivo had clandestinely put three packages of wool in front of her house and her niece Mara Pavlova had taken them home for spinning.

Then it was Anuhla's turn to be interrogated. She admitted that she had given Mara Pavlova the wool for spinning that belonged to the patrician Marin Đurđević (Giorgi). Anuhla claimed that the wool was not infected because it was kept in a special chest. When her daughter became sick, Anuhla started worrying about the wool in her home that belonged to others. Her son Đivo, who was healthy, gave the wool to Mara Pavlova. Anuhla added that she had more wool at home that belonged to Marin Radaljević. Mara Pavlova testified that she had taken the wool from Anuhla because Anuhla had persuaded her that the wool was not infected and that her son Đivo was healthy. Mara Pavlova stated that she had already spun a significant quantity of the wool that she had taken home.

The sentence was pronounced on 22 June 1528, with Luka Nikolin Bunić (Bona) presiding over the health officials, five of whom were present and two of whom were absent. Anuhla Nikolina and Mara Pavlova were sentenced to be tied and led through the city along the usual path, taken to the column of shame (the *berlina*), and branded with hot irons as a reminder of their trespassing and offence: *et ivi siano bulate a questo per memoria del loro exzeso e delicto.*[24] By giving the wool from her infected home for spinning, Anuhla had committed a serious offence. Wool was considered very dangerous for the transmission of plague. It is not surprising that such a harsh sentence, cruel from our point of view, severe even for the sixteenth century, was pronounced, even as the ink was barely dry on the regulation that dealt with this type of offence.

The lives of these two women were spared because their offence had been immediately reported to the health officials, which reduced the possibility of further infection.

Although it is never mentioned in the sources, the Ragusans were aware of the link between the plague and the poor that had been identified in Italian cities (see Chapter 4). This was partly the excuse for treating the resanati from the lower social classes harshly. At the same time, the health officials could not find an excuse to bring the full force of the plague control measures against the patricians. Also, we should not forget that one of the objectives of the plague control measures was to preserve the economy of Dubrovnik.

These very strict and utterly menacing regulations, all adopted in a very short period, must have caused dissatisfaction and even shock and unrest in all levels of society, including among the patricians. The strict character of these regulations was due to the reappearance of the plague infection. In the foreword of the last regulation in the *Libro deli Signori Chazamorbi*, the health officials acknowledge the severity of the plague legislation. Perhaps realizing that they had gone too far, they quickly adopted a new regulation that gave the opportunity to all the offenders to avoid severe punishment. The nature of the new regulation is very pragmatic: its role was to act as a kind of temporary amnesty and replace previous threats of penalties. On 20 June 1528, the health officials announced that, from their daily experience, they had concluded that the sporadic cases of plague that had reappeared were due to infected goods. Therefore, they decided henceforth to leave a big chest in the Church of St Mary the Great, into which everyone would be able to deposit previously concealed, unwashed, un-aired items and items that were still suspected of being infected.[25]

Priests, monks, nuns, and persons from every walk of life were all warned specifically that if they knew of the existence of such items, they could attach a label indicating the source of infection and bring them to the church to be cleaned. To make sure that people would not avoid performing such a useful deed out of fear of being punished, it was announced that persons who brought infected items would not be punished and the goods would be disinfected at the expense of the commune.[26] The threat of penalties was lifted for a period of ten days. However, should infected items be found after this grace period, the offenders would be dealt with according to the Statutes of Dubrovnik, the recent decrees, the laws and regulations of the Health Office.[27]

On 22 June 1528, according to the letter found in the big chest left in the Church of St Mary the Great, the health officials elected, behind closed doors, a reputable priest, Marino de Benedictis, rector of the Church of St Peter and St Lawrence, and gave him the authority to secretly pronounce infected and unclean any object belonging to any person of any rank, status, or condition.[28] The health officials announced publicly that anyone who wanted to leave a message about infected goods could do so by divulging it to the priest Marino de Benedictis. It was promised that the name of such a person would be kept secret and that the items would be sent to the rocky islet of St Andrew to be cleaned and would later be returned to their owners. The last lines of the regulation were written in a particularly friendly and cordial tone. In order to eradicate plague and its consequences, the health officials, in a benevolent frame of mind, exhorted everyone who knew anything about infected goods to report them.[29]

OFFENCES OF PRIESTS AND NUNS

In the same manuscript, there are also several cases that illustrate the health officials' treatment of priests and nuns. On 20 June 1527, during the worst plague attack, the health officials ordered the priests Nikola B. Crivaldi and Pavle Vukašinović, as well as Nikola Barneo, to pay one hundred hyperperi and to be banished from Dubrovnik for two years if they ventured out of their homes without permission.[30] This sentence was pronounced in agreement with and with the permission of the archbishop of Dubrovnik. From this case, we gather that priests did not always obey the plague control measures. Therefore, they received a strict conditional sentence. During the investigation process in the trials conducted by the health officials, priests were often summoned as credible witnesses. The health officials obviously made an effort to show consideration for the priests in order to be able to count on their cooperation in the future.

However, the priest Pavle Vukašinović, also known as Tamparica, was seen walking around the city without a guard in spite of the prohibition by the health officials and without any respect for their edict. To put a stop to such disobedience in the future, especially during the time of great mortality from pestilence, the health officials emphasized that this time around, and within eight days, the priest had to pay one hundred hyperperi for the silver ornaments of the relics in the cathedral of St Mary, and if he turned a deaf ear, his fine would be doubled. The health officials made clear again that this decision was made in the presence of and with the permission of the archbishop's vicar, who was summoned to act as an extra judge together with the health officials. The involvement of the ecclesiastical authorities is also apparent in the fact that the monetary fine was granted to the cathedral of Dubrovnik.[31] On 18 August 1527, the priest Nikola Aligretto was warned that he would have to pay a fine of one hundred hyperperi and be imprisoned for six months if he did not obey the order of the health officials to stay confined in his home until the 18 September 1527. This decision was also made with the permission of the archbishop's vicar.[32]

From a very short text registered on 21 September 1527, one gets the impression that the health officials treated the nuns in the convents infected by plague with much less consideration than the priests. The nuns were ordered to hand over the keys of their convent by the next day. Otherwise, the health officials threatened to enclose them with a sealed wall and stop the delivery of food and other necessities of life.[33] Was this decision the result of the misunderstandings between these convents and the health officials that had gradually piled up or was the above threat just the last straw in the otherwise harsh treatment of the nuns? The aim of the health officials was probably to protect the nuns but the wording of their pronouncement is threatening and disrespectful. The archival sources do not mention anything else regarding the fate of these nuns but we can easily imagine that they were compelled to submit to the authority of the health officials. Some convents evidently had contacts with people in the city, while others were completely closed off from the rest of the world. In these isolated convents, the infection did not penetrate the thick stone walls.

On 8 and 10 January 1528, the health officials interrogated Maruša, the nun from St Elias above Pile. They asked her if she had visited the house of Pavle Krizmanović, who had died of plague the day before. Maruša stated that she had been in that house three times in the last few days but just to ask how Pavle was doing. She said that she had not touched anything and if anyone said that she had, she offered to have her hands cut off. She said that she did not know if there were infected items in Pavle's house but she knew that a girl had died of plague and another one living in the house had survived. After the interrogation, Maruša was taken to a place between the inner and the outer city wall. In the meantime, the health officials learned from Dominka, Pavle's aunt, that Maruša had dined and slept in Pavle's house. During the interrogation two days later, Maruša admitted that she possessed some items belonging to Pavle's brother that she had cleaned. Asked if she had gone to the city after Pavle's death, she acknowledged that she had attended the holy mass at the Franciscan church and from there she wanted to go to the Dominican church when she was stopped near the fish market by the messengers of the health officials, who took her to the place between the walls.[34] Four days later, Maruša was sentenced to stand for fifteen minutes at the *berlina* and then to be taken on the ritual round of the city on a donkey. At Pile, she was to be tied to a column and branded with three hot irons on her cheeks and then taken by the gravediggers to the island of Lokrum together with all the items found in her room. In their explanation of the sentence, the health officials stated that Maruša had disregarded their proclamations and the rules imposed by them, and therefore, as an example to others, she could not remain unpunished.[35]

The unfortunate Maruša had completely overlooked the plague protection measures. Moreover, on the first day, she had given false testimony. Her fear of strict punishment was probably stronger than her love of truth. We can always wonder whether her offences were due to disobedience or ignorance. There is no mention of the fact that the health officials sentenced the nun in agreement with the Church dignitaries, as was prescribed for the priests. Neither is there any mention that the vicar of the archbishop was present, nor that he took part in the trial. This kind of treatment is definitely a result of the inferior social status of women, and especially the nuns, in the Ragusan society. The aim of the health officials was for Maruša to serve as an example to others, to threaten and to warn, and Maruša's permanently disfigured face would serve as an admonition.

In those times of crisis, there was a single example of improper behaviour among the priests. Every priest who had to hear confessions and perform last rites in quarantine found himself in a situation equally dangerous to that of the plague doctor, the barber, the scribe, and the gravediggers. These duties were tantamount to a death sentence. The *Libro deli Signori Chazamorbi* registers a range of offences, including the following one of a single priest. The events in the quarantine compound on the island of Lokrum show that, at the end of 1527, the health officials could no longer control the situation. On 27 November 1527, the patrician Pompej Marinov Gundulić (Gondola), delegated by the health officials to guard the infected on the island, complained to the health officials about the priest Miho and the barber Ilija de Gemia, who were also serving on Lokrum. The priest and the barber tried forcefully to take the communal rowboat that was at the disposal of Pompej. The barber Ilija, stating that he had to obey the priest Miho and not Pompej, wanted to take the oars that were housed in Pompej's house. The barber tried to enter Pompej's house by force and threatened that he was going to infect Pompej with the plague. Pompej said that the priest and the barber, who were armed, irrupted into the house of Božo, the messenger of the health officials, with such force that the mother of Vukas, also a messenger of the health officials, became sick. Pompej also reported that Mara, the wife of Marin the fisherman, complained about the behaviour of the priest Miho who had insulted her with rude words and brutal acts; that he had also beaten Lucija in front of the monastery on Lokrum; and that he had, several times, violently attacked the female servant of Mihajlo Rastić (Resti) and a certain Mada. Each accusation was borne out by three witnesses. Although these offences were serious, the decision of the health officials is not registered.[36] It has to be emphasized that in the whole manuscript, which covers thirty years, this is the only case of an offence of this nature committed by a priest. Living in fear of death and shaken by the circumstances, this priest appears to have forgotten the rules of his calling.

During plague crises, most priests remained faithful to their calling and cooperated fully with the authorities to curb the spreading of disease (see Chapter 8).[37] However, the above examples demonstrate that the relations between secular and religious authorities could be full of tensions and contradictions. Still, as we have seen above, in all the plague control measures, the health officials and the Senate had the last word.

The health officials noticed quite early that their port city was a particular target for the plague because the most diverse goods, from all over the Mediterranean and beyond, were unloaded in the port of Dubrovnik. This awareness urged them to improve the plague control measures and it also convinced them that they had to control the movement of all citizens including priests, monks, and nuns. After a few initial misunderstandings, secular and Church authorities each settled into their own role and respected the regulations and responsibilities upon which they had agreed. Secular authorities wholeheartedly supported all joint charitable actions in order to deserve divine protection for the whole community. Moreover, the patricians recognized the exceptional value of religious celebrations for the promotion of their political ideas and used them to their advantage to inform the citizens about the plague control measures and impose new plague control regulations. After every plague attack on the Republic, the Councils cooperated with the Church authorities to add to the yearly calendar yet another major religious festival in which the "liberation of Dubrovnik from disease and the recovery of pristine health" were celebrated.[38] As Samuel Cohn noted regarding sixteenth-century Italy, "Church and State were bound together in mutual support against a common enemy."[39] In Dubrovnik, a high level of cooperation between secular and religious authorities was demonstrated in their mutual effort to combat plague. The Church was, indeed, a careful observer of the plague. It encouraged the clergy to respect the plague protection measures of the government because of their practical value. For the secular authorities, controlling plague was a matter of administrative skill and political willpower. In concert with the government, the clergy had no choice but to courageously shoulder the burdens imposed by plague.

As in other cities, physicians serving in Dubrovnik did not participate in bridging the differences between secular authorities and the Church. As foreigners employed by the community, the physicians were not empowered to intervene. Moreover, except for rare exceptions, during the epidemics, they were mostly absent. The physicians also had their own problems to cope with – principally a decline in their reputation and social standing due to their impotence in dealing with plague. Medical theories of plague transmission were based on classical authorities that did not foresee that plague could be transmissible from person to person. This fact caused a huge intellectual problem for physicians and delayed their learning from their own observations. Most of them considered that plague was the result of corrupt air but they allowed that plague could also spread outwards from the place of its origin, by contagion alone. Thus, an epidemic in one city might derive immediately from the air whilst in another contagion might be the cause. Such a compromise, proposed in the sixteenth century, permitted the physicians to combine miasmatic and contagionist views and gave them the opportunity to argue about the factors involved in every particular plague outbreak.[40]

In principle, the health officials, as the executive branch of the secular authorities, the Church, and the physicians, each of them in their particular fields, complemented each other's activities. Due to the preeminence of secular authorities in Dubrovnik, if they occasionally disagreed, it did not lead to conflicts that could not be resolved. In sum, to survive in the threatening circumstances of a plague outbreak, they all needed each other's assistance and support.

In 1527, the trial proceedings of the health officials lasted up to a year. However, in the latter part of 1528, apparently aware of the fact that their reputation would depend on their efficiency as trial judges, the health officials hastened the process and wrapped up the trials in a few days. Since the strictest coercion measures did not eliminate the concealment of infected goods, the health officials decided to step back and change their strategy. Frustrated by the results of their previous endeavours, they decided to use a more conciliatory tone with the citizens. They left behind the scare tactics likely to irritate, and by focusing more on the results than on the punishment, they started limiting their repressive measures. Physical attacks on their assistants may also have given the health officials a hint. Tolerating infringements of the regulations meant risking greater disaster and yet, it was essential to temper the rigours of the law with charity and humanity.

The plague control measures were always unpopular, often threatening, and sometimes even counterproductive. Implemented in a nightmarish atmosphere of alarm and death, they were difficult to observe because they infringed on the freedoms of the citizens and often endangered their livelihood. As authorities began recording deaths and burials, inspecting merchandise, and controlling many aspects of trade, they gained more detailed information about their citizens: the plague control measures brought along a much tighter control of many aspects of citizens' lives. Although the broadened judicial powers were not the original objective of the stringent plague legislation, they certainly became their by-product.

It seems that by 1528, the health officials were in a state of utter despair because the plague epidemic resisted all the measures that they had undertaken to fight it. It turned out that it was simply not a neat phenomenon that could be easily controlled with containment measures. Still, the escalation of repressive measures was short-lived and the authorities soon replaced it with a softer, more humane approach. Everything we know about the characteristics of the Ragusan society points to the fact that repression, in and of itself, was not the purpose of the implementation of strict plague control measures. The eradication of plague was still the health officials' primary concern. The Ragusan experience exemplifies the possibilities and the limitations of both the plague control measures and of state coercion in early modern Europe.

PLAGUE EXPERIENCE IN SEVILLE AND TURIN

Kristy Wilson Bowers studied the plague restrictions of the rural areas in the vicinity of Seville in 1582. She quotes the case of Diego Escobar, the wine merchant, who lived in an infected community. He had a substantial quantity of wine that he wanted to sell in Seville. In order to achieve that, he first moved from his infected community to a healthy one. After a certain time of residence there, he petitioned the local judge for an official declaration of his health. Armed with that document, he gained permission to enter the city of Seville. He stayed there for a few weeks before deciding to bring his wine to the city. By that time, the wine had been sitting outside the city for more than forty days and he received permission from both the doctor who examined it and the ad hoc health commission to bring the wine into the city. Diego, the wine merchant, thus circumvented the plague legislation and was able to continue trading. It seems that many citizens of the area around Seville took advantage of such arrangements and obtained individual exemptions from the ad hoc health commissions. Bowers argues that the ad hoc health officials in Seville successfully negotiated a balance between medical concerns and the economic interests of their citizens. She also states that such exemptions empowered residents, allowed trade to continue, and dissipated popular resistance to plague restrictions, travel bans, and quarantine. Such arrangements seem to have been possible because there were only sporadic cases of plague in smaller communities surrounding Seville, while the city remained unaffected.[41]

No evidence has been found that individual exemptions were ever granted in Dubrovnik. Such decisions would actually have run counter to the philosophy of Ragusan political culture. Always afraid of favouring an individual or a group, the Ragusans avoided making any personal exceptions. Furthermore, in the case of Dubrovnik in 1526–28, when the city was hit with the plague much harder than the countryside, such administrative accommodation would hardly have been justified.

In their microhistory of Seville, covering a three-year period at the beginning of the 1580s, Alexandra Parma Cook and Noble David Cook focus on the city government and its handling of successive waves of crises, including preparations for war and a failed uprising of the Moriscos, the converted Muslims of Spain. The councillors were forced to face not only a plague outbreak but also drought, crop failure, locust infestation, and epidemics of influenza and typhus. Through all these emergencies, the governor and the councillors maintained the air of normality and continued performing their duties conscientiously to ensure the survival of the citizens. When plague appeared in 1581–82, the physicians tried to deny it, even when faced with the plague buboes, the typical symptoms of plague. A plague epidemic was much too scary a prospect. The government asked several physicians to confirm the diagnosis. When plague could no longer be denied, the infected communities were cut off. Trade and travel bans were imposed. Anyone not complying with the orders would be punished. Cook and Cook explain, "People of 'quality' were condemned to serve four years in the galleys without salary, while those of low 'quality' received the same punishment and two hundred lashes."[42] Luckily, the 1581–82 outbreak of plague in Seville was a rather mild one and it did not cause the social system to break down.

Sandra Cavallo has examined the cost of plague control measures in Turin during the 1598–99 plague outbreak. The city of fifteen thousand inhabitants had spent 125,000 *scudi* to combat plague, while only 15,000 *scudi* entered the city coffers every year. This enormous sum of money was mostly spent on quarantine, feeding three thousand people from the public purse, and the after-plague cleansing program that employed more than two hundred people. With every passing day, civic authorities were increasingly concerned with the number of people to feed, rather than with the plague and the number of the dead. Considering the high cost of plague protection measures and the burden they represented for the city, Cavallo shows no enthusiasm for the plague control program. She concludes that long after the disappearance of the plague, the city remained isolated and its inhabitants endured unemployment and poverty.[43] One can always wonder what the cost to the people of Turin would have been if measures to fight plague had not been undertaken.

Conclusion

In 1377, the aristocratic city-state of Dubrovnik, situated on the Dalmatian Adriatic coast of present-day Croatia, became the first government in the world to formulate, develop, and apply the concept of quarantine. This legislation, which proposes a novel approach to plague, including the concepts of incubation and healthy carriers, demonstrates that the Ragusan Major Council believed that plague was a communicable disease. It was predicated on the idea that the government was justified in controlling the space and the movement of the few in the interest of the common good.

In 1390, Dubrovnik established the earliest recorded Health Office, an important landmark in the history of plague containment. The early plague control regulations, examined in the State Archives of Dubrovnik, covering the period from 1377 to 1400, bear witness to that significant event. The health officials had to apply, enforce, and control the implementation of plague control regulations that the Ragusan Councils promulgated on a regular basis as a defensive shield against recurrent plague outbreaks. In 1397, the Major Council decided that the plague control officials, as they were then called, would, in the future, be elected by the Minor Council, which would be allowed to elect as many officials as necessary. The Health Office was thus transformed from a regular, but still ad hoc, to a permanent office. Since 1397, these officials were elected in January, together with most of the public officials of the Ragusan state.

Why did the Health Office in Dubrovnik become permanent at a time when this office was either non-existent or temporary in other cities? In short, it was because of the Ragusan political culture. Ragusans always instituted a temporary office first and then, a few years later, if it suited their needs, they made it permanent. In the case of the health officials, because of the perceived urgency to act, the need for a permanent office was recognized in 1397. Once adopted, the plague control measures were strictly and consistently implemented and the Health Office was maintained at all times, whether or not the danger of plague was imminent. This was necessary because Dubrovnik was situated on the frontier of the Ottoman Empire, from where the plague arrived. The attitude of the Ragusan government was proactive. It considered plague as a survival issue that affected the whole society.

In 1426, the Major Council adopted a regulation concerning the election of the health officials. It stipulated that they had to serve without pay and that neither the members of the Minor Council nor the Civil Court should be elected to serve as *Cazamorti*, the name used for the health officials in the fifteenth century. This decision was based on the fact that the office of the Cazamorti was very demanding. Another reason was to avoid the concentration of power in the hands of a few, something that the Ragusan Councils very carefully monitored at all times. From 1390 until 1426, the Cazamorti were elected by the Minor Council and, after that date, by the Major Council, as was the practice with the majority of the Ragusan state officials.

In 1457, the status of the Cazamorti underwent a significant change. The Senate referred to them as salaried officials of the state. That meant that they no longer served without pay. Unfortunately, the amounts they were paid have not been registered. This new status is an acknowledgment of the importance of their office and the high esteem in which the Cazamorti were held in Dubrovnik. In order to ensure maximal efficiency, their terms of office were staggered during yearly elections so that new officials served together with those who had started six months earlier. From 1390 until 1457, the Minor Council was responsible for giving the Cazamorti specific instructions. After 1457, that role was taken over by the Senate. Since the Cazamorti were of crucial significance for the survival of the Ragusan Republic, they were recruited exclusively from the most reputable patrician families, usually at the age of forty or fifty. Once elected, they could not refuse to serve, even if they ran the risk of not surviving until the end of their term. In the second half of the fifteenth century, it took at least twenty-seven years of experience in the Major Council to be elected to this office, which served as a steppingstone to the inner circle of power.

During the particularly deadly 1482 plague epidemic, new regulations were issued concerning the obligations of the Cazamorti. Other regulations dealt with infected items, decontamination, and especially with the danger posed by gravediggers, who could transmit plague through their contact with infected patients and their belongings. The spreading of plague through contaminated items became one of the health officials' major preoccupations. Thus, in December 1482, two gravediggers were sentenced to death by hanging for stealing from the quarantine compound. This was the first time anyone in Dubrovnik was executed for contravening plague control measures. Such a harsh sentence definitely constituted an escalation of repressive measures. Why did the two gravediggers have to lose their lives? Was it the result of the health officials' utmost concern with the spreading of infection, or were the two gravediggers, who obviously belonged to the lowest social class and were not protected by a confraternity or any other institution, easy prey, in a way? Were the frustrated Cazamorti looking for a scapegoat? Plague obviously created social tensions that the governing patricians found difficult to reconcile.

Over time, the duties of the Cazamorti became more complex and demanded more coordination with the authorities as well as the assistants that were assigned to the Cazamorti who supervised plague doctors, barbers, priests, guards, gravediggers, and laundresses in quarantine compounds. The Ragusan Republic bestowed wide-ranging judicial and executive powers on the health officials in matters concerning plague control. However, the legislative power remained the domain of the Councils. The Senate watched over the health officials to make sure that they did not use their extensive authority to get rid of their political adversaries. Furthermore, when serious violations of plague control measures occurred, the health officials acted as trial judges who had to punish delinquents. As a result of the 1526–27 calamitous plague outbreak, relations among all social groups in the Republic were changed. The trials registered in the *Libro deli Signori Chazamorbi* corroborate these transformations. During each epidemic recurrence, new, more stringent plague control measures were adopted. Thus, each successive plague outbreak became a new milestone in the development of the plague protection legislation and necessitated major modifications. This was particularly evident in 1527.

Among other duties, the health officials also investigated where people went, with whom they associated, items they touched, and where the goods they bought had originated. When people became sick, they had to report their illness to the health officials, who asked the physicians to diagnose the disease. If the patient died, the body could not be buried without the permission of the health officials, who had to decide where, when, and in which way the remains could be inhumed. If the patient survived the plague, he was subjected to more social control. Members of the lower class who survived the plague especially faced a widespread mistrust and stigma. By deploying unprecedented plague

control measures and investing considerable financial resources, the government gained an enormous amount of information about its citizens. This kind
of control affected the relations between the health officials, the Church, and
common citizens. Because of the dominance of secular authorities in Dubrovnik, as far as plague control measures were concerned, the health officials and
the Senate always had the last word, and all citizens, including the clergy, had
to obey. In most situations, secular authorities and the Church acted as partners against the plague – their common enemy.

One could say that the trials against those who contravened the plague control measures were conducted in an authoritative and sometimes even cruel
manner, especially when the plague survivors, also known as the *resanati*, from
the disadvantaged social classes, such as the gravediggers and the laundresses,
were concerned. Truth be told, this was the characteristic of the penal system
of the time, not only in Dubrovnik, but also elsewhere. Strict sentences were
likely meant to be deterrents and serve as warnings to other citizens. Feared
and envied at the same time, the plague survivors posed a particular problem
for the authorities. Since no one knew if they could still potentially transmit
the plague, the authorities aimed to control all the movements and social contacts of the *resanati*. But above all, for a minimal pay, the health officials utilized the survivors' resistance to plague and used them as plague workers. The
plague survivors were forced to transport and bury the dead. Handling contaminated items was also among their duties.

One could certainly claim that objectionable differences existed in the type
of punishment decreed for common citizens on the one hand and the patricians
on the other. When caught with contaminated items in their own houses, most
of the patricians still insisted that their goods were not dangerous. The health
officials protected members of their own social class and they had significant
difficulties prosecuting and punishing other patricians. After all, Dubrovnik
was an aristocratic Republic. Furthermore, the Ragusans were aware of the link
between the plague and the poor that had been identified in Italian cities. This
represented a considerable stumbling block for the health officials. Because of
this link between the plague and the poor, they could not find an excuse to bring
the full force of the plague control measures against the patricians. As a cul-
mination of state repression, the health officials, frustrated with long trials of
recalcitrant citizens, drafted the draconian regulation of November 1527, according to which, at least on paper, all social classes became equal. However,
the health officials quickly realized that they had gone too far and retracted the

strict repressive measures. A ten-day amnesty for all was announced. The draconian regulation was never adopted by the Councils and there is no evidence that it was ever applied.

In the aftermath of the 1527 plague outbreak, the judicial powers of the health officials were extended and punitive measures were redoubled. This was definitely a major change. Five more people were sentenced to death for spreading plague – one was a servant, three were guards of infected clothing, and the fourth one was an employee of the Health Office. Did such measures scare people into obedience? Could they save lives or did they endanger them even more? Seven death sentences were pronounced during the most pernicious plague outbreaks in 1482 and 1527 and are linked to only one incident in 1482, one in 1527, and one in 1528. Facing what seemed like a never-ending epidemic, the officials were most likely exhausted and probably felt quite helpless. After being surrounded by death on a daily basis for such a long time, they had likely become desensitized to it. Sadly, gravediggers were also sentenced to death in other afflicted cities, including Geneva in 1530 and Venice in 1576.

Why was Dubrovnik, despite all Ragusan efforts, and a lengthy experience with plague control measures, not able to avoid the 1527 plague outbreak? The arrival of a contaminated ship from the Levant, a constant source of plague, is the most likely cause of the 1527 outbreak. Another possible cause could have been the increased virulence of the plague pathogen circulating in the Adriatic in the 1520s due to massive army movements of the French and the Spanish. Finally, we must emphasize that epidemics could not be completely avoided at a time when the aetiology and the pathology of plague remained unknown.

One might also wonder whether the patricians at some point no longer cared about stopping plague and instead wanted to assert their power at any cost. This hypothesis has to be vigorously rejected because Ragusan patricians maintained stable relations with the commoners, some of whom had become even richer than the patricians through trade. These wealthy merchants shared with the patricians the interest in the common good and other civic ideals of the Republic. In sum, they were more interested in imitating the patricians' lifestyle than in taking over power. The sixteenth century was still the so-called golden age of Dubrovnik. Thus, everything we know about the characteristics of the Ragusan society leads us to conclude that, in 1527, the main motivation of the patricians was fear of plague and its recurrence. Moreover, during an epidemic, the threat of an enemy attack from outside – from the Ottomans or the Venetians – was always present, as was the threat of economic and social collapse.

Conflicts, between two factions of patricians occurred only in the seventeenth century. The Republic slowly turned into an oligarchy and the city experienced a serious decline after the 1667 earthquake.

The Councils and the patricians, as a group, perceived fighting plague as a survival issue for the whole state. They were, therefore, wholeheartedly interested in plague management. From their point of view, combating plague, ensuring the survival and the stability of the state, as well as securing the protection of the Ragusan economy, was all part of the same goal. They were not in a position to care about one issue without considering the rest. The state, the people, the economy – they all had to be rescued, and the responsibility for doing so rested squarely on the shoulders of this small group of men. Strict social control was certainly a by-product of plague control measures but it cannot be said that the plague laws were instituted to keep the patricians in power. As other historians have argued, in the big Italian cities, for example, with thousands of the poor, the plague control measures had become a method of controlling the destitute and the undesirable. This was not the case in Dubrovnik, which always had a small population and could not afford thousands of victims. Thus, the Ragusans continued to fight the plague. They co-existed as best they could with the Ottomans and the Venetians, as well as a host of other states, and they managed to stay masters of the Republic until 1808.

It was the senators' role to worry about social peace. They, therefore, consistently chose to promulgate the most sensitive and the most unpopular regulations themselves. It is important to emphasize that the Senate always offered its unconditional support, both financial and moral, to plague control measures, and shared with the health officials the responsibility for the most unpopular anti-plague actions. This is significant because, in some northern Italian cities, as Richard Palmer has shown, the lack of political will was the most frequent reason for the failure of plague control measures. The Senate also kept an eye on the relations among patricians. Acutely aware that the health officials could abuse their authority and send their political rivals into quarantine, the Senate made the decisions about the patricians and gave the health officials permission to rule over all other social classes.

The Ragusan health officials were convinced of the communicable nature of the plague. Despite all the medical and religious theories prevalent at that time, they put the isolation of the sick and the suspects at the core of their protection measures. The words *miasma* and *corrupt air*, often cited by physicians as causes of plague, have not been used at all in any of the Ragusan sources. Moreover, in the *Libro deli Signori Chazamorbi*, the word *infection*, although it did not have the same meaning it has now, was used more than thirty times. The physicians serving in Dubrovnik, once they had diagnosed the first cases of plague, were usually allowed a leave of absence until the epidemic had abated. They could thus play only a secondary role in plague protection.

The health officials were aware of the fact that their city was situated at the crossroads of trade routes of different civilizations, and they sensed that the Ragusans were exposed to a higher than normal risk of contracting plague. That awareness demanded extra caution. In 1440, Diversis reported that plague epidemics in Dubrovnik had a shorter duration because of the decisive measures undertaken by the Ragusan Councils. The health officials had no medical training but they were experienced administrators whose pragmatic stance was based on their experience. This emphasizes the distinctively mediaeval and early modern nature of the Dubrovnik phenomenon. It assumes a shared consensus among the elite as to what plague was, as well as a pre-modern understanding that it was their social status that would guarantee social order in a crisis of this kind.

What was it about Dubrovnik that made it a forerunner of plague control measures? First of all, the plague control measures were firmly rooted in the social, environmental, economic, and political structures of Dubrovnik. It was a wealthy and ambitious city with a centralized government that maintained full control of the state apparatus and encouraged the actions of the health officials. Providing health care for all was an important part of the Ragusan identity based on the political ideals of liberty, prosperity, stability, longevity, and social tolerance. Those ideals, as well as the Ragusan Christian identity, included keeping the state free of epidemics. The patricians realized that a healthy population would be their greatest asset. Notably, in this fiercely independent Republic, as in other city-states in northern Italy, the community feeling was more developed than in countries governed by a feudal lord. As a result, plague control measures were primarily developed in city-states. It seems that large states would have had neither the financial resources nor the level of control of the city-states to institute such measures.

From the earliest times, the wealthy Ragusan state demonstrated a preoccupation with cleanliness and hygienic living conditions for all citizens. It worked to maintain cesspools, lay stone-paved streets, and replace wooden with stone houses, for example. Early in its history, Dubrovnik established institutions and infrastructure to improve and maintain the health of its citizens. The first pharmacy was established in 1317 and the first hospital opened three decades later in 1347. A grain depository was set up in 1410; urban garbage collection began in 1415; the aqueduct and water fountains were built in 1420; the orphanage opened in 1432; and the sewage system functioned as early as 1436. Since the 1280s, the city regularly employed physicians, surgeons, and pharmacists to take care of all citizens. As Susan Mosher Stuard has emphasized, health care in Dubrovnik was a right extended to all. It was not a charitable handout.

Second, we should not forget that, geographically, Dubrovnik was very close to the Ottoman-controlled territories from where the plague arrived. Since the Ottoman Empire did not apply any plague laws, the proximity of the Ottoman frontier was an additional factor that propelled Dubrovnik to act.

Third, in comparison with northern Italian cities, such as Venice or Florence, Dubrovnik had a small population that it was determined to protect. The Ragusans were always acutely aware of their limited biological pool.

Fourth, in order to survive, the Ragusans also had to protect their economic prosperity. Therefore, they could not close down the city and stop trading; that would have led to their financial ruin. Faced with such contradictory demands, a society that valued conservatism, pragmatism, and continuity, adopted a pragmatic solution: it embraced the plague control measures that permitted trading to continue but on a smaller scale.

In Italy, religious orders and confraternities took over the care of plague victims. In Dubrovnik, this was not an option. Suspicious of voluntary citizens' associations, which could develop into parallel lines of power, secular authorities in Dubrovnik dominated the Church and controlled the confraternities. Delegating their powers to the religious communities was out of the question. The government financed and organized health care at all times and especially during the plague outbreaks. Because epidemics also posed a threat to law and order, the Ragusan authorities preferred to keep all the control in their hands.

Finally, plague control measures were never popular. They were always resisted because they limited individual freedom and they interfered with citizens' economic interests. Moreover, to be sent all alone into quarantine and remain separated from loved ones was certainly frightening. The anti-plague measures were often threatening, sometimes counterproductive, and, at times, they even endangered the lives of the citizens they claimed to protect. Implemented as they were under frightening circumstances of fear and death, it is no wonder that they were difficult to obey. However, at a time when the aetiology and the pathology of plague were completely unknown, they seem to have contributed to the reduction of the scale and duration of the epidemics. The Dubrovnik experience is of remarkable historical interest because this bold precedent in government intervention was permanent, rigorous, and wide-ranging. At the same time, it demonstrated the possibilities but also the limitations of state intervention in health and sanitation.

More than five hundred years later, we have to wonder whether the health officials contributed to the fact that after 1533 Dubrovnik was never again levelled by a great plague. The courage of these unwilling heroes was admirable: with no scientific knowledge at their disposal, they faced an invisible but formidable enemy. The cities on the Apennine Peninsula were subjected to two more waves of deadly plague epidemics – one in 1575–78 and another in 1630. But Dubrovnik was spared both of them. Was Dubrovnik unaffected by these outbreaks because of the actions of the health officials? Or was the city simply lucky to be bypassed by successive upsurges of infection? Recent historiography on the plague in early modern Europe has confirmed that the eventual disappearance of plague can be ascribed to the success of the quarantine model: hence the significance of the precocious Ragusan precedent.

While they saved their families and their homeland in an altogether innovative way at that point in time, the Ragusans also helped many other people near and far away. Dubrovnik maintained lively trade relations with cities on both sides of the Adriatic Sea. Considering how difficult, time-consuming, and uncomfortable travel was, it is amazing to find out how much the people of that era travelled. Vibrant contacts between cities lead us to believe that government officials on both sides of the Adriatic were aware of the plague control measures that other cities implemented. Further research in the archives of particular cities, especially Venice, is necessary to shed light on this point. Each city, according to its geographical position, its type of government, economic situation, and available financial resources, decided which plague control measures to implement. The rigour of plague laws also depended in no small measure on the political willpower of those who governed and on the perceived urgency to act.

Since the Black Death in 1348, plague became endemic in the Mediterranean and Western Europe and remained a permanent fact of life of the early modern world, recurring in virulent onslaughts for over 350 years. From 1377 until 1530, during the crucial 153 years of the most frequent plague epidemics, Dubrovnik, in order to ensure the survival of its people and its state, continued to develop ever more sophisticated plague control measures.

The plague control measures applied in Dubrovnik became standard practice in many other cities across Europe by the sixteenth and seventeenth centuries. Northern Italian cities are widely recognized as precursors of health measures in Europe. While Milan established a sanitary cordon in 1400 and Venice was a forerunner in establishing the first hospital for plague victims in 1423, Dubrovnik led the way with the promulgation of quarantine legislation in 1377 and the establishment of the first Health Office in 1390. The Ragusan concerns of the past resemble our own present-day debates about fighting SARS, AIDS, bird flu, and the Ebola virus. All these issues are reflected in the plague control measures of mediaeval and Renaissance Dubrovnik.

Appendices

The State Archives of Dubrovnik

The State Archives of Dubrovnik are among the best preserved in Europe. They are the most important source not only for the study of the Ragusan Republic but also for the vast regions of the Mediterranean, the Balkan hinterland, the Middle East, England, and even America, with which Dubrovnik maintained commercial and political relations during more than eight centuries. The Archives constitute, therefore, the most valuable cultural heritage of Dubrovnik.[1]

THE BEGINNINGS OF THE RAGUSAN ARCHIVES

The Archives contain several hundred charters, bulls, privileges, and contracts negotiated with other cities and states from the year 1022 onward.[2] These documents were jealously protected because they guaranteed the Ragusan citizens' legal security in international relations. As early as 1023, the canon Petar acted as notary in Dubrovnik. However, the Archives were established in 1277–78 when Thomasinus de Savere (Sauere) from Reggio in Lombardy, who had obtained his diploma from a university, probably in Bologna, was hired by the government as the first professional notary public. His title was *iuratus notarius communis*, sworn notary of the commune. The need for the services of a professional notary arose since, in 1275, the government had decided that all transactions of loans of more than ten *hyperperi* had to be based on a contract written by a notary. By this decision, the government wanted to promote trade and ensure its legal framework. *Magister* Thomasinus started the first notary books, *Debita Notariae*, *Diversa Notariae*, *Diversa Cancellariae*, and *Testamenta*, which were kept continuously until the end of the Republic in 1808. He organized the Archives and performed the duties of notary, scribe, and chancellor.

With the founding of the Archives, notary books became property of the state.[3] In court, the chancellor's role was to assist the judges. During the deliberations of the governing Councils, he took notes of the proceedings. In 1285, Thomasinus probably realized that he had too much work to do so he continued to perform his duties of chancellor while the duties of notary were executed by a priest, *presbyter* Johannes, who performed these duties until 1292. Johannes was succeeded by *diaconus* Andrija Benešić (Benessa), a priest from a Ragusan noble family, who carried out the duties of notary of the government until 1324. In the Middle Ages, all the notaries and chancellors who followed were professionally trained foreigners from Italy.[4] In his work, *Opis slavnoga grada Dubrovnika* (Description of the illustrious city of Dubrovnik), written in 1440, Philippus de Diversis, describes the duties of chancellors, notaries, and scribes who keep the books and emphasizes the significance of their profession.[5] Since 1297, it is easy to follow the names of the chancellors because they are mentioned in the deliberations of the Major Council that employed them.[6] This practice was continued until 1808.[7]

DOCUMENTS FROM 1272 UNTIL 1808

Written by notaries and chancellors, the deliberations of the Ragusan Councils, court decisions, and private legal documents contained in bound books constitute the biggest part of the Archives. These documents guaranteed the legal security of citizens in internal relations. The most important documents were written on parchment paper. Damaged documents were copied and bound again. In 1910, Josip Gelčić catalogued the archival material. He organized it into ninety-two series that occupy more than seven kilometres of shelves.[8] The series include seven thousand bound books and a further one hundred thousand separate acts. Information pertaining to medicine and public health is scattered throughout this vast bulk of records.

For the sake of convenience, all the documents in the State Archives of Dubrovnik can be divided into four groups. The first group consists of the proceedings of the three Councils that governed the city. They are subdivided into *Acta Consilii Maioris* (the Major Council), *Acta Minoris Consilii* (the Minor Council), and *Acta Consilii Rogatorum* (the Senate). The resolutions of the Senate constitute a very abundant series, which, for example, for the period of

1555 to 1595, consists of six thousand pages. The Senate often revised the documents that contained a potentially embarrassing or dangerous content concerning foreign relations. That means that many valuable documents have been destroyed, especially the *Secreta Rogatorum* (the Secret Documents of the Senate). The most important revisions happened in 1358, when the Venetian rule ended, and in 1807, before the end of the Republic. The records of the deliberations of the three Councils constitute an indispensable source for the study of public health in Dubrovnik, although their contents are not primarily medical but a chronological listing of the Councils' decisions on a variety of matters over a period of five hundred years. Nevertheless, in an incidental manner, they constitute a unique source of medico-historical information.

The instructions of the Ragusan Senate to its consuls in the Eastern and Western Mediterranean can be found in the *Lettere di Levante* and the *Lettere di Ponente*, which also belong to this group. The *Acta Sanctae Mariae Maioris*, also called *Acta et Diplomata*, which includes the correspondence of Dubrovnik's consuls, foreign envoys, and private persons, is also part of this group. It is one of the oldest series in the Archives and covers the period from the eleventh to the nineteenth centuries.

The second group of documents deals with the financial matters of the Ragusan Republic. These reports are a valuable source for the analysis of food prices and other imported and exported goods, including medicines. Some of these sources can be used to determine food prices during epidemics. The most important series from this group of documents are the *Salinaria*, the *Grassia*, and the *Libro di cassa pubblica*, which cover purchases and sales of salt, grain, and other foodstuffs. Further, two series, the *Naula et securitates* and the *Liber navigiorum*, record all aspects of maritime trade. Relevant information concerning public health can also be gathered from the *Liber statutorum doane*, the Ragusan customs statute book, which covers the period from 1277 until 1808.

The third group includes collections of public laws, tribunal sentences, cadastral surveys, and the development of the Ragusan Chancery. It consists of the earliest codification of Dubrovnik's laws, the *Liber statutorum* (The statute book) from 1272, and its continuations, the *Liber omnium reformationum* (1335–1410), the *Liber viridis*, (1358–1460), and the *Liber croceus* (1460–1803). The last laws of the Republic, from 1791 to 1808, are recorded in the *Parti dei Pregadi*.[9]

The fourth group of documents, including wills (*Testamenta*), contracts of sale, marriage and dowry contracts, and debtors' books (*Debita Notariae*),

Diversis on the Import and Export Trade in Dubrovnik

Those who establish and found the most renowned cities want their cities to benefit from being conveniently located; if a city is not strategically located on land and near sea, it suffers various inconveniences. With the aid of these two locational factors, however, produce and goods arrive easily as do building materials, items that all citizens need. From their own territory, from foreign lands and from far away nations, items are brought to these cities over land on animals and carried on ships with great ease. Dubrovnik abounds with these advantages. It occupies part of the territory on land, wherefrom every day travelling by land, a wondrous multitude of people flows, bringing on horses or other animals, or carrying on their own backs, everything that is necessary and useful for people's needs or for trade. Peasants arriving from the vicinity of the city, whether Ragusan citizens or not, bring cabbage, flowers, the freshest fruit of the season, chickens, eggs, pigs, rabbits, and everything else that is necessary for the nutrition of living beings. The peasants from areas further away bring honey, fish, wood planks, coal, rough woollen fabric (*raša*), furs, boat covers that they call *celegas*, wooden contraptions for making bread, and devices for washing linen fabrics for weavers, and, last but not least, they bring many animals, the meat of which humans eat. Others arriving by land are mostly merchants who bring gold, silver, lead, crimson, pepper, wax, and many other items of great value from Adrianopolis (today Edirne), from Rascia (today Serbia), particularly from Novo Brdo, and from Bosnia. The city of Dubrovnik equally enjoys a maritime location that brings numerous advantages. Since Dubrovnik is inhabited by numerous dwellers and cannot feed its inhabitants with what its own soil produces, nor from what is brought by land, nor is it possible to get building materials, every day wheat, millet, barley, leguminous plants, oil, salted meat and fish, olives, nuts, fruit, chestnuts, cheese, sugar, spices, sweets, remedies, wool, cloth, linen, corals, salt, and countless other types of merchandise, as well as a large quantity of gold ducats, are brought by sea from Italy, the most flourishing and most bountiful with all kinds of goods; namely from Venice, Marche, Apulia, Abruzzo, Fermo, Pesaro, Recanati, Ancona, and Rimini to which various goods for trading are transported from Toscana, mostly from Florence, and are then shipped to Dubrovnik; from Manfredonia, Ortona, Lecce, Vasto, Monopoli, Bari, Barletta, Trani, and also Naples; from Sicily, that is, from Palermo or Panormo, from Syracuse and other Sicilian cities; from the Aragon Kingdom, as, for example, from Barcelona and Valencia and other localities from this kingdom; from Greece, for example from Arta, Patras, Valona, and many other regions; wood, beams, stone, bricks, nails, iron, lime, roof tiles, and other items necessary for construction are also brought. Those who bring goods and merchandise by land take away from Dubrovnik large quantities of salt, linen, cotton and silk fabrics, glass jars, and many other items useful for living and for profit. Those who arrive by sea take away gold, silver, lead, wax, furs, pepper, fabrics, corals, and gold ducats – everyone, of course, takes what he considers more useful, more advantageous, and more convenient. First of all, the city of Dubrovnik enjoys an excellent location, and now we can discuss other things.[1]

The Testament of Angelo de Leticia

In the name of the Lord, Amen. In the Lord's year 1348, on 5 May, I, Angelo de Leticia, being of sound mind, compose my last will as follows. First of all, 500 *hyperperi* should be given for what has been unfairly charged, and from that amount, 4 orphaned daughters of good men should get married and each of them should be given 50 hyperperi. Further, 100 hyperperi should be given for the construction of the hospital but if the construction does not start within two years, this amount should be given for the clothing of the poor, to be decided by the executors of my will. Further, from the amount of 100 hyperperi a church of the Annunciation of the Virgin Mary should be built on Mount Krstac (Cresta), on the way to Ombla, and it should be built as fast as possible.[1] Further, I want my wife Draže to have all my possessions, houses, vineyards, and land, and all the furniture, as long as she lives, and after her death it should be as written below. Further, I want my house where I lived, with everything in it, including the arms and all the bedding, to be given to Nikola, the son of my son Radoš, when Nikola reaches 18 and becomes of age, but only if he is a good man. Should he be insolent and lead a bad life, nothing should be given to him and I let my executors take care of that. But should this boy die before he reaches adulthood or should he lead a bad life, I want my executors to sell all the arms and everything in the house and this house should be given to the Franciscan monastery forever, under the condition that they cannot sell it, donate it, or exchange it, or sell it in any way or under any pretext, but that they should take the rent from this house and pray to God for my soul. Further, if there is no one left of my heirs, I want the terrain that I own in front of Sir Nikola Lukarević (Luchari) to be sold in 6 years and I want 9 annual rents from that amount to be given for the construction of the church of Saint Blaise on Placa.[2] Further, 500 hyperperi should be given to the Franciscan friars for the construction of their monastery. Further, 200 hyperperi should be given to the Dominican friars for the construction of their monastery. Further, 1,100 hyperperi should be given for the construction of the bell tower of the church of Saint Mary the Great.[3] Further, let my executors spend 200 hyperperi for the roof of the church of Saint Stephen. Further, let 50 hyperperi be set aside for the furnishing of Saint Peter the Great. Further, 50 hyperperi should be given for the furnishing of the monastery of Saint Andrew in Kaštel. Further, 50 hyperperi should be given to the monastery of Saint Bartholomew for the furnishing of its church. Further, 25 hyperperi should be given for the furnishing of the monastery of Saint Simon. Further, 25 hyperperi should be given to Saint Mary in Kaštel for the furnishing of the monastery.[4] Further, 25 hyperperi should be given to Saint Thomas for the furnishing of the monastery. Further, 25 hyperperi should be given to the Lokrum Benedictines for the clothing of poor old people, and if there is anything left from that amount, I want it to be given according to the best judgment of my executors. Further, I want the house that belonged to my father to be given to Saint James in Višnjica forever, and it cannot be sold or mortgaged or exchanged in any way and under no pretext but those who serve in that church should take the rent of the house.[5] Further, I want and command that my vineyard in Župa, which borders that of Dražena, should be given to that church which I ordered to be built in the name of Annunciation, to provide a permanent income for the priest who will serve there. He should be asked to celebrate two holy masses a week for my soul. I want this priest to be of my language, and if none should be found, let him be a man of the people as best judged by those who are always competent in this matter.[6] Further, after the death of my wife Draža, I want the vineyard in Župa, in Mandaljena, to be given to my daughter Srđana. Further, after the death of my wife, I want my vineyard in Ombla to be divided in half and given to the monasteries of Saint Andrew in Kaštel and of Saint Thomas in Pustijerna. Further, I want Draža to have, over and above her dowry, 600 hyperperi and all the silver tableware and the gold earrings. Further, Bilča, the daughter of Đurađ from Kotor, should be given 300 hyperperi. Further, all the companions who were with Sir Vlaho Budačić (Bodaça) should be given 100 hyperperi. Further, Toma de Viçiano should be given 100 hyperperi for our ship which perished. Further, my executors should give 50 hyperperi for the soul of Dobre Sorkočević (Sorgo). Further, the sons of Mato Đurđević (Georgi) should be given 50 hyperperi. Further, the son of Nikola Gučetić (Goçe) should be given 25 hyperperi. Further, I want the executors of my will to give 25 hyperperi for the soul of Vita Đurđević (Georgi). Further, 4 men should go to Rome at the moment of the great pardon and each of them should be given 25 hyperperi. Further, a priest should be sent to Saint Angelo de Monte, to Saint Nicholas in Bari, and to Saint Mary del Casale near Brindisi, and for his effort he should given 20 hyperperi.[7] Further, a priest should be sent to Saint James of Compostela in Galicia, and for his effort he should be given 100 hyperperi. Further, the cloth manufacturer Çavio in Venice should be given 6 hyperperi. Further, Saint Anthony the Abbot (monastery) should be given 5 hyperperi. Further, 5 hyperperi should be given for the tithe and the *primitia*.[8] Further, the Franciscan friars should be given (money) for 1,000 holy masses. Further, the Dominicans should be given (money) for 500 holy masses. Further, all the priests of the Ragusan district should be given (money) for 500 holy masses. Further, the Lokrum Benedictines should be given (money) for 250 holy masses. Further, the Franciscans at Daksa should be given (money) for 100 holy masses. Further, the Benedictine monastery in Pakljena and the priest of Saint Stephen should be given (money) for 100 holy masses.[9] Further, don Pijero de Tascha should be given 10 hyperperi. Further, don Lovro should be given 36 hyperperi for a chalice. Further, 40 hyperperi should be given for the clothing of 50 poor persons. Further, each local or foreign repentant woman should be given 6 *grossi*. Further, each convent should be given 5 hyperperi and the convent of Saint Clare should be given 10 hyperperi. Further, for 25 hyperperi a missal should be bought for a whole liturgical year and given to the church of Saint Barbara for singing of masses. Further, I want the debt of 310 hyperperi owed to me by Nale de Cherça to be free and forgiven by God. Further, Frane and Pero de Miriçacha owe me 1,328 hyperperi and they have kept my money for 3 years, so if they want to give a gift, let them give it, and if they do not want to, let it be according to their goodwill and the notary document. Further, I want and command that all my debtors registered in my notebook be verified according to outstanding debts. Further, since I owe 50 hyperperi to the sons of Nikola de Pobrat, according to the testament of their father, let it all be settled, and to that effect there is a notary document in the name of Todor de Bodaça in the amount of 1,000 hyperperi, which should be given to those young men. Further, 50 hyperperi should be given to Jela, the mother of my son's illegitimate son. Further, Marinče Çombal should be given 5 hyperperi. Further, Andrija, the son of Tolan, should be given 10 hyperperi. Further, Paskuša, the daughter of Marino Spataro, should be given 20 hyperperi for Marko Spataro. Further, Domanja and Grga de Scrigna should be given 20 hyperperi. Further, 2 ducats should be given for a pair of stockings for each executor. Further, Frane and Petar, the Miriçacha sons, should be given 1,300 hyperperi and more than that if they wish to have it. Further, after the death of my wife Draža, if there are no heirs of mine, I want everything that is found that belongs to me to be given by the grace of God by my executors according to their best judgment. For this testament I name the following as executors and trustees: don Lovre Bratoslavov, my wife Draža, Ðivo Tudišić (de Theodoysi), Nikola Marinov de Volço, Marin Nikolin Menčetić (de Mençe), and Angelo de Maxi. Further, since my testament is finished, I want everything to stay in the hands of my executors as long as there are two of them left. Then, if the testament should come into the hands of the treasurers of Saint Mary, let them be the executors of my movables. And if all my executors should, God forbid, die, the treasurers of Saint Mary should be the executors of my whole testament. The witnesses are Domena de Sriça and Mihoje Kačić.[10]

Testament of Angelo de Leticia 5 May 1348
(fol. 2 v)
In nomine domini amen. Anno domini MIIIcXLVIII, mense madii die V intrante. Eo Angelo de Leticia faço meo testamento con bona et sana mente mia cosi acendo inprima sia dato per malcollecto perperi Vc delli quali dicti deneri sia marita de IIII orphane fili de boni homini, et sia li dati per L per ciasche duna. Ancora sia dato perperi C per lavorero delo spedale veramente che se lo spedale non se començasse a lavorare infra II anni che questi perperi C sia dato investire de poveri secondo che mellio parra ali mey pitropi. Ancora de questi denari sia lavorata una ecclesia in lo monte de Cresteç nela via Dorubla ad honore de Santa Maria anunciata, e sia lavorata lo piu tosto che porra. Anchora si vollio che tutte le mee possessioni si case come vigne e le tere et tutte massariçie de casa Draxe uxor mea in soa vita posseda et pola morte soa vada secondo chome sera scritto. Anchora si vollio che la casa mia in la quale io habitai con tucta la camera et con tucte l'arme dela casa mia et tucto fronininto (?) del mio lecto deli mia camera sia dato a Nicola filliolo del filliolo meo Radas a tempo quando sera in XVIII anni inplena etade. Veramente se lo fante fosse bono homo, et se lo fante fosse de mala foça et tenesse rea via non li sia dato niente, et questo lasso a prouedere a li pitropi mey. Et se lo fante morisse avanti de ço che per venisse a quolla etade che scripta, overo che tenesse mala via vollio che le arme et tucte cose sia vendute per mano deli mey pitropi e sia dato per deo secondo che mellio parra al mey pitropi, e la casa predicta sia data alo convento deli frari menori prope cualmente con questa condictione che nola possa vender ne donare (fol. 3) ne cambiare ne vendere per modo ne per ingegno se no atorle lofitto dela dicta casa e pregare dio per anima mea. Ancora vol-

lio che lo terreno che aço in fronte de ser Nicola de Lucharo, se non remanisse nessuno de li mey herede si vollio che sia venduto de mofina (?) vi (?) am (?) et none a nançi et de questi denari sia dato per lo lavorero de la ecclexia de Santo Blaxio la quale si lavora in plaça perperi CC. Anchora sia dato perperi Vc a frari menori per lavorero delo loco deli frari predicti. Ancora sia dato per-peri IIc a frari predicatori per lavorero dello locho. Ancora sia data perperi C per lavorero delo campanile de Santa Maria maçore. Ancora sia spesso per mano deli mey pitropi perperi IIc per la coperta della ecclesia de Santo Ste-phano. Ancora sia perperi L in fare a riconçare Santo Petro maçore. Ancora sia dato alo monestero de Santo Andrea de Castello perperi L per conçar lo mo-nastero. Ancora sia dato alo monastero de Santo Bartholome perperi L per conçare la ecclexia. Ancora sia dato alo monastero de Santo Symeone perperi XXV per conçare lo monastero. Ancora sia dato a Santa Maria de Castello per-peri XXV per conçar lo monastero. Ancora sia dato a Santo Thome perperi XXV per conçatura delo monastero. Ancora sia dato perperi XX (cassatum: V) ala Cromena per vestimento delli vetrani poveri et se alcuna cosa remanesse de questi vollio che sia dati la vmellio parra a mey pitropi. Ancora vollio che la casa che fo de mio pare aprio de vita de bachance sia data a Santo Iacobo de Vesniça prope civitate, et che non se possa vendere ne impegnare ne cambiare per modo ne per ingegnio se non l'afficto sia tolto per man de quelli che offi-çiara la dicta ecclexia. Ancora si vollio et commando che sia data la mia vigna de Breno la qual confina con Drasenuo sia data a quella ecclexia che aço com-mandato a lavorare a nome de Santa Maria anunciata, che sia per so reditaço perpetualmente a quello preuede che la officiara et sia tenuto per debito de dire due messe la semana per anima mea, et questo preuede (fol. 3 v) vollio che sia delo lignaço meo et se non se trovasse nessuno e ello sia messo alcuno de Pouelo preuede lo mellio che paresse aglli che avera a fare per questo facto perpetualmente. Ancora vollio che la vigna de Breno, la quale aperuo de Santa Maria Magdalena sia data a Serga mia fillia depo la morte de mia uxor Draxe. Ancora la mia vigna d'Ombla dopo l'obito dela mia uxore sia data la metade alo monastero de Santo Andrea de Castello e l'altra metade sia data alo mo-nastero de Santo Thoma de Pusterla. Ancora vollio che li sia donati perperi VIc a Draxe sopra la soa dota et tucto lo vascellame d'argento et çercelli d'auro. An-cora sia dato a Bilçe fillia de Çora de Cottoranio perperi IIIc. Ancora sia data a tucta la compagna che fo chon ser Blaxio de Bodaça perperi C. Ancora sia dato a Thoma de Viciano perperi C per fallo de raxon nostre. Ancora sia data per l'anima de Dobre de Sorgo perperi L chelli dea li miei pitropi. Ancora sia dato alli filli de Matheo de Çorçi perperi L. Ancora sia dato ali fillioli de Nicola de Goçe perperi XXV. Ancora sia dato per anima de Vita de Çorçi perperi XXV, et sia dati per mano deli mei pitropi. Ancora sia mandati IIII homini ad Roma quando sera la perdonança grande et sia dato perperi XXV per çaschuno. Ancora sia mandato uno preuede a Santo Angelo de Monte et Santo Nicola de Bari et a Santa Maria delo Casale in Brindiçio et sia li dati perperi XX per soa fatigha. Ancora sia mandato uno preuede a Santo Iacobo de Galiçia et sia li dati perperi C per soa fatigha. Anchora sia dato in Venesia a Çani çimator perperi XVII. Ancora sia dato ad Antoni de Barbaria perperi VI in Venexia. Ancora sia dato per decima et primitia perperi V. Ancora sia dato messe mille ali frari minori. Ancora sia dato messe Vc a frari predicatori. Ancora sia dato messe Vc a tucti li preuedi dela terra. Ancora sia dato ali monaçi preuedi della Cromena messe CCL. Ancora sia dato alli frati menori Daxa messe C. (fol. 4) Ancora sia dato a Peclina et allo preuede de Santo Stefano messe C. Ancora sia dato a don Piero de Tascha perperi X. Ancora sia dato a dom Laure per caliçe I perperi XXXVI. Ancora sia dati perperi XL investire de poveri L. Ancora sia dato per çascheduna remita dentro et de fori della terra a grossi VI. Ancora sia dato per çascheduno monastero de monache a perperis V et alle pulselle perperi X. Ancora sia comprato uno libro de messe de tucto tanto per perperi XXV et sia dato in Santa Barbara per cantare messa. Ancora vollio che lo debito che me de dare Nalede Cherça çoe perperi IIIcX et oni debito che me de dare sia libero e francho da dio e dami. Ancora me de dare Frane et Pero de Miriçacha fratelli perperi MIIIcXXVIII et sia tenuti III anni li mei denari et se me uorra fare alcuno dono et eli dea et se non vorra sia in bontade loro e una carta de notaro. Ancora vollio et commando che tucti li mei debitori che sono scritti in lo mio quaterno si de dare chome de reçevere si vollio che sia cretto (!). Ancora si sia debitore alli fillioli de Nicola de Pobratta perperi L per lo testamento de loro pare ogne raxon facta et aço I carta de notaro sopra Thodoro de Bodaça de perperi M, la quale carta sia de questi fanti predicti. Ancora sia dato perperi L ad Helena matre delo bastardo de mio fillio. Ancora sia dato a Marinçe Çombal perperi V. Ancora sia dato ad Andrea fillio de Tollano perperi X. Ancora sia data a Paschussa fillia de Marino spataro per Marcho spatero perperi XX. Ancora sia dato a Domagna et Ghergo de Scrigna perperi XXX. Ancora sia dato per çascheduno pitropi ducati II per I pitropo per uno par de calçe. Ancora sive de dare Frane et Piero fillio de Miriçacha perperi MIIIc et delo pro quanto la plaxera. Ancora vollio che doppo la morte de Draxe uxor mia non se trovasse viro nessuno delo mio rede, vollio che tucto che se trovasse delo mio facto sia data per deo secondo che mellio parra ali mey pitropi. (fol. 4 v) Et sopraço constituische pitropi et comessarii mei: don Lauro de Barattosclavo, Draxe mollier mea et Çive de Theodoysi et Nicola fillio de Marino de Volço et Marino fillio de Nicola de Mençe (cassatum: Crexe) et Angelo de Maxi. Anchora vollio che siando complito lo (cassatum: mie) testamento de tucto lo dimissorio per man deli mey pitropi fine in che durira II et poi si vegna lo testamento in mano de li thesaureri de Santa Maria chelli sia pitropi dello facto della possessione. Et se tucta li pitropi morisse ço che deo non faça sia pitropi de tucto lo meo testamento li predicti thesaureri de Santa Maria. Questi son testimoni: Domena de Sriça et Michoe Caçich.[11]

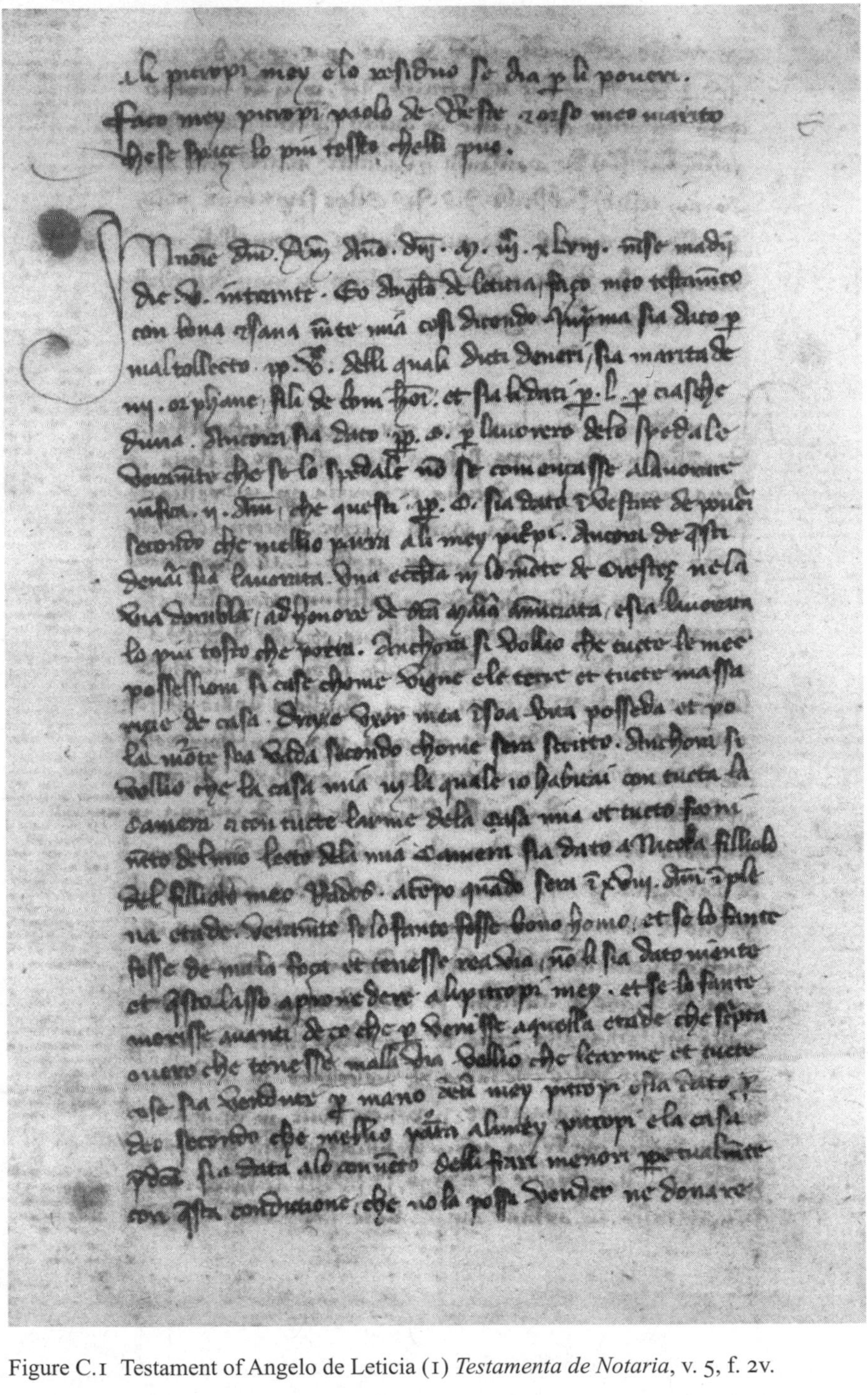

Figure C.1 Testament of Angelo de Leticia (1) *Testamenta de Notaria*, v. 5, f. 2v.

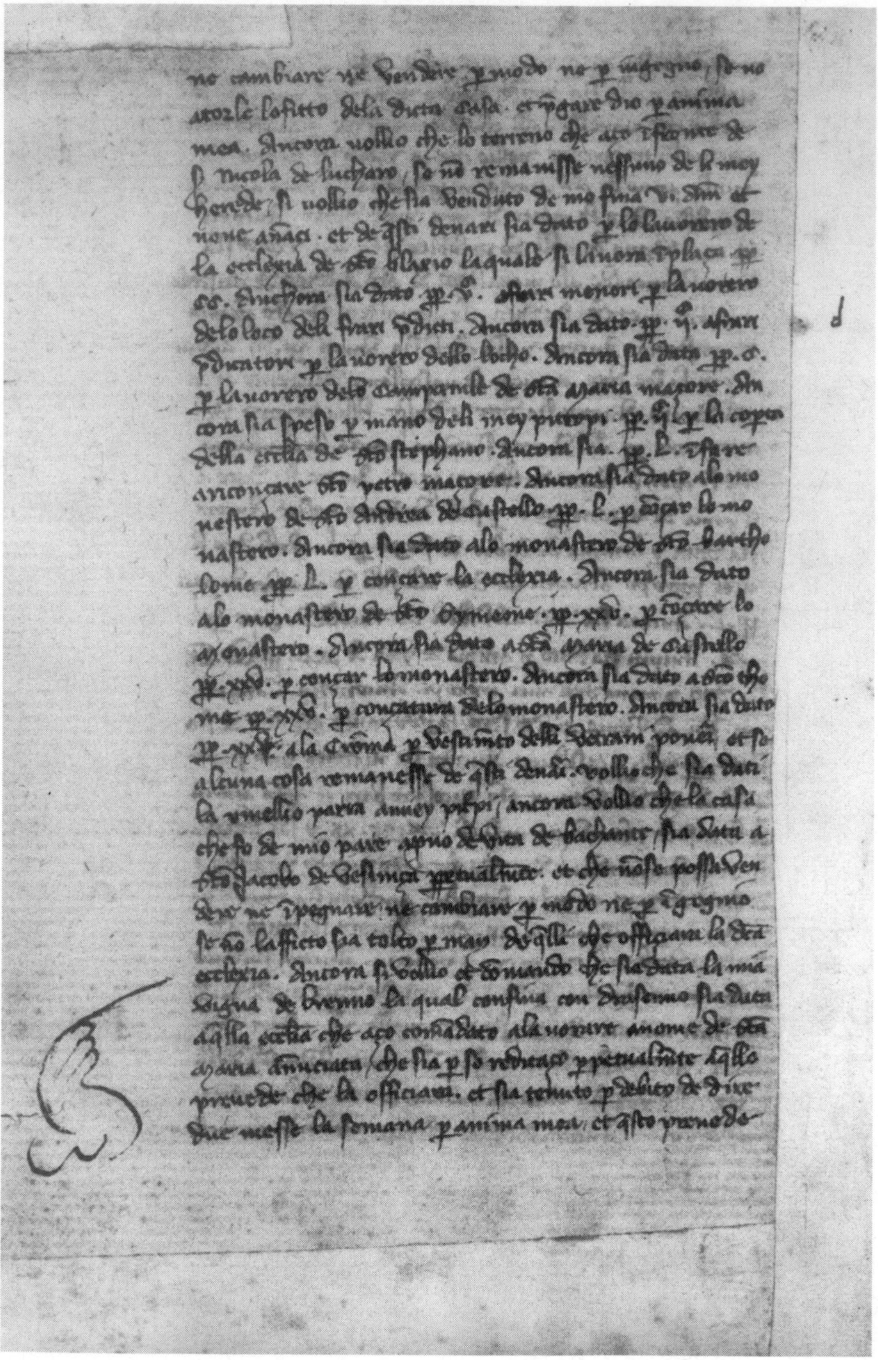

Figure C.2 Testament of Angelo de Leticia (2) *Testamenta de Notaria*, v. 5, f. 3

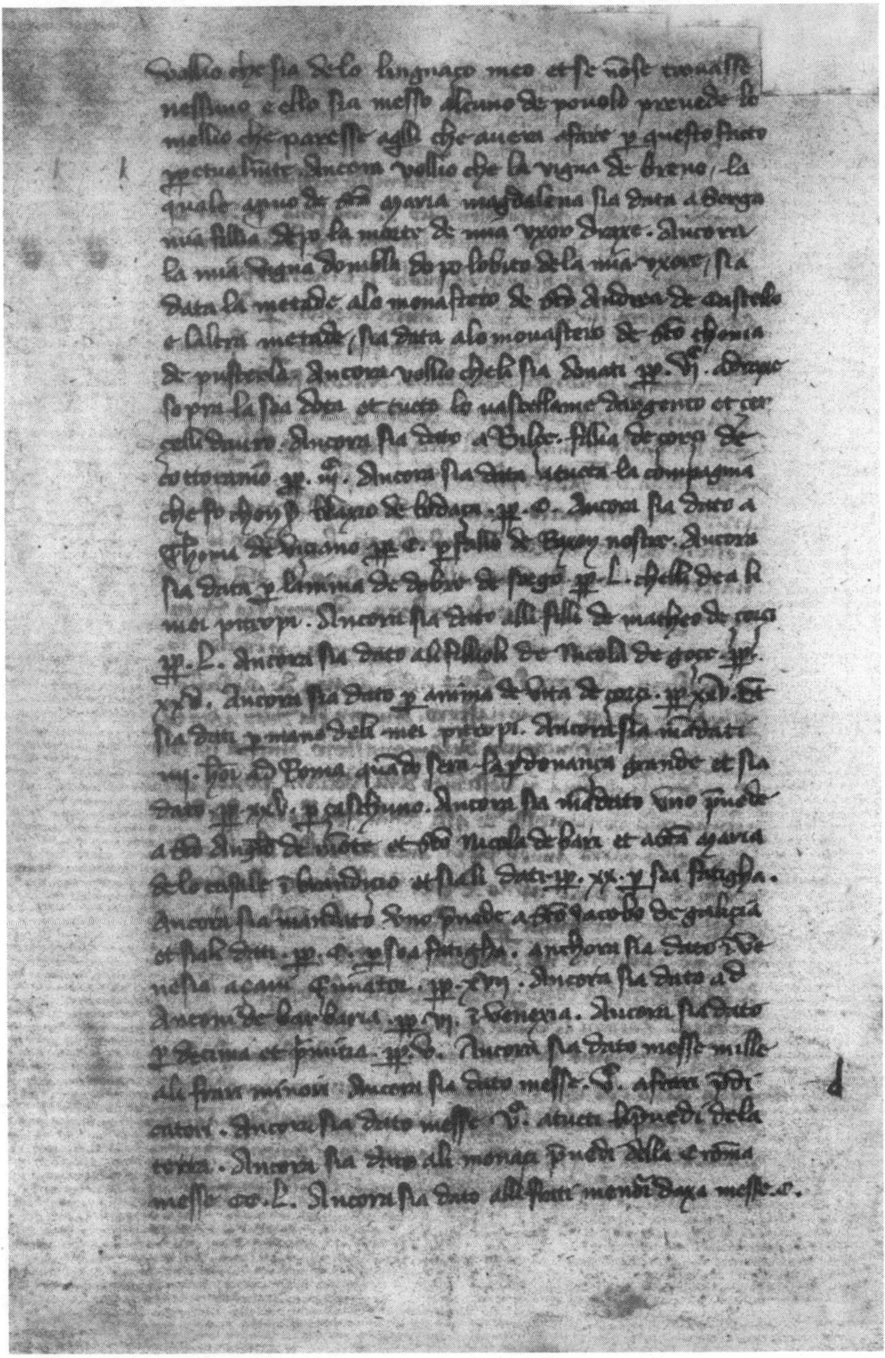

Figure C.3 Testament of Angelo de Leticia (3) *Testamenta de Notaria*, v. 5, f. 3v.

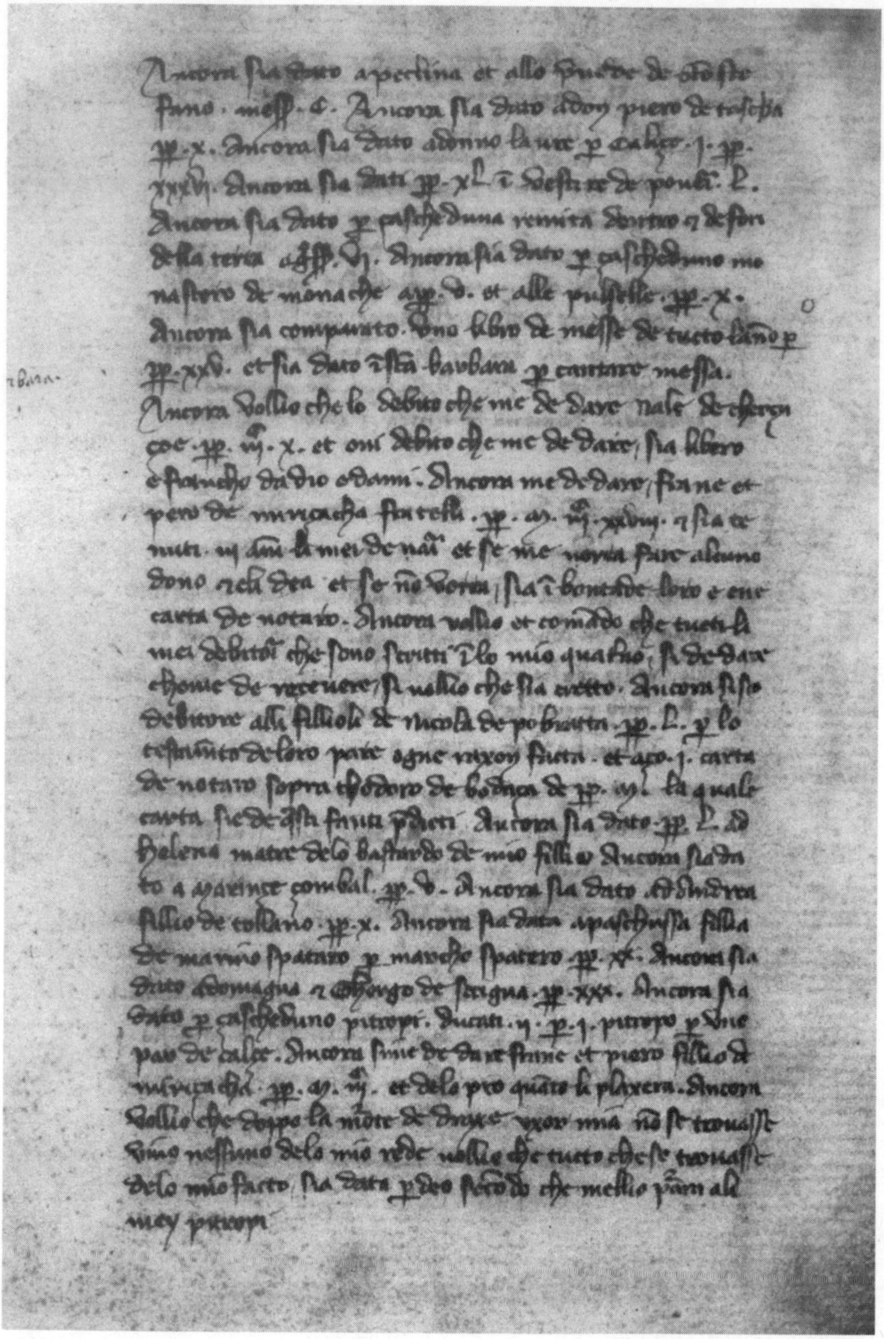

Figure C.4 Testament of Angelo de Leticia (4) *Testamenta de Notaria*, v. 5, f. 4

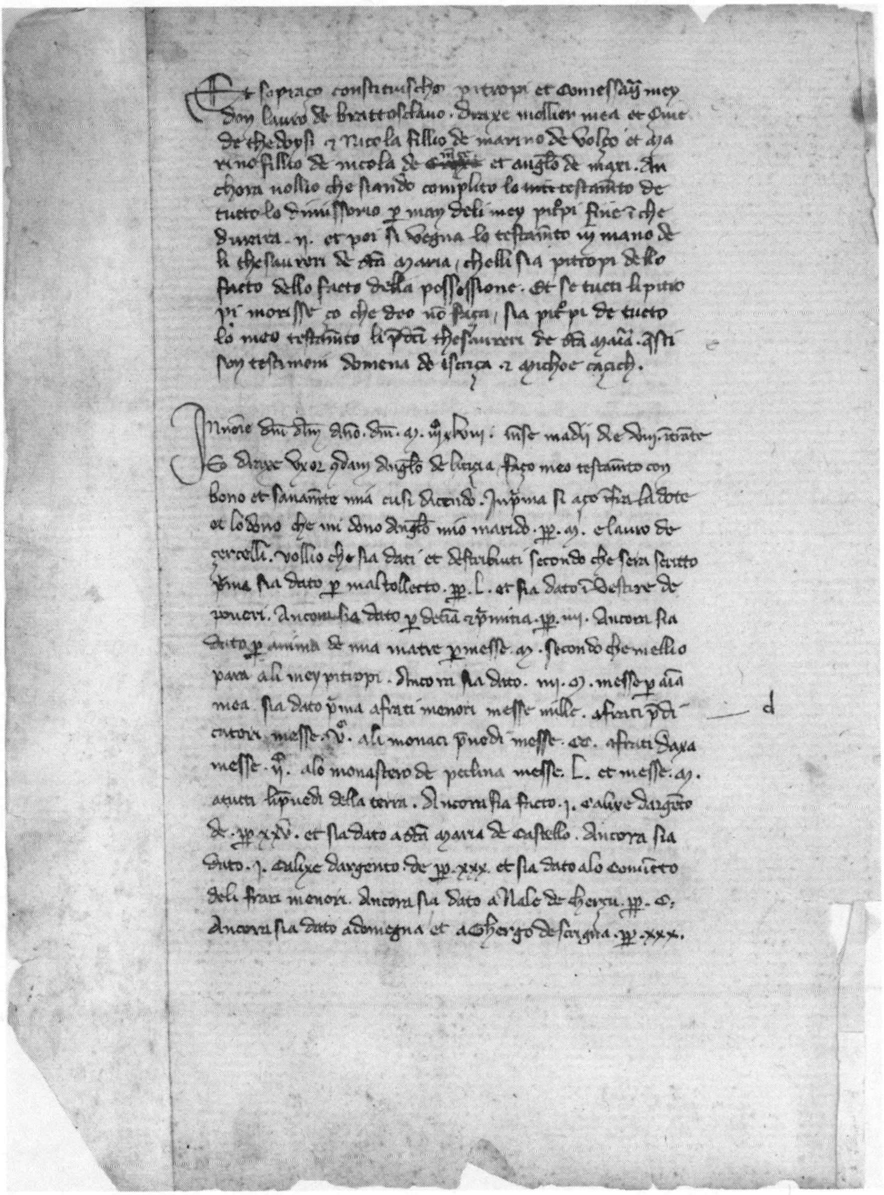

Figure C.5 Testament of Angelo de Leticia (5) *Testamenta de Notaria*, v. 5, f. 4v

Notes

INTRODUCTION

1 Grmek, "Le concept d'infection," 9–54.
2 See Appendix A for the description of the materials that can be found in the State Archives of Dubrovnik.
3 "DOM / Heu mors omnia truncas / MDXXVII crudiore peste / Vita peregrinatio / Fugaces dies." Bazala, *Pregled*, 36–7.
4 Harrison, *Contagion*, 12.
5 This book is a completely revised and substantially expanded edition of a work by Zlata Blažina Tomić published by the Institute for the Historical Sciences of the Croatian Academy of Arts and Sciences in Dubrovnik in 2007. Several new chapters, as well as an updated and enlarged bibliography, have been added to the English edition.

CHAPTER ONE

1 Diversis was the rector of the grammatical school in Dubrovnik from 1434 to 1440. Originally from Lucca, Italy, he came to Dubrovnik from Venice, attracted by a salary of 450 to 540 *hyperperi* per year and paid lodging. His work, written in the style of "city praises," very accurately documents the architecture, political system, and the customs of fifteenth-century Dubrovnik. Diversis, *Opis*, 43–58; 143–54.
2 Diversis, *Opis*, 91, 174; 85, 170; 131, 200.
3 See *Tajna diplomacija u Dubrovniku u XVI. stoljeću.*
4 Diversis, *Opis*, 120; 193.
5 Janeković-Römer, *Okvir*, 9.
6 The diplomatic correspondence and laws such as the Statute, *Liber viridis*, *Liber croceus*, and others were written in classical or mediaeval Latin. This was the language of official usage. *Materno linguagio* or the Croatian mother tongue was spoken by all the social classes in the city and on the territory of the Ragusan Republic. Until the end of the fifteen century, the patricians also used *lingua vetus Ragusea* or *lingua latina Ragusea*, the age-old local Romance speech. Archival records show that the Croatian language, *in idyomate materno* or *dalmatico* was also spoken in the Councils in the sixteenth century (Janeković-Römer, *Okvir slobode*, 343–4; Janeković-Römer, "Gradation," 118–19). When talking about

their local Romance speech, Diversis notes that the Ragusans speak a language that "we the Latins" cannot understand: *bread* is *pen*, *father* is *teta*, *house* is *chexa*, *to do* is *fachir* (Diversis, *Opis*, 72–3; 161). About the development of the Croatian language in Dubrovnik, see also Harris, *Dubrovnik*, 247–9.

7 Foretić, *Povijest*, 1:31–6; Krekić, *Dubrovnik in the 14th*, 115; Harris, *Dubrovnik*, 27–32, 247–8.

8 "Freedom could designate the autonomy under the protection of royal power, or, the very sovereignty of the city state; it could mean free life under republican institutions, or, the institutions themselves, or, the Republic itself." Kunčević, "On Ragusan *Libertas*," 68–9; Janeković-Römer, *Okvir*, 21.

9 Diversis, *Opis*, 65; 156.

10 Razzi, *La storia di Raugia*, 121–5; Krekić, "La navigation," 129–30; Carter, *Dubrovnik*, 9; Harris, *Dubrovnik*, 19–21.

11 Lučić, "Najstarija zemljišna knjiga," 57–64; Marinković, "Territorial," 7–23.

12 Beritić, "Stonske utvrde," 297–354; Beritić, "Stonske utvrde 2," 71–152.

13 Foretić, *Povijest*, 1: 95–9, 123; Harris, *Dubrovnik*, 43–58; Marinović, "Pravni," 277–96; Dabelić, "Samostan," 297–315.

14 Diversis, *Opis*, 119–20; 193.

15 Kaznačić-Hrdalo, "Dioba i ubikacija," 19–22; Kurtović, "Motivi," 117–18; Zovko, "Metode," 30–43.

16 Diversis, *Opis*, 120; 193; Krekić, *Dubrovnik in the 14th*, 54.

17 Obad, Dokoza, and Martinović, *Južne granice*, 1–104.

18 Mitić, "Imigracijska politika," 133–44; Mitić, *Dubrovačka država*, 52–3.

19 Šundrica, "O darovima u dubrovačkoj diplomaciji," 427; Hrabak, *Izvoz žitarica iz Osmanlijskog carstva*, 531; Stulli, *Povijest Dubrovačke Republike*, 59; Krivošić, *Stanovništvo Dubrovnika*, 51; Vekarić, "The Population of the Dubrovnik Republic," 7–28; Vekarić, *Vlastela*, 1: table 39, p. 145, 224–320; Harris, *Dubrovnik*, 290.

20 Constantine VII Porphyrogenitus (909–959), the Byzantine emperor and historian, states that Dubrovnik was founded in the seventh century by fugitives from the destroyed Epidaurum (nowadays Cavtat) fleeing north. Constantine VII Porphyrogenitus, *De administrando imperio*, 128; Novak, *Povijest*, 1–84; Harris, *Dubrovnik*, 23–5; Carter, *Dubrovnik*, 39–45.

21 It seems that the harbour of Dubrovnik, situated forty nautical miles north of Budva, and forty-five miles south of Lumbarda on the island of Korčula, was the logical stopover between the two as it represented the distance covered in one day of navigation in Roman times. Ničetić, *Povijest*, 67–74.

22 It was a basilica – with a nave and two aisles, one apse, a dome – that was demolished in the 1667 earthquake. In the vicinity, on Bunićeva poljana, a defence wall, consisting of late Roman and early mediaeval levels, probably from the sixth century, was discovered. Coins from third century BC were also recovered at this site (Stošić, "Research," 326–35; Žile, "Archaeological Findings," 73–92). See also Harris, *Dubrovnik*, 27–9, 221; "Novije znanstvene spoznaje," 5–275.

23 Our Lady of Sigurata, name derived from *Transfiguratio Christi*. Peković and Žile, *Ranosrednjovjekovna crkva Sigurata*, 1–40.

24 Lučić, "Povijest," 6–139.

25 Krasić and Razzi, *Povijest*, 22–5; Foretić, *Povijest*, 1:17–31; Klaić, *Povijest Hrvata u ranom*, 335; Harris, *Dubrovnik*, 41.

26 To determine the size and the exact appearance of the church, Željko Peković used computer reconstruction of sculpted stone fragments, ornamented with typical Croatian lacework from the tenth century. The author claims that the church was renovated and refurbished for the investiture in 998 of Vital Gučetić (Goze), the first Ragusan archbishop. When the archbishop was given metropolitan authority in 1022, a new cathedral was built. Peković's findings demonstrate that the church of St Peter the Great was a building of stunning beauty with the largest amount of stone ornamentation in an early mediaeval church anywhere in Dalmatia, or, for that matter, in Europe (Peković, "Prva katedrala"). See also Peković, *Crkva Sv. Petra Velikog.*

27 Foretić, *Povijest,* 1:33.

28 "Da Stagno a Raguso, o come altri dice, Ragusah (Ragusa) trenta miglia. Sono Dalmati che hanno navi da corso, gente prode e risoluta. Questa e ultima citta della Croazia" (El Idrisi, *Libro del re Ruggero,* 108; qtd. in Lučić, "Povijest," 65). El Idrisi lived at the court of the Norman ruler in Palermo.

29 Rastić, *Chronica,* 52–74; Tadić, "Dubrovnik," 633–5; Krekić, *Dubrovnik in the 14th,* 12–5; Carter, *Dubrovnik,* 74; Harris, *Dubrovnik,* 38–9.

30 The purpose of the Statute was to "harmonize discrepancies, suppress superfluities, fill in omissions, elucidate obscurities and confusions, so that nothing superfluous, obscure, insignificant or captious should remain in them." The first book specifies the duties of the count and his vicar, the treasurers of St Mary, the archbishop, and the guards as well as various types of dues to which they were each entitled. The second book records the oaths and salaries of state officials. It includes salaries prescribed for diplomats in various cities with which Dubrovnik maintained trade relations. The third contains the law of civil procedure and determines the rules for court cases between Ragusans and the citizens of other Dalmatian cities. The voluminous fourth book deals in a particularly systematic way with laws of marriage, including family and inheritance laws. The fifth defines property rights, building laws, and land tenure. The sixth constitutes the criminal code and contains miscellaneous regulations including the illegal import of wine (*Statut grada Dubrovnika,* 81). By the wealth of its content, the Statute of 1272, one of the oldest documents of an Eastern Adriatic commune, is one of the most valuable documents not only in Croatia but in all of Europe (Prlender, *Crkva,* 231).

31 *Knjiga odredaba,* 3–8.

32 Ragusans had a tendency to name their law books according to the colour of their cover. Thus we get *Liber viridis* (Green book), which covers the period from 1358 to 1460. Its continuation is called *Liber croceus* (Yellow book), which consists of laws from 1460 to 1803, almost until the end of the Republic. These books list regulations chronologically and are not organized by subject as was the Statute Book of 1272. Foretić, *Povijest,* 1:121–2; Carter, *Dubrovnik,* 587–91; Harris, *Dubrovnik,* 123–5.

33 On the Ragusan presence in Venice and the Venetians in Dubrovnik, see Krekić, *Unequal Rivals*; and Ćoralić, "The Ragusans in Venice," 15–57. For centuries, Venice and Dubrovnik maintained an ambivalent relationship based on thorough knowledge of each other's activities. The positive aspect of their relationship was based on everything they shared as two aristocratic republics with a strong Catholic tradition, both surrounded by autocratic neighbours and threatened by an expansionist Ottoman Empire with utterly different political, social, and

religious traditions. The negative aspect of the Dubrovnik-Venice relationship was based on a constant trade rivalry in the Adriatic and the Mediterranean. Stereotypes existed on both sides. Venice considered Dubrovnik to be a small but annoying rival with powerful friends – namely, the Ottomans and the pope – that it was better not to touch. According to Ragusan mythology, Venice was "scheming day and night to destroy their city." This is obviously an exaggerated statement but it reflects the permanent insecurity of Dubrovnik. As Dubrovnik was situated just south of its Dalmatian possessions, it was normal for Venice to remain interested in what was going on in that city. However, on several occasions, Venice tried to occupy some of the Ragusan islands but without success. Kunčević, "Dubrovačka slika Venecije," 9–37.

34 This shows that membership in the Major Council was not yet compulsory for all the nobles. Foretić, *Povijest*, 1:122.

35 "The title *Ser* appeared in the fourteenth century and was used only for rare individuals of particular eminence. After 1358, this title was used for all the senators. In the fifteenth century, it was used for all the members of the Major Council. Moreover, in order to emphasize their patrician heritage, even parents called their children *Ser* (for boys) and *Donna* (for girls)." Janeković-Römer, *Okvir*, 246.

36 Rheubottom, *Age, Marriage*, 51.

37 "Nati legiptime ex his stirpibus nobiles appellantur, et non alii." Diversis, *Opis*, 65–6; 157.

38 Harris, *Dubrovnik*, 127–9.

39 At the time of the closure of the Major Council, the noble circle represented more than 40 percent of the overall population. Vekarić, "The Proportion of the Ragusan Nobility," 14.

40 Vekarić, *Vlastela*, 1:145, 225–6.

41 "Sit perpetuo privatus omnibus consiliis, officiis et beneficiis communis Ragusii." *Liber croceus, caput* 18; *Acta Consilii Maioris*, v. 12, f. 68v.

42 Other Dalmatian cities, and even Venice, were more lenient. In Venice, only the father's origin counted. In some cities, even the illegitimate sons of patricians were accepted into nobility, but in Dubrovnik, it was not the case. The Ragusans were willing to marry their daughters with patricians from Dalmatian cities because they shared common roots and culture. However, very high Ragusan dowries posed a real obstacle for patrician women from other Dalmatian cities: few fathers could afford to pay them if they wanted their daughters to marry Ragusan patricians. Janeković-Römer, *Okvir*, 69–73.

43 The patricians, in keeping with their "gentlemanly" behaviour, never mentioned this event in the deliberations of the Major Council or in any other official documents. Fully aware of the importance of their future relations with Venice, they immediately sent their envoys to the city on the lagoon to patch things up. From the letters that were written to him later, it seems that the relations with the former Venetian count remained cordial. Janeković-Römer, *Višegradski ugovor*, 87–8; Harris, *Dubrovnik*, 67.

44 Originally, the king wanted to appoint the count of Dubrovnik from among his own trusted men. Since the Ragusans wanted to avoid this at all costs, they continued negotiating after the treaty was signed. On 3 January 1359, the king granted the Ragusans the right to choose their own count as long as he was not Venetian. Janeković-Römer, *Višegradski ugovor*, 80–5; Foretić, *Povijest*, 1:131–51; Harris, *Dubrovnik*, 62–76.

NOTES TO PAGES 18-19

45 The Treaty of Višegrad is considered as one of the most important documents of Croatian history. The political union of Dubrovnik with Dalmatia and Croatia contributed in the long run to the national integration of Croatian lands. Janeković-Römer, *Višegradski ugovor*, 139–41; Klaić, *Povijest Hrvata u razvijenom*, 630; Mitić, "Kada," 487–93. See also Pešorda-Vardić, "The Crown, the King," 7–29.

46 Čizmić, *Državni grb*, 8–27.

47 To elect the rector it sometimes took many ballots over several sessions of the Major Council. Absenteeism among patricians was rampant but most members showed up to elect the rector for the month of February when the Feast of St Blaise, the most solemn state holiday of the Ragusan Republic, was celebrated. On that occasion, they wanted only the most respected candidates to be elected. Patricians older than seventy were not fined for not attending the sessions of the Major Council. Rheubottom, *Age, Marriage*, 139; Janeković-Römer, *Okvir*, 119, 127–30; *Liber viridis, caput* 465; Harris, *Dubrovnik*, 133.

48 This term was officially adopted in 1441. Foretić, *Povijest*, 1:137.

49 *Liber viridis, caput*, 459; Foretić, *Povijest*, 2:353; Mustać, "Dubrovačko human-ističko školstvo," 43; Lonza, "Na marginama," 7–32.

50 Harris, *Dubrovnik*, 196–7, 201–8. Women were mostly confined to the home. They were allowed out only to go to church. They were usually betrothed at the age of seventeen and married three years later. A marriage contract was signed between families and the amount of dowry determined but the young people barely saw each other before the wedding. The average age of men at marriage was thirty-three. Women wielded some power through their female family con-nections. On rare occasions, a woman, usually when widowed, was able to take over and manage her husband's business (Rheubottom, *Age, Marriage*, 80–4; Janeković-Römer, *Rod i grad*, 48, 55–97, 126–37; Janeković-Römer, "Noble Women," 143–6; Janeković-Römer, *Okvir*, 192–211). Concerning wedding cus-toms, see Diversis, *Opis*, 121–6; 194–7. See also Kotruljević, *Libro del arte dela mercatura*, 320–5.

51 The archival book *Speculum Maioris Consilii* (Mirror of the Major Council) is a register of all the public functions of the Republic that lists the names of all the officials elected since 1440. Since 1455, all the entrants to the Major Council and their age of entry were recorded. *Speculum Maioris Consilii*, series 21.1, v. 1 (1440–1499).

52 Rheubottom has established a list of 813 male patricians who were politically ac-tive between 1440 and 1490. The Major Council met about 50 times a year and transacted more than 250 items of business. In 1470, on average, 127 patricians per session were present. The total number of patricians, male and female, has been estimated at 1,700 in the year 1300, almost 2,000 in 1500, 1,234 in 1600, and only about 300 in 1800. Rheubottom, *Age, Marriage*, Appendix C, 175–91; Vekarić, *Vlastela*, 1: table 39, 145, 248.

53 On every occasion, the Major Council had to grant permission to the Minor Council to go ahead with the elections. Most of the officials of the Republic were elected for a year and could not be re-elected before another two years had elapsed. Rheubottom, *Age, Marriage*, 33–6, 47; Janeković-Römer, *Okvir*, 96–106; Harris, *Dubrovnik*, 134–6.

54 The inscription, *Obliti privatorum publica curate* (Forget private matters and look after public ones), stood above the entrance reminding the councillors to

put public interests first and to perform their duties honourably. Lonza, "Obliti," 25–47.

55 The positions outside the city were unpopular because they were unpleasant, boring, and brought minimal financial benefit. Ston, for example, was outright dangerous because of malaria. Several researchers have reached the conclusion that there were no truly lucrative offices in the Ragusan Republic. In contrast with Venice, the election to an office could not transform an individual's future. As a result, cheating during the elections was not widespread. Rather, the Ragusan political life was characterized by overlapping jurisdictions and multiple offices designed to disperse power. *Liber viridis, caput* 65; Lonza, "Election," 39–40; Janeković-Römer, *Okvir*, 159–69; Rheubottom, *Age, Marriage*, 39, 41.

56 For example, the rector had to be at least fifty; the guards of the fortresses were between thirty and fifty years of age. The first election to an office usually came several years after entering the Major Council. The offices reserved for young men – such as supervisor of the aqueduct, of the roads or the sewers, scribe at the customs house or officer at the mint – were meant to give young men some practical experience in government. A true *cursus honorum* existed, the sequence in which offices were held by the individuals over the course of their career. Janeković-Römer, *Okvir*, 121–7.

57 In the eighteenth century, there was another demographic crisis, and again, out of necessity, elected officials tended to be younger. However, the most prestigious officials were elected among the senators who were liable to be very old. Janeković-Römer, *Okvir*, 120.

58 Diversis points out that Ragusans of both sexes attend mass every day and are par ticularly generous in their almsgiving. Diversis, *Opis*, 91; 174.

59 "The walls are not built of stone extracted from the ground but ... from living rock carved with the greatest care and polished with the greatest attention ... Vaults in the form of an arcade rise halfway up walls in which are carved the faces of different animals. The roof is of lead. The church has three doors ... At the summit rises the high altar, covered by a beautiful ciborium on four pillars and adorned with a gorgeous altar-piece or icon of silver. Beside the altar is to be found the stone throne on which the lord archbishop sits when he hears or celebrates mass ... The whole church is paved with living rock of different colours ... All the windows, both great and small, are made of stained glass depicting the saints ... On pillars above the side aisles vaults are built, above one of which a chapel is constructed ... On the basis of all this, I could say that the chief and metropolitan church is the most magnificent and most beautiful of all" (Harris, *Dubrovnik*, 222–3). Outside the city there were the Benedictine monasteries on the islands of Lokrum and St Andrew as well as that of St James in Višnjica; the Franciscan monasteries on the island of Daksa, in Slano, at Pridvorje in Konavle, in Ombla; the Dominican Monastery of the Holy Cross in Gruž, and many others. In Dubrovnik, Diversis mentions the churches of St Blaise, Sts Peter, Lawrence and Andrew – the three martyrs from Kotor, St Stephen, and of course the churches and monasteries of the Franciscans and Dominicans (Diversis, *Opis*, 44–53; 143–9).

60 The Dominicans came to Dubrovnik in 1225, the Franciscans in 1227. The Dominicans started building their church and monastery in 1304 while the Franciscans moved inside the city walls in 1317 and then started building their complex. Both the Dominican and the Franciscan monasteries have a lovely cloister, a

marvel of Gothic-Renaissance architecture, with a fountain and a garden in the middle. The Romanesque cathedral was built upon the Byzantine basilica dating from the seventh to eighth centuries. The Romanesque cathedral was destroyed in the 1667 earthquake and has been rebuilt as a Baroque church. The original Church of St Blaise was situated near the location of the St Clare convent and the Pile gate. After the 1348 plague pandemic, it was rebuilt in its current location in the centre of the city as a votive church against the plague. That church was damaged in the 1667 earthquake but was repaired. It burned down on 24 May 1706 and was rebuilt in the Baroque style by the Venetian architect Marino Gropelli and reopened in 1715. At the end of the sixteenth century there were forty-seven churches, two monasteries, and eight convents in Dubrovnik. Ostojić, "Benedikt-inci," 113–83; Ničetić, "O otoku," 339–64; Lupis, "Benediktinci," 317–37; Pejić, "Zapadno," 669–86; Žile, "Kameni," 445–515; Peković, "Nastanak," 517–76; Harris, *Dubrovnik*, 456n68; Razzi, *La storia*, 76, 123, 128, 139–45, 160, 173–5.

61 Kunčević, "Retorika," 191–204.

62 Janeković-Römer, "Gradation," 125–6.

63 Wherever the Ragusan merchants established their colonies in the Balkan hinterland, they also built their churches and brought their priests as well as Dominican, Franciscan, and Benedictine friars from Dubrovnik. They thus maintained a Catholic presence on the Ottoman occupied territories. Furthermore, they cooperated closely with the Franciscan friars of Bosnia and often defended their rights as well as those of the Catholics of Bosnia at the Porte in Istanbul. Molnár, *Le Saint-Siège*, 50–8, 126–32, 136–9.

64 In the tenth century, the archbishop played an important role in the life of the commune of Dubrovnik. At the beginning of the eleventh century, a balance of power existed between secular and ecclesiastical authorities. Soon after that, the power tilted toward secular authorities. Prlender, *Crkva*, 310–11.

65 The archbishop was entitled to certain revenues from the Ragusan merchant ships that transported grain or salt. He was also entitled to a part of the fish caught around Lastovo and Korčula but his share was not big – it was equal to a share of one sailor on those ships. It is impossible to ascertain what his income was but it is known that many candidates declined the honour because of insufficient income. Prlender, *Crkva*, 234–5.

66 Moreover, in 1303, the Minor Council and the Venetian count imposed on the Benedictine monastery on Lokrum three procurators and a lawyer. In 1313, the Minor Council decided that no one was allowed to lease land from a monastery without it being first evaluated by two expert witnesses. Prlender, *Crkva*, 246, 251–6.

67 Prlender, *Crkva*, 309–11.

68 *Liber viridis, caput* 129; *Annales Ragusini Anonymi item Nicolai de Ragnina*, 233.

69 Janeković-Römer, *Višegradski ugovor*, 101–2.

70 Diversis, *Opis*, 85; 170.

71 Janeković-Römer, *Okvir*, 211–12; Harris, *Dubrovnik*, 220–3.

72 In the sixteenth century, the Republic even went as far as undertaking a diplomatic action in the Vatican in order to obtain from the pope the right to limit the nun's dowry to ninety *hyperperi*. Such limitations dealt a heavy blow to the nuns' already low living standard. Janeković-Römer, *Okvir*, 204. ·

73 After the age of twelve, a daughter's consent was necessary. A girl could also

enter the convent without the consent of her father who had to give his daughter "a nun's dowry," which was usually very little – her bed, her clothes, her prayer book, and not much else. In his testament, he could leave his daughter living in the convent anything he wanted. However, that right was thwarted in the first half of the fourteenth century when the Councils decided that monks and nuns could not inherit real estate (Prlender, *Crkva*, 239–49). In 1426, the Major Council reduced the nun's dowry to ten hyperperi (*Liber viridis, caput* 209). The convents were overcrowded with girls who had no desire for religious life. The convent was usually the solution for the patrician father who could not afford a dowry, especially if he had several daughters. In fifteenth-century Dubrovnik, the standard dotal sum was 2,600 hyperperi. Of that sum, 1,000 hyperperi was designated for the bride's clothing and jewellery. A further 1,600 hyperperi went to the husband who had the use of this money but the capital was to keep the widow and provide for her heirs. This sum was sufficient to support the widow in food and necessities for 32 years, obtain the leasehold on over 50 shops or houses, or commission 37 boats and the services of 185 sailors for voyages (Rheubottom, *Age, Marriage*, 82–3; Janeković-Römer, *Okvir*, 204–5.

74 Janeković-Römer, *Okvir*, 215–17).

75 Janeković-Römer, "Nasilje," 35–9; Janeković-Römer, "Noble Women," 158–9.

76 A young man entering priesthood could still inherit his share of property from his parents. His share was equal to the share of his brothers, and the parents were allowed to leave him a gift of not more than fifty hyperperi. Young men entering the monastery had to write a will but they were not allowed to leave any real estate to the Church. In the 1340s, it was decided that young men entering the mendicant orders of St Francis or St Dominic could not inherit any real estate. In 1408, it was decided to elect three procurators, one each for the Franciscans, the Dominicans, and the convent of St Clare. From then on, the treasuries of the monasteries would have three keys, two to be held by the procurators, and one to be held in the monastery. Prlender, *Crkva*, 252–6.

77 In 1333, the number of treasurers was increased from two to three. Since 1500, instead of being elected for life, the treasurers served for a three-year period. In 1512, this period was extended to five years. From the sixteenth century, the size and the number of trusts forced the treasurers to assemble once a week and decide on the distribution of charitable funds. Buklijaš and Benyovsky. "Domus Christi," 82–6, 106; Janeković-Römer, *Okvir*, 213; Vojnović, "Državni rizničari," 1–101.

78 It took on average 24.5 years to be elected procurator of the convent of St Clare, 26.2 years to become procurator of the Dominican monastery, 29 years to become procurator of the Church of St Blaise, and 35.8 years to occupy the position of the procurator of the Hospedal Grande, while it took only 33.1 years to be elected rector of the Republic. Rheubottom, *Age, Marriage*, 45–6.

79 Prlender, *Crkva*, 291; *Liber viridis, caput* 338.

80 Diversis, *Opis*, 49; 146.

81 Janeković-Römer, *Okvir*, 223.

82 Janeković-Römer, *Okvir*, 213–18; Vojnović, "O državnom ustrojstvu," 24–67; Vojnović, "Crkva i država," I:32–142; II:1–91; Tadić, *Pisma i uputstva*, 27.

83 Lonza, *Kazalište*, 229–66. Similarly, in Venice, the relic of St Mark was taken to the doge, not to the bishop or the patriarch. The doge built the Church of St Mark as his private chapel and placed the relic in it. It seems that both in Venice and in

Dubrovnik, the government's control of the Church had its roots in the Byzantine tradition (Lane, *Venice*, 88, 394).

84 Čremošnik, "Dubrovački pečati," 32–7; Harris, *Dubrovnik*, 131. In the eighteenth century, the white flag with the inscription LIBERTAS (freedom) was used (Foretić, *Povijest*, 1:151).

85 The Ragusan Republic revered St Blaise and avoided erecting a monument to any of its citizens. Miho Pracat (ca 1522–1607), the ship captain from Lopud, is the only Ragusan citizen who has been honoured with a bronze bust that stands in the courtyard of the Rector's Palace. This is because he left all of his considerable fortune to the Republic and was a generous contributor to many charities during his life. Kisić and Lupis, *Miho Pracat*, 37–80; Harris, *Dubrovnik*, 195.

86 For the feast day of St Blaise, the most important religious and state holiday, several patricians were elected to guard the relics during the celebration and ensure their security. The feast day of St Blaise started with the deafening noise of firing cannons, beating drums, and ringing of church bells heard in the early morning. The celebration included the vigil on 2 February, a military parade, a religious procession, and solemn high mass in the cathedral on the morning of 3 February and popular entertainment in the afternoon. Lonza, *Kazalište*, 364–83.

87 "St Blaise is the defender of Ragusan freedom sent by God. He is the leader of the celestial army that defends the walls of Dubrovnik. According to the rhetoric used by the Ragusan diplomats in the fifteenth century, the very survival of the city became the miraculous proof of "God's mercy," which protects the city like the most powerful shield against "deceitful Venetians," "evil Patarenes," and "Turkish infidels" who are scheming day and night to destroy the Republic." Kunčević, "O dubrovačkoj," 37, 40.

88 According to the same logic, the Major Council decided in 1451 that the rector could, if he wished, personally carry the relics of St Blaise in the procession. In other words, he was allowed to take them from the hands of the archbishop. Janeković-Römer, "Public Rituals," 20.

89 "On the feast day of St Blaise in 1588, 111 relics of saints, mounted in silver, were brought to the cathedral. More of them were available but there were no monks to carry them. Many of these relics were apparently procured by Ragusan merchants who had bought them from the Ottomans on the occupied territories of Bosnia. Although the relics were held in churches, senior senators insisted on keeping the key for them. It is said that when the Florentines asked the Ragusan Senate to give them the arm of St John the Baptist held in the Dubrovnik cathedral, the Senate replied that Dubrovnik, situated on the border with the infidels, needed those relics much more than Florence, which is not in such danger, which lives content and secure in peace, and which enjoys the protection of count Cosimo, a wise and devout ruler." Razzi, *La storia*, 176–8.

90 Two to three hundred armed soldiers took part in the military parade. It was included not only to make the feast day of St Blaise more solemn but also to show military readiness to defend the territory of the Republic. Mitić, "Organizacija," 113.

91 Diversis, *Opis*, 93–4; 175–7; Razzi, *La storia*, 135–9; Foretić, *Povijest*, 1:48; Belamarić, "Sveti Vlaho," 703–31; Janeković-Römer, "Public Rituals," 14–22; Janeković-Römer, *Okvir*, 374–7; Lonza, *Kazalište*, 357–83; Kunčević, "O dubrovačkoj," 36–40; Harris, *Dubrovnik*, 237–41.

92 Because of the distance from the city, this arrangement suited the government.

Krekić, *Dubrovnik, a Mediterranean Urban Society, 1300–1600*; See also Voje, *Poslovna uspešnost*.

117 In the fourteenth century, the Ragusans built more than 120 new trade ships and the whole fleet had more than 2,700 mariners. In the fifteenth century, the merchant fleet continued to grow in number and size reaching its peak tonnage in the sixteenth century. At that time the total value of the Dubrovnik fleet was about 675,000 to 700,000 ducats. Luetić, "Dubrovačka međunarodna," 67; Luetić, "Dubrovački galijun," 130; Tadić, *Španija i Dubrovnik*, 32–3; Tadić, "Organizacija," 27–33; Foretić, "Dubrovnik," 267; Vekarić, S., "Dubrovačka trgovačka flota," 427–32; Tadić, "Le port de Raguse," 9–20.

118 A variety of ships was built in Dubrovnik: a *grip* was a smaller merchant ship that had a reputation of being very fast; a *caravel* and a *brigantine* were larger while the carrack, also called *nava* or galleon, was huge. At its peak, in the sixteenth century, the Ragusans probably owned a merchant fleet similar in tonnage to that of Venice (Vekarić, "Vrste," 19–42; Vekarić, *Naši jedrenjaci*, 261; Luetić, *Pomorci i jedrenjaci*, 227–9; Lane, *Venice*, 381–4; Harris, *Dubrovnik*, 164). On 18 September 1577, Serafino Razzi went to visit a huge Ragusan ship docked at Vasto in Italy that had a crew of 140 and carried 1,900 kilograms of grain. He admired its size, design, and equipment. He also mentions that Ragusan ships navigate in almost all the inhabited parts of the world (Razzi, *Viaggi in Abruzzo*, 240–3; Razzi, *La storia*, 182).

119 The carrack had a high forecastle and stern castle, a very big square mainsail on the main mast, a square topsail above the crow's nest, a square sail on a mast rising from the forecastle, and one or two lateen-rigged masts aft. Luetić, "Dubrovački galijun," 129–41.

120 A considerable expatriate community of Ragusans lived in London. However, in the 1540s, this vigorous trade was abruptly cut off because of insecurity of the sea route caused by wars and a prohibition imposed by England on the export of wool via Flanders. This prohibition concerned the Italians and included the Ragusans. The Ragusans protested but to no avail. Then, on 28 January 1558, the Ragusan government wrote a protest note to Queen Mary Tudor, which the Ragusan merchants in London were supposed to deliver. They were instructed to say to the Queen that they are not Italian, that their homeland is on the other side of the Adriatic and that their language is as different from Italian as is Italian from English. Foretić, *Povijest*, 2:44–5; Harris, *Dubrovnik*, 169–70.

121 Lentić, "Zlatarstvo," in *Zlatno doba*, 384, 389; Kisić, "Pomorska," 242–9; Kisić, *Zavjetne slike*, 5–14; Lupis, "Zavjetne," 230–4.

122 To reduce the financial risk, the ownership of the ship was divided by means of *karats*, which represented a share of 1/24. The ownership of the cargo could be divided the same way. Both ships and cargo could be insured and the Ragusans launched a dynamic maritime insurance business. Harris, *Dubrovnik*, 165–6, 179.

123 The trade treaty with Messina was signed in 1283 and the first consulate was established there in 1390. By the end of the sixteenth century, there were eleven consulates in Sicily, among them in Syracuse (1390), Trapani (1475), Agrigento (1504), Milazzo (1511), and Castellamare (1574). The consuls were elected among the most eminent people in Dubrovnik. In the fourteenth century, they were elected by the Minor Council and, later on, by the Senate. Not only did the consuls have full control of the Ragusan ships in their ports, but they also served

as judges in cases of misunderstanding among sailors and merchants. The consul did not have a salary but he collected from the ships a consular tax, based on the value of the merchandise imported or exported. It was his duty to report to the Ragusan government the value of the cargo of all Ragusan ships. The authorities used this information for tax purposes. There were consulates on the western side of the Adriatic in many port cities, including Ancona, Bari, Barletta, Crotone, Otranto, and, of course, Venice, where there was a large Ragusan expatriate community. Other consulates were in the ports of Alexandria, Istanbul, Malta, and Salonika. Sometimes the consuls were local people. Among them were honorary consuls in Alicante, Barcelona, Cadiz, Cartagena, Malaga, Tarragona, Valencia, and on the islands of Mallorca, Menorca, and Ibiza. Mitić, "Dubrovački konzularni predstavnici," 99–102; Mitić, "Prilog proučavanju," 113–19; Stuard, *A State*, 206; Mitić, "Dubrovački konzulati," 598.

124 For a map of Ragusan consulates in the sixteenth century, see Mitić, *Dubrovačka država*, 128–9. Foreign countries also had their representatives in Dubrovnik (Mitić, "Predstavnici stranih država," 382–93; Lonza, *Kazalište vlasti*, 159–65).

125 In 1386–87, an arch was built for each berth. At the end of the fifteenth century, the arches were closed off with a wall for the protection of the warships housed inside. Whenever a vessel was launched, the wall of the archway had to be knocked down and then rebuilt when the ship returned into its berth. Nowadays, the Arsenal houses the City Café under its three remaining arches. One was sealed with a wall. Harris, *Dubrovnik*, 294.

126 Krekić, "Le port," 655, 659–61.

127 In 1409, a Small Arsenal for three ships was added. Ničetić, *Povijest*, 140; Harris, *Dubrovnik*, 278; Prijatelj, *Dubrovačko slikarstvo*, 22–6, illustrations nos. 36, 39, and 40.

128 Prijatelj, *Dubrovačko slikarstvo*, 23–4, illustration nos. 39 and 40. Diversis describes the Arsenal "with beautiful triremes and biremes" and mentions how impressed he was with the speed with which the Ragusans readied their trireme warships in times of need (Diversis, *Opis*, 55, 150; 100–6, 180–3).

129 In just two and a half years, a northern wall, twenty-two metres high and four metres thick, was built between the eastern gate of Ploče and the Minčeta Tower. Harris, *Dubrovnik*, 291.

130 Blažina Tomić, *Uloga javnih zdravstvenih službenika*, 48–53.

131 The archival series *Acta Turcarum*, held in the State Archives of Dubrovnik, contains 182 receipts of the tribute paid to the Ottomans by Dubrovnik from 1458 to 1804. Since the Ragusan tribute was considered a personal gift to the sultan – that is, to his private treasury – almost all of the original documents are in the form of sultan's edict or firman. The transcripts and translations of the original, mainly into Croatian, and less often into Italian, are also preserved. The receipts were transcribed by the scribes at the Porte or by the dragomans of the Ragusan Republic who also provided the translations. The receipt contains the following information: type and amount of money delivered as tribute; names of the Ragusan patricians who delivered it; the period covered by the payment; date of payment; place and date of the receipt. In 1442, Dubrovnik paid the equivalent of 1,000 gold ducats in silverware; in 1458, 1,500 gold ducats in cash; in 1481, 12,500 gold ducats; from 1703, it paid the tribute every third year; from 1804, the Ottomans agreed to be paid every five years. Miović, "Turske priznanice," 53–77;

Biegman, *The Turco-Ragusan Relationship*, 126–50; See also Miović, *Dubrovačka Republika u spisima osmanskih sultana*.

132 Prlender, "Diplomacija," 186.

133 Janeković-Römer, "Gradation," 129; Janeković-Römer, "O poslaničkoj," 193–204.

134 The Ragusan envoys travelled by land, usually via Niš, Sofia, and Adrianople (nowadays Edirne) to Istanbul. This risky journey took about a month. Their departure from Dubrovnik was a solemn affair. After attending mass, they greeted the rector and the Minor Council, and on their way out of the city, they turned around and bowed towards the Church of St Blaise, asking for the blessing of their patron saint on their difficult journey. Once they left the territory of the Republic, they faced many trials, including brigands and robbers on the road, difficult terrain and uncomfortable inns, and plague-infected areas (Miović, *Dubrovačka diplomacija*, 21–80). Concerning the protocol of departure of the *poklisari* from Dubrovnik, see Lonza, *Kazalište vlasti*, 152–9; Razzi, *La storia*, 181–2.

135 The dragomans were highly trained professionals who had studied Ottoman Turkish, Arabic, and Persian at the expense of the Ragusan state. For a year or two, they were trained in Dubrovnik by an Armenian or other Christian subject from Istanbul, a salaried employee of the government. Later, they continued their studies for several years in Adrianople (today Edirne) and finally in Istanbul. Mastering the art of sophisticated conversation was an important goal of Ragusan diplomacy because the negotiations often turned into competitions in erudition and oratory skills. Miović-Perić, "Dragomans," 81–94; Miović-Perić, "Dnevnik," 93–8, 114; Miović, "Diplomatic Relations," 192–8; Efendić, "Dragomani," 158–61; Krizman, *O dubrovačkoj*, 118–26.

136 The Chancery clerks translated the Ottoman documents into Croatian, or sometimes into Italian, assisted the Ragusan authorities with writing letters to various Ottoman dignitaries, and were responsible for the state correspondence with the neighbouring rulers. The clerks in the Slavic Chancery transcribed texts from "Slavic letters [cyrillic] into Latin alphabet" and they also composed documents in the Slavic languages. Čremošnik, "Postanak i razvoj," 73–84.

137 Miović and Selmani, "Turska kancelarija," 235–40.

138 Even when Ottoman representatives in Bosnia were persons of Bosnian origin, the mastery of the dragomans was still crucial because agreements were written in Turkish that only the dragomans could verify. Miović, "Beylerbey of Bosnia," 39–44, 54–8; Šundrica, "O darovima," 53–7.

139 Many of the gifts – marzipan, fruit syrups, and sweets ("confetti") – were prepared in the pharmacies of Dubrovnik. In 1515, the Senate proclaimed the regulation against luxury. At weddings, it was forbidden to serve marzipan, made with cane sugar and almonds. However, the apothecaries were allowed to prepare it for medicinal purposes and as gifts sent by the Republic to foreign dignitaries, especially the Ottomans in Bosnia (Kesterčanek, "Iz povijesti farmacije," 250; Kesterčanek, "Roko Fasano," 268). Concerning gifts as part of foreign policy, see Lonza, *Kazalište vlasti*, 203–27.

140 Harris, *Dubrovnik*, 352; Šundrica, *Tajna kutija II*, 269–78.

141 Tadić, *Španija i Dubrovnik*, 32–3; Božić, *Dubrovnik i Turska*, 131–205, 341–4; Krekić, *Dubrovnik (Raguse) et le Levant*, 67–8; Foretić, *Povijest Dubrovnika*,

1:320–25; 2:7–48; Popović, *Turska i Dubrovnik*, 9–176; Stulli, "Dubrovačka Republika u XV i XVI stoljeću," 16–8; Stulli, *Povijest Dubrovačke Republike*, 47–66; Stulli, "Kronologija važnijih zbivanja," 283–299; Miović-Perić, *Na razmeđu*, 13–25; For relations with the Ottomans from 1684 to 1699, see Zlatar, *Between the Double Eagle*, 1–214.

142 Kunčević, "Retorika," 210; Kunčević, "Janus-faced," 110–18 .

143 Prlender, "Diplomacija," 190; Miović, "Diplomatic Relations," 189–91; Krizman, *O dubrovačkoj*, 159–64.

144 Vekarić, *Vlastela*, 1:334.

CHAPTER TWO

1 See Little, *Plague and the End of Antiquity*, xi, 3–32, 99–118.

2 Grmek, "Les conséquences," 792–4.

3 Coined in the nineteenth century by Justus F.C. Hecker, *Black Death* is the term used for the plague pandemic of 1347–50. In the fourteenth century, Ragusan and other archival sources mention the terms *prima* or *tertia mortalitas, pestilencia*, or simply *infirmitas* (illness). With time, the number of terms increases, especially in Latin: *plaga, pestis, pestilentia, febris pestilentialis, contagium pestilentiale, morbus pestiferum*; in Italian: *peste, peste bubonica, peste orientale, pestilenza, contagio, moria*; in French: *fléau, peste*; in English: pest, pestilence, plague; in German: *Plage, Pest, Pestilenz, Menschen-Pest*; in Spanish: *pest, pestilencia*; in Croatian: *kuga, čuma, morija*; in Turkish: *ta'un*; in Russian: *čuma, bubonaja čuma*. Frari, *Della peste*, 41; Skok, *Etimologijski rječnik*, 2:222; Dols, *The Black Death*, 315–16; Poljanec, *Rusko-hrvatski*, 983.

4 Le Roy Ladurie, *The Mind and Method*, 44, 62–71; Biraben, *Les hommes*, 1:156–85; Hecker, *Die Grossen Volkskrankheiten*, 21, 52–55; Benedictow, *The Black Death*, 380–4.

5 Musis, "Historia de morbo," 26–59.

6 Siegfried, *Itinéraires de contagions*, 114; Ziegler, *The Black Death*, 43.

7 Howard-Jones, "Kitasato, Yersin", 23–7; Mollaret and Brossollet, *Yersin*, 164–6.

8 It has been argued that the Black Death constitutes a major watershed in the development of Europe that brought about the transformation of society in economic, technological, cultural, and religious terms. Herlihy, *The Black Death*, 39–81.

9 The Ottomans were familiar with contagion, but did not necessarily accept it as their main etiological explanation for plague. The difficulty with the concept of contagion grew out of the larger moral and theological problem of how a merciful and benevolent God could bring upon mankind a scourge that killed one individual after another regardless or their good or evil deeds. The concept of miasma was more widely accepted. The Ottomans must have been aware of quarantine measures applied by their neighbours in the Mediterranean basin, but they first used the quarantine on their side of the border only in the nineteenth century. Shefer-Mossensohn, *Ottoman Medicine*, 173–8.

10 Miasma, meaning pollution in Greek, was considered to be a noxious vapour filled with particles from decomposed matter believed to cause diseases. Hippocrates, *Hippocratic Writings*, 78–9, 213, 260–2, 265–7; Cipolla, *Miasmas and Diseases*, 4–6; Nutton, "Humoralism," 1:281–91; Hannaway, "Environment," 295–6.

11 Grmek, "Le concept," 15; Siegel, *Galen's System*, 196–359; Temkin, *Galenism*, 124; Campbell, *The Black Death*, 44; Pelling, "Contagion/Germ Theory/Specificity," 311–15.

12 The third plague pandemic started in Canton, southern China in 1894 and quickly spread to Hong Kong. It reached Bombay in 1896 and Vietnam in 1898. In 1900, ships spread it to Honolulu, San Francisco and Sydney, Australia. At that time, bacteriological and microbiological methods had advanced to such a degree that it was finally possible to identify the plague pathogen. Alexandre Yersin, the Swiss bacteriologist from the Pasteur Institute in Paris, stationed in Vietnam, asked to be sent to Hong Kong to help fight the epidemic. After being in Hong Kong for barely five days, Yersin managed to identify the plague pathogen. On 20 June 1894, he discovered and correctly identified a rod-shaped, Gram-negative plague bacillus. Originally named *Pasteurella pestis*, in 1971, the plague pathogen was finally renamed *Yersinia pestis* in honour of its discoverer. See Mollaret and Brossollet, *Yersin*; Mohr, *Plague and Fire*; Chase, *Barbary Plague*; Eschenberg, *Plague Ports*. From 1954 to 1997, human plague was recorded in thirty-eight countries, seven of which – Brazil, Democratic Republic of the Congo, Madagascar, Myanmar, Peru, United States, and Vietnam – were affected virtually every year. From 1985 to 2003, over forty-three thousand human cases were reported to the World Health Organization by twenty-five countries. World Health Organization, *Plague Manual*, 18–25; Pollitzer, *The Plague*, 16–67.

13 Hirst, *The Conquest of Plague*, 244.

14 The proventriculus is a muscular dilatation of the foregut in most mandibulate insects. It is armed internally with chitinous (horny) teeth or plates for grinding food. These teeth act as a valve that permits blood to flow into the stomach, but it cannot escape. Hirst, *The Conquest of Plague*, 184–5; Pollitzer and Meyer, "The Ecology of Plague," 461–5.

15 Simond analyzed the fleas on the rats that had suffered from plague and the fleabites of the plague patients. When both showed the presence of the plague bacillus, he knew that he had discovered the mechanism of plague transmission from rodents to humans. Simond performed an experiment on two rats, one plague-infected and the other healthy. The cages prevented physical contact between the two rodents, but their open grillwork let the fleas hop back and forth. When the infected rat died, the fleas deserted its corpse and jumped through the bars to the healthy rat in the neighbouring cage. Within six days, the second rat died, too, its blood brimming with plague bacteria. Mollaret and Brossollet, *Yersin*, 194–5.

16 Carmichael, "Bubonic Plague," 628–31.

17 Shrewsbury, *A History of Bubonic Plague*, 5.

18 Viseltear, "The Pneumonic Plague Epidemic," 40–1; Hirst, *The Conquest of Plague*, 222; Pollitzer, *The Plague*, 424; Butler, *Plague*, 73–83; Meyer, "Pneumonic Plague," 249–61; Dennis and Campbell, "Plague and Other Yersinia Infections," 980–5.

19 Bazala, "Calendarium pestis," 55–65; Diversis, *Opis*, 116; 190. While many authors report massive population flight from infected cities, Shona Kelly Wray, basing her research on testaments of 1348 Bologna, maintains that most people stayed and continued functioning as they had always done. Wray, *Communities*, 261–4.

20 Slack, "The Disappearance of Plague," 475–6; Ell, "Immunity," 879.
21 Christensen gives Venice as an example. He claims that after 1550, when the Health Office was fully operational, Venice was spared the outbreaks that ravaged other Italian cities (Christensen, "Appearance and Disappearance of Plague," 19–21). This is not entirely true. Venice may have been spared some plague epidemics, but from 1575 to 1578 and in 1630, it was ravaged, like the rest of Italy. See Chapter 6 for the disappearance of plague from Dubrovnik.
22 Corradi, *Annali*, 3:71.
23 Cohn, *Cultures of Plague*, 181.
24 From 1740 until 1871, a military sanitary cordon existed along a thousand-mile frontier of the Austro-Hungarian Empire with the Ottoman Empire. Rothenberg, "The Austrian," 18–23.
25 George Christakos and his interdisciplinary team, for example, developed a sophisticated mathematical model of the spatial and temporal dissemination of the Black Death from 1347 to 1351 through different parts of Europe at different seasons (Christakos et al., *Interdisciplinary Public Health Reasoning*, 223, 230); Michel Drancourt and his colleagues at the University of Marseilles, including historians, archaeologists, and microbiologists, were able to recover *Yersinia pestis* DNA from the dental core of human remains identified as having died of plague in the 1720 Marseilles epidemic. They were subsequently able to recover *Yersinia pestis* DNA from the fourteenth-century mass graves of plague victims in Montpellier (Drancourt et al., "Detection of 400-year-old *Yersinia pestis* DDNANA in Human Dental Pulp," 12637–40; Raoult et al., "Molecular Identification," 12880–3; Aboudharam et al., "La mémoire des dents," 207–16; McCormick, "Toward a Molecular History of Justinianic Pandemic," 290–312). *Yersinia pestis* DNA has also been detected in the dental core of two skeletons from Aschheim, Upper Bavaria dating from the time of Justinian's plague in the sixth century (Wiechmann and Grupe, "Detection of *Yersinia Pestis* DNA," 48–55). In 2011, scientists revealed that they have sequenced the DNA of *Yersinia pestis* extracted from the dental pulp and bones of one hundred skeletons buried during the 1348 epidemic in East Smithfield plague pits in London. These results prove that Black Death was indeed caused by *Yersinia pestis* and that the genome of the bacterium is practically identical to the modern one present around the world today (Bos et al., "A Draft Genome of *Yersinia pestis*").
26 Theilmann and Cate, "A Plague of Plagues," 371–93.
27 Walløe, "Medieval and Modern Bubonic Plague," 67–8; Carniel, "Plague Today," 120–1; Ell, "Immunity as a Factor," 868.
28 The Ragusan Anonymous chronicler was probably a friar who lived in the fifteenth century while Nikola Ragnina (1494–1582) was a Ragusan patrician and author of the Annals of Ragusa. Serafino Razzi (1531–1611) was a Dominican friar from Lucca who was sent to Dubrovnik to reorganize the Dominican monastery. While in Dubrovnik, he made an effort to learn as much as possible about the city and upon his return to Lucca in 1595, published his history of Ragusa. Chroniclers usually copied some of their information from older extant documents. *Annales Ragusini Anonymi item Nicolai de Ragnina*, v–x; Razzi, *La storia*, 7.
29 Biraben, *Les hommes et la peste*, 1:54; Grmek, "Pregled," 178–84; Ravančić, *Crna smrt*, 61–220; Ravančić, *Vrijeme umiranja*, 71–134.

30 According to Nikola Ragnina, 273 patricians and 10,300 commoners perished in
    the most horrendous and most cruel plague epidemic. *Annales Ragusini Anonymi
    item Nicolai de Ragnina*, 227–8.

31 Ragusan chroniclers cite exceptionally high mortality rates for this first plague
    outbreak in Dubrovnik. Serafino Razzi reports that 173 patricians and 7,300 com-
    moners lost their lives (Razzi, *La storia*, 42). The Anonymous chronicler states
    that it was "not plague but the wrath of God" that killed 170 patricians, 300 "peo-
    ple of good repute" and 1,000 commoners (*Annales Ragusini Anonymi item Nico-
    lai de Ragnina*, 39).

32 Krivošić, *Stanovništvo Dubrovnika*, 37–8.

33 *Casata* is an enlarged nuclear family, roughly a household, with a strong sense of
    belonging. It consists of five to six members, the parents, their children, and the
    family of the first-born son. Vekarić, *Vlastela*, 1:129–37, 145, 236.

34 Ravančić, *Crna smrt*, 80–3, 117, 128–33, 180–91; Ravančić, *Vrijeme umiranja*,
    81–3.

35 Ravančić, *Crna smrt*, 196–203; Ravančić, *Vrijeme umiranja*, 122–9.

36 Stuard, *A State of Deference*, 82–7.

37 For religious practices and private devotion in Venice during the plague of 1576,
    see Preto, *Peste*, 76–89.

38 Palmer, "The Control," 280–314.

39 Testamentum Andree quondam Nicolai de Dersa (Držić), *Testamenta de Notaria*,
    v. 34, f. 56v; Testamentum quondam Petri filii quondam Blasii Nicole de Dersa,
    Testamenta de Notaria, v. 34, f. 124v–125, as cited by Lučić, "Arhivska građa o
    kugi," 55–7.

40 Raukar, *Hrvatsko*, 245–6, 338, 352–64; Janeković-Römer, "*Pro anima mea*,"
    25–33.

41 Razzi, *La storia*, 42.

42 *Testamenta de Notaria*, v. 5, f. 2v-4.

43 At the end of the fifteenth century, Džore Držić, the uncle of the famous Ragusan
    comedy writer Marin Držić (1508–1567), was abbot of the Church of the Annun-
    ciation.

44 Marshall, "Manipulating," 511–18.

45 Janeković-Römer, "Na razmeđi," 5–6; Boeckl, *Images*, 73.

46 "Et anchora vollio, che se acatti 1. crocisso, che costi perperi LXXX et che se
    metta ali frari predichatori aprono al altare grande, et anchora voilio che se acatti
    l. ancona che sia in essa designada la maestade et che sia posta soura; allo croci-
    fisso ali frari Predicatori." *Testamenta de Notaria* 10-1, v. 5, f. 9v, as cited by Ra-
    vančić, *Crna smrt*, 249–51.

47 Gamulin, *The Painted Crucifixes*, 31–2; Ivančević, *Art Treasures*, 85, 106; Clif-
    ford, "Dubrovnik," 155–6; Harris, *Dubrovnik*, 272.

48 Jeremić and Tadić, *Prilozi*, 1:68; Vekarić, *Vlastela*, 1:234.

49 The Anonymous chronicler briefly mentions that this plague outbreak, which had
    originated in Alexandria, began on 15 January and lasted for a year. Nicola Ragn-
    ina states that the outbreak began on 15 May and lasted for a year. It spread so fu-
    riously that it did not spare even half of the people in most places. It targeted
    mostly men, the rich and the young, and few women. *Annales Ragusini Anonymi
    item Nicolai de Ragnina*, 41, 233.

50 *Annales Ragusini Anonymi item Nicolai de Ragnina*, 234. In 1363, there were
    293 registered testaments (Jeremić and Tadić, *Prilozi*, 1:68).
51 *Monumenta Ragusina* 3:265.
52 *Annales Ragusini Anonymi item Nicolai de Ragnina*, 235–6. Judging by the num-
    ber of testaments for these years, 66 in 1371, 73 in 1372, 11 in 1373, and 15 in
    1374, it would seem that there were only two plague outbreaks. Unfortunately,
    this information cannot be compared with the decisions of the Ragusan Councils
    because the proceedings for the years 1368 to 1378 have not been preserved (Je-
    remić and Tadić, *Prilozi*, 1:69; Ravančić, *Crna smrt*, 210–12).
53 Jeremić and Tadić, *Prilozi*, 1:69–70; *Odluke dubrovačkih vijeća*, 188; *Annales
    Ragusini Anonymi item Nicolai de Ragnina*, 49, 241.
54 *Reformationes*, v. 30, f. 67.
55 *Reformationes*, v. 31, f. 62v–f. 63.
56 Chroniclers cite high mortality rates for 1400 that must be exaggerated. If they
    were true, no one would have remained alive in Dubrovnik. Razzi, *La storia*, 42;
    Annales Ragusini Anonymi item Nicolai de Ragnina, 54, 246.
57 According to Richard John Palmer, this is the first known Venetian attempt to
    deal with the spread of disease by contagion and is interesting in a number of
    ways. First, the whole tone of the document, with its lengthy self-justification, in-
    dicates the novelty of such action as far as Venice is concerned. Second, whilst
    Ragusa was singled out in a retaliatory way, there is no indication that other
    plague centres were similarly isolated. Palmer, *The Control of Plague*, 36.
58 Harrison, *Contagion*, 13.
59 Vekarić, *Vlastela*, 1:236.
60 *Annales Ragusini Anonymi item Nicolai de Ragnina*, 54, 248. There were 106
    testaments in 1416, 60 in 1417, and only 28 in 1418. Jeremić and Tadić, *Prilozi*,
    1:71.
61 Jeremić and Tadić, *Prilozi*, 2:28.
62 Jeremić and Tadić, *Prilozi*, 1:71–2; *Annales Ragusini Anonymi item Nicolai de
    Ragnina*, 249.
63 *Acta Minoris Consilii*, v. 4, f. 114v. On 3 April 1428, Marin Nikolin Gučetić was
    allowed to return to Dubrovnik with those two ships (*Acta Minoris Consilii*, v. 4,
    f. 151v).
64 Jeremić and Tadić, *Prilozi*, 1:72–4.
65 Providimentum et ordines Regiminis et custodie civitatis Ragusii firmati ut infra
    in consilio Rogatorum ex dubio pestifere contagionis, *Acta Consilii Rogatorum*,
    v. 4, f. 249–254v.
66 Jeremić and Tadić, *Prilozi*, 2:28.
67 Jeremić and Tadić, *Prilozi*, 1:75.
68 *Annales Ragusini Anonymi item Nicolai de Ragnina*, 252; Jeremić and Tadić,
    Prilozi, 1: 75–6; Providimentum et ordines Regiminis et custodie civitatis Ra-
    gusii firmati in consilio Rogatorum heri et hodie ob dubium pestis, *Acta Consilii
    Rogatorum*, v. 6, f. 122–128, 131, 134, 136v. There were 127 registered testa-
    ments in 1437 (Vekarić, *Vlastela*, 1:241).
69 Vekarić, *Vlastela*, 1: table 39, p. 145, 241.
70 There were 150 testaments in 1457 and only 71 in 1458. Vekarić, *Vlastela*, 1:246.
71 Jeremić and Tadić, *Prilozi*, 1:78–81.

72 Jeremić and Tadić, *Prilozi*, 1:82–4.
73 *Annales Ragusini Anonymi item Nicolai de Ragnina*, 66, 262.
74 Marshall, "Manipulating," 496.
75 Badurina, "Sakralna arhitektura," in *Zlatno doba Dubrovnika*, 325; Demori-Staničić, "Uvod," 185; Buconić Gović, *Dubrovačke crkvice*, 26–31; Lupis, "Nove spoznaje," 94–6. Sheila Barker argues that the beauty of St Sebastian's almost naked young body may have had a therapeutic effect for Renaissance viewers. Some plague tractates recommended seeking pleasure through the senses in order to stay healthy by, for example, spending time in gardens with fragrant herbs or looking at precious substances such as gold, silver, and gemstones, and wearing such substances. The author compares St Sebastian's perfect body with those precious substances and concludes that his body may have been regarded as a form of visual medicine. Barker, "Making," 123–4.
76 Boeckl, *Images*, 53; Mormando, "Introduction," 30–2.
77 Jeremić and Tadić, *Prilozi*, 1:85–90; Razzi, *La storia*, 64; *Annales Ragusini Anonymi item Nicolai de Ragnina*, 73, 266. There were 184 testaments in 1482, 159 in 1483, and only 60 in 1484 (Vekarić, *Vlastela*, 1:247).
78 Sanudo, "Odnošaji," 5:6; Hrabak, "Kuga," 25.
79 About pilgrimage see Raukar, *Hrvatsko*, 351–61; Šanjek, *Crkva*, 254–5. The chroniclers Serafino Razzi, the Anonymous, and Nikola Ragnina, all report that the plague, which was brought to Dubrovnik by the pilgrims who were returning from Rome, was not severe. The Anonymous chronicler adds that it lasted two months, and 1,500 ducats were spent from the public treasury to combat it. He notes that all the suspects were sent, under guard, into confinement at Polače on the island of Mljet (Razzi, *La storia*, 69; *Annales Ragusini Anonymi item Nicolai de Ragnina*, 83, 272).
80 Razzi, *La Storia*, 74; *Annales Ragusini Anonymi item Nicolai de Ragnina*, 98, 276.
81 Lupis, "Oltarna," 117–20.
82 Since 1968, the church has belonged to the parish of the Holy Cross and is administered by the Dominican friars. The authors wish to thank Dr Vinicije Lupis, head of the Pilar Institute in Dubrovnik, for providing them with the valuable data pertaining to the history of the Church of the Annunciation.
83 Jeremić and Tadić, *Prilozi*, 1:96; *Acta Consilii Rogatorum*, v. 39, f. 18–18v.
84 *Testamenta de Notaria*, v. 34–5. This information was graciously provided to the authors by Mr Zoran Perović, archivist at the State Archives of Dubrovnik.
85 The *Libro deli Signori Chazamorbi* is written in black ink on paper. The manuscript, 340 x 222 mm, is protected with a soft parchment paper cover, somewhat damaged by humidity. The spine of the cover has been strengthened with sheep leather. Twenty-one fascicles made up of six leaves each are bound together. Every paper leaf has been folded into four pages. The same type of paper has been used throughout with the same filigreed ornamentation consisting of a decorated sphere. Six leaves, mostly unrelated to the subject matter of the manuscript, have been inserted into the book. The ink from one side of the paper has seeped to the other side, which has also been written on as a clean sheet making the transcription of the text, written in barely legible humanistic cursive script, even more challenging. The reader gets the impression that the records were mostly written in a great hurry, without any concern for calligraphy. The authors grate-

fully acknowledge the contribution of Dr Vinicije Lupis, director of the Ivo Pilar Institute in Dubrovnik, to the description of this manuscript. *Libro deli Signori Chazamorbi*, forthcoming.

86 The existence of a round stamp, 22 mm in diameter, with the barely visible image of St Blaise imprinted at the end of the letter, is of particular interest. On the edges of the seal impression, one can read the word *Ragusii* – of Ragusa. This seal belongs to the group of the so-called official hagiographic seals, of which there must have been hundreds. Gregor Čremošnik states that only six have been found so far: the oldest is from 1396, and the most recent from 1503. He emphasizes that the 1503 seal resembles the Ragusan dinar (*grossus*) coin with the image of St Blaise in the centre and the words *S. Blasius – Ragusii* written on the edges (Čremošnik, "Dubrovački pečati," 31–47). We have compared the 1503 seal with the 1528 one in the *Libro deli Signori Chazamorbi* and have come to the conclusion that both seals belong to the same category. Thus the one in the *A tergo* part of the manuscript represents the seventh small seal of the Ragusan authorities extant in the State Archives of Dubrovnik. Such seals were frequently used on court summons, as well as on instructions to officials and to private persons sent to outlying areas of the Republic. Although the manuscript has already been validated from the point of view of palaeograhy, diplomatics, and linguistics, this seal further confirms its authenticity (Batelli, *Lezioni di paleografia*, 32–54; Bischoff, *Latin Palaeography*, 145–9; Brown, *A Guide to Western Historical Scripts*, 74).

87 *Libro deli Signori Chazamorbi, a tergo*, f. 1, 3, 77, 81, 82, 115, 119v–120, 131v, 135.

88 Cf. Meiss, *Painting*, 165.

89 For example, the painting *Mater Misericordiae*, from the Church of Our Lady of Mercy in the Gorica neighbourhood of Dubrovnik, shows the Mother of God who, with her hands, opens up her wide protective mantle and exposes small, kneeling human figures under it. With their hands clasped in prayer, these figures are shown crowding around Mary's legs. The Mother of God with the faithful under her protective cloak wears a medallion with the image of Christ around her neck. This painting was the central part of the triptych of the main altar in the church that received many offerings from sailors. This central painting is held in the Museum of the Rector's Palace while the other two parts of the triptych remain in the Church of Our Lady of Mercy. Gjukić-Bender, "Poliptih," 214–20; cf. "La Vierge au grand manteau," Delumeau, *Rassurer*, 210–13, 241–8, 261–80.

90 Palmer, *Control*, 297–8.

91 Worcester, "Saint Roch," 156; Hopkins, "Combating," 138–40, 142–5.

92 Marshall, "Manipulating," 170.

93 Demori-Staničić, "Uvod," 185–90; Lupis, "Nove," 94–6; For the cult of St Roch in Lubeck and Nuremberg, see Dormeier, "Saints," 161–86.

94 Worcester, "Saint Roch," 153, 168–70.

95 Vanzan Marchini, *Rotte*, 30–1; Stevens, "The Lazaretti," 42.

96 *Acta Minoris Consilii*, v. 35, f. 216v.

97 Buconić Gović, *Dubrovačke crkvice*, 157–62.

98 Lisičar, *Lopud*, 37.

99 *Annales Ragusini Anonymi item Nicolai de Ragnina*, 102, 283–4.

100 Razzi, *La storia*, 80; Jeremić and Tadić, *Prilozi*, 1:97.

101 Badurina, "Sakralna arhitektura," in *Zlatno doba Dubrovnika*, 327–8; Buconić Gović, *Dubrovačke crkvice*, 42–3.
102 *Acta Consilii Rogatorum*, v. 41, f. 232.
103 Razzi, *La storia*, 80. See also Chapter 6, p. 164.
104 In 1558, he signed a contract with Luka Matković, a stonemason from Gruž, for some decorative stone fragments for the Church of St Roch. In 1564, he received from Jacques de Spinis d'Orléans, a French sculptor, works that had been ordered for the church. Kesterčanek, "Roko Fasano," 271; Badurina, "Sakralna arhitektura," in *Zlatno doba Dubrovnika*, 328–9; Buconić Gović, *Dubrovačke crkvice*, 63–6; Lonza, *Kazalište*, 279–86.
105 *Annales Ragusini Anonymi item Nicolai de Ragnina*, 283–4; Razzi, *La storia*, 95.
106 Vekarić, "The Population of the Dubrovnik Republic," 7–28; Vekarić, *Vlastela*, 1:145, 257.
107 Marković, "Slikarstvo," in *Zlatno doba Dubrovnika*, 357.
108 Marković, "Slikarstvo," in *Zlatno doba Dubrovnika*, 361; Demori-Staničić, "Lik," 195–200.
109 Marković, "Slikarstvo," in *Zlatno doba Dubrovnika*, 362; Lupis, *Sakralna*, 118; Lupis, *Ston*, 23–5; Lupis, *Trstenica*, 24–5. For other famous votive paintings of sixteenth century Dubrovnik, see Chapter 1.
110 Demori-Staničić, "Uvod," 174.
111 Miović, *Na razmeđu*, 132.
112 Jeremić and Tadić, *Prilozi*, 1:100–1, 3: 106–7.
113 Jeremić and Tadić, *Prilozi*, 1:102.

CHAPTER THREE

1 As mentioned in Chapter 1, the Ragusan patricians did not trust the confraternities with the task of providing health care. They did not want any "parallel channel" of power in Dubrovnik and preferred to offer these services through the institutions of the state. Providing health care for all was part of the political philosophy of the aristocratic republics in the Mediterranean. Their governments pursued the common good, which included keeping their inhabitants free of disease.
2 In the early Middle Ages, monastic medicine, together with secular medicine, played a significant role in treating the sick. Croatian archival sources from this early period are scarce. However, there is an important text from the eleventh century in the *Supetarski kartular* that states that Petar Crni (Peter the Black), the abbot of the Benedictine monastery in Poljice, founded in 1089, cured the pig keeper who had smallpox and to thank the abbot, the pig keeper agreed to become a slave of the monastery. The document is held in the Treasury of the Split Cathedral. Novak, *Supetarski kartular*, 106.
3 Ferngren, *Medicine*, 141–2.
4 On the cultivation of gardens, see the poem by Walahfrid Strabo (died 849), abbot of Reichenau on Lake Constance in southwestern Germany. Wallis, *Medieval Medicine*, 98–109; Šišić, "The Gardens," 99–122; Nodilo, "Vrt," 383–95.
5 However, according to the principle that the Church abhors blood – *Ecclesia abhorret a sanguine* – the Council of Le Mans in 1247 forbade the priests from participating in any surgical intervention on the human body that required cauterization or incision of the wounds. With these limitations, monastic and clerical

medicine gradually lost their significance. Amundsen, "Medieval Canon Law," 22–44; Blažina Tomić, *Historical Development*, 36–7; Ell, "The Two Medicines," 16–17.

6 Jeremić and Tadić, *Prilozi*, 2:161–4; Velnić, "Ljerkarna," 13–15; Foretić, "Opće prilike," 36–38. The Franciscan and Dominican monasteries in Dubrovnik maintained large libraries of medical and scientific books, among other subjects, that contributed to their scholarship. Unfortunately, both libraries suffered in the earthquake of 1667 and the fire that followed. The Dominicans still possess a library with over two hundred medical and pharmaceutical books dating from the fifteenth and later centuries (Krasić, *Zdravstvena*, 83–129; Šanjek, *Dominikanci*, 95–9; Šanjek, "The Studies," 9–24).

7 Miličić, "Počeci," 70.

8 Tartalja, "Znameniti," 78; Tartalja, "Dubrovačko," 23–34.

9 In the fourteenth century, most of the pharmacists were foreigners, usually from Italy. At the end of fifteenth century and into the sixteenth century, there were already many Ragusans serving as pharmacists. Jeremić and Tadić, *Prilozi*, 2:148, 154.

10 *Monumenta Ragusina* 2:50, 1:54, as cited by Ravančić, *Crna smrt*, 141–2.

11 Ordo super erectione novi hospitali et eius regimine, *Liber croceus*, *caput* 258: 287–90; Jeremić and Tadić, *Prilozi*, 2:164–6, 3:173–7. See also Krekić, "Images," V: 6, 12, 18–20.

12 Bishop Sormano spent more than six months in Dubrovnik. His report is also an excellent source of information about the cultural heritage of Dubrovnik at that time. He mentions seventy-three churches and eleven monasteries with a detailed account of their altars, paintings, and other inventory. Badurina, "Likovnost," 280–1.

13 Cf. Henderson, "Healing the Body," 216; Henderson, *The Renaissance Hospital*, 113–85.

14 David Rheubottom found that, in the fifteenth century, to be elected to the office of the trustees of the city hospital, *Procuratori del hospedal grande*, it took 35.8 years after admission to the Major Council, which places it in the first place among 56 public offices of the Republic. For the sake of comparison, a trustee of the orphanage needed, on average, nineteen years in the Major Council to be elected. Rheubottom, *Age, Marriage*, 43–6.

15 Buklijaš, "Domus Christi," 81–107. Before *Hospedal de Misericordia*, there was an orphanage situated in the convent of St Clare since 1290 (Diversis, *Opis*, 62; 154; Jeremić and Tadić, *Prilozi*, 2:178–95; Janeković-Römer, "Nasilje zakona," 30–2; Ferri, "Dubrovački hospitali," 58–66).

16 Janeković-Römer, *Rod*, 116–19; Jeremić and Tadić, *Prilozi*, 1:129–30, 2:199–204; Vekarić, *Vlastela*, 1:124–8.

17 Stuard, *A State of Deference*, 48–9; Stuard, "A Communal Program," 141–2.

18 Palmer, "Physicians and the State," 47.

19 *Spisi*, 14, 48, 64, 112, 123, 138, 176, 268, 273; Jeremić and Tadić, *Prilozi*, 2:7; Grmek, "Medicina," 326; Grmek, "Les médecins communaux," 11–12.

20 Jeremić and Tadić, *Prilozi*, 2:7–60, 137–44, 3:123–54; Bačić, *Stazama*, 9–125; Blažina Tomić, "The Status of the Medical Profession," 18–50. Jurica Bačić studied the fourteenth-century archival sources and was able to add several physicians and surgeons who are not mentioned in Jeremić and Tadić. It is fairly possible

that more medical men who served in Dubrovnik could be found for the remaining centuries.

21 For example, when his contract was not renewed in 1400, Andreas de Pellagiis from Bari stayed in the city and in August 1402 was allowed to take care of a patient from Koločep; although his contract had expired in 1455, and inspite of his advanced age, Thomasius de Papia agreed to go to Bosnia in 1458 to take care of the Bosnian duke Vladislav. Jeremić and Tadić, *Prilozi*, 2:19, 27.

22 Croatian surgeons and physicians: Johannes de Tragurio – Ivan from Trogir, 1375–80; Michael de Catharo 1483–84; Franciscus Marci Marcolinovich from Ston, 1506–26; Johannes Mednich – Ivan Mednić from Kotor, 1526–29; Thoma Natalis Budislavich, 1580–1608; Spanish surgeons: Jacobus Catellanus from Barcelona, 1486–1500; Johannes de Hyspania, 1482–84; Franciscus from Valencia, 1497; Jaymus Cattelanus de Villa Nova, 1506; Antonius Hispanus, 1510; and Jacobus Hispanus, 1524; French physicians: Gaudenzio Mureto Gallus, 1584–87; and Jacobo Riscarolo from Nice, 1588; Greek physicians: Andreas Constantinopolitanus in 1458, probably a refugee after the fall of Constantinople; and Emanuel Marulla from Corfu, 1465; physicians and surgeons of Jewish origin: Isac Hebreus, Judeus, 1324; Benedictus, olim Judeus, 1354; Amatus Lusitanus, 1557–58; Abraham Hebreus, 1558–90; Josephus Salama 1575–92; and Samuel Abeatar 1588–1607.

23 Jeremić and Tadić, *Prilozi*, 2:12, 24, 26–7, 32, 35, 46.

24 "Sedet autem dominus Rector sub architectis palatii in medio medicorum, nisi ibi fuerint qui altioris gradus vel dignitatis." Diversis, *Opis*, 93; 175–6. For further descriptions of the celebrations of St Blaise feast, see Janeković-Römer, *Okvir*, 299–303, 374–7; Lonza, *Kazalište vlasti*, 357–83.

25 Jacobus de Gondovaldis from Ferrara, *artium et medicine doctor*, was present in Dubrovnik during the plague outbreak of 1416 and 1430. In 1416, while he served as rector of the school, he advised the Senate to concentrate on prevention by isolating the infected. In 1430, when he served as a *physicus*, he suggested that the belongings of the plague victims should be burned to eradicate the disease. Jeremić and Tadić, *Prilozi*, 2:28.

26 Diversis, *Opis*, 127; 198; See also Lonza, "State Funerals," 71–89.

27 The terms used for surgeons were: *medicus plagarum, cirologus, medicus in arte cirologie, ciroicus, cirusicus medicus cirogye, cirurgicus, cerusicus, cyrogichus, ciroychus, medicus cirurgicus, chirurgus, medicus chyrurgus, medicus pestis, medicus fracturam*, and *infirmitatem membrorum genitalium*. Jeremić and Tadić, *Prilozi*, 2:7–60, 137–44, 3:123–54; Bačić, *Stazama*, 9–125.

28 A doctorate in surgery was granted by Bologna, Pavia, Padua, and other Italian universities from medieval times. Palmer, "Physicians and Surgeons," 453.

29 For surgical anaesthesia by soporific sponge, see Wallis, *Medieval Medicine*, 315–16.

30 Siraisi, *Medieval*, 153–77; Cipolla, *Public Health*, 3–7; Park, "Medicine," 79–82. For the description of the removal of bladder stones, the operation for cataract, see Wallis, *Medieval Medicine*, 306–15.

31 Miasma, meaning pollution in Greek, was considered to be a noxious vapour filled with particles from decomposed matter believed to cause diseases. Hippocrates, *Hippocratic Writings*, 78–9, 213, 260–2, 265–7; Cipolla, *Miasmas and*

Diseases, 4–6; Nutton, "Humoralism," 1:281–91; Hannaway, "Environment," 295–6.

32 Pelling, "Contagion/Germ Theory/Specificity," 311–15.

33 Compare John of Burgundy's Treatise *De epidemia* composed around 1365. Wallis, *Medieval Medicine*, 422–9.

34 One of them was Jacobus Rizo who was employed by Dubrovnik in 1527 but was quickly exposed, tried, and expelled from the city (see Chapter 6).

35 In Italian towns, the same situation prevailed. They all hired *medici condotti* – town physicians – brought from outside. In the sixteenth century, as the number of physicians increased, the big cities like Venice educated their own doctors and did not need to bring them from outside. From then on, the physicians in Venice were private. The system of *medici condotti* remained in smaller towns and more isolated communities. Barber-surgeons performed minor operations, including bleeding and cupping, applying leeches, and pulling teeth. Palmer, "Physicians and the State," 48–9; Park, "Medicine," 80.

36 *Spičar* was a Ragusan name for pharmacists, from the Latin *speciarius*. Blažina Tomić, "The Status," 18–50.

37 In the fourteenth century, the term *syndicus* denoted any representative of the government entrusted with a special duty. In the fifteenth century, the term came to denote the officials elected by the Senate to supervise the local authorities outside the city. Lonza, *Pod plaštem pravde*, 76–7.

38 *Odluke veća*, 1:37–8.

39 "Perché siamo consciadi che se trovara a Bologna de boni medesi," *Lettere di Levante*, series 27.1, v. 2, f. 3; Bačić, *Stazama*, 89.

40 "Qui teneatur medicare dominum archiepiscopum ragusinum et eius familia, dominum comitem presentem et futuros et eorum familias, cancelarium et eius familiam, omnes religiosos et religiosas Ragusii, et indifferenter omnes homines masculos et feminas civitatis Ragusii et eius districtus, sine aliquo pretio." Bačić, *Stazama*, 33.

41 For example, the contract of the physician Tomas scr Bone de Nomais de Furlivio, signed in 1363, included the same clause. Jeremić and Tadić, *Prilozi*, 2:15, 3:133.

42 Pullan, *Rich and Poor*, 63–83; Carmichael, *Epidemic Diseases*, 142.

43 Jeremić and Tadić, *Prilozi*, 2:35, 3:140.

44 Buklijaš and Benyovsky, "Domus Christi," 103.

45 In comparison with other professions, Giovanni Ventura was not badly remunerated at all. University professors usually earned less than two hundred florins a year, although some received as much as one thousand florins a year. The mayor was paid five hundred forty florins a year. Of course, the question remains how much should a man be paid for a job where he had to risk his life every day. Cipolla, "A Plague Doctor," 66–72.

46 Pullan, *Rich and Poor*, 239–86, 431–43.

47 *Theriac* is derived from Greek meaning "pertaining to wild animals." It was known since Galen's times as a remedy against snakebites in which the flesh of vipers was an important ingredient. Kesterčanek, "Roko Fasano," 267–76; Remington, *Practice of Pharmacy*, 1893; Nockels Fabbri, "Treating Medieval Plague," 248–52; Wallis, *Medieval Medicine*, 176–7.

48 "In minori consilio, captum fuit, quod nullus medicus, tam physicus quam
     ciroicus, sallariatus communis possit exercere aliquos mercationes Ragusii, neque
     habere societatem cum aliquo speciario." *Monumenta Ragusina*, 2:332; Blažina
     Tomić, *Historical Development*, 44; Bazala, *Pregled*, 44–62.
49 Jeremić and Tadić, *Prilozi*, 2:15; Bačić, *Stazama*, 105.
50 Ravančić, *Život u krčmama*, 67.
51 Lonza, *Pod plaštem pravde*, 229; *Statut grada Dubrovnika*, VI, 3:327.
52 The criminal records for the years 1425 to 1429 have been lost. Buklijaš, *"Per
     relationem,"* 52–3.
53 Ruggiero, "The Cooperation of Physicians," 156–66.
54 Jeremić and Tadić, *Prilozi*, 2:7–60, 3:123–54.
55 Mahnken, *Dubrovački patricijat*, 101–2.
56 Diversis, *Opis*, 107; 184.
57 Čremošnik, "Postanak i razvoj," 82. For salaries of surgeons and physicians
     working in the lazaretto during the 1555–58 plague outbreak in Venice, see
     Stevens, "The Lazaretti," 114–16.
58 For example, Jacobus de Salgheriis from Padua died in Dubrovnik in 1424 and
     left a library of 114 titles; Johannes Petrus from Verona died in Dubrovnik in
     1464 and left 21 books and an inventory of all his possessions. Bačić, *Stazama*,
     115–24; Jeremić and Tadić, *Prilozi*, 2:37–8, 3:142, 205–16.
59 Stuard, "A Communal Program," 134–5.
60 Jeremić and Tadić, *Prilozi*, 2:38–9.
61 Jeremić and Tadić, *Prilozi*, 2:41–2.
62 For example, the contract of Jaymus Cattelanus de Villa Nova in 1508, Vincen-
     tius de Novaria in 1518, and Bartholomeus de Vegetiis in 1524. Jeremić and
     Tadić, *Prilozi*, 2:46, 48, 49.
63 Nutton, "Continuity," 33; Palmer, "Physicians and the State," 51–6; See also
     Table 3.1.
64 Park, *Doctors*, 4, 34–40. In 1355, Petrarch (Francesco Petrarca), the Italian poet,
     wrote an invective against physicians: "These are vulgar people, who take fees,
     poke their noses into urine and excrement, lie and quarrel, and whose vaunted au-
     thorities are pagans like Galen, or free-thinking Muslims like Averroes. Doctors
     are intellectually beneath contempt; to top it all, they are not much good at heal-
     ing" (Wallis, *Medieval Medicine*, 531–7).
65 Gelcich, *Delle istituzioni*, 37.
66 Jeremić and Tadić, *Prilozi*, 2:35.
67 Blažina Tomić, *Historical Development*, 44–7, 90.
68 Jeremić and Tadić, *Prilozi*, 2:13–14; Bačić, *Stazama*, 112–13; Bačić, "Magister
     Kristofor," 108.
69 "Ex primorum numero unum notabo, qui cirurgicus fuit vocatus magister Jo-
     hannes de Aldoardis de Papia optimus quidem, ut fama praedicat, suae artis medi-
     cus, huic facto seni provisio omni vita elargita fuit" (Diversis, *Opis*, 106–8;
     183–4). "Magister Johannes de Papia, alias de Aldoardis, medicus cerusicus, in-
     cepit servire dicto communi die XXIV mensis julii 1376 et habere debet duc. auri
     II C quolibet anno in tribus paghis. Die XXIV mensis februarii anno 1415 (cap-
     tum fuit) de faciendo provisionem magistro Johanni de Papia quam die vixerit
     suorum et pro honore rei publicae nostrae" (*Diversa Cancellariae*, v. 25, f. 24, f.

167v; *Reformationes*, v. 34, f. 28; *Acta Consilii Maioris*, f. 29, f. 111v, f. 119v, 139v).

70 "Die IX mensis madii MCCCCLVIII ... Hoc faciendo ad exemplar eius genitoris magistri Johannis de Papia, qui propter suam fidelitatem ... de dando ipsi magistro Thome in sustentatione vite sue et pro nutrimento suo illorum pauchorum dierum, quibus habet vivere, iperperos ducentos omni anno, quousque vixerit." Jeremić and Tadić, *Prilozi*, 3:137–8.

71 "Alteri meo tempore id ipsum decreverunt, cui nomen erat magister Johannes de Teolo Patavus cirurgicus quidem. Nam cum non tantum senio quam egritudinibus gravaretur, quibus pro maiori parte vel iacebat, aut domi residebat, sueque impotentiae conscius Senatui renunciasset, decreto Generalis consilii proponente suadenteque Minori quinquaginta ducatorum provisio vitalis fuit illi definita." Diversis, *Opis*, 108; 184–5; Jeremić and Tadić, *Prilozi*, 2:30; Blažina Tomić, *Historical Development*, 46, 53.

72 Diversis, *Opis*, 106; 184.

73 Stevens, "The Lazaretti," 116.

74 Four such contracts from 1305 to 1313 have been preserved. Čremošnik, "Nekoliko ljekarskih," 43–5.

75 For contracts between patients and healers, and breach of contract, in early modern Bologna, see Pomata, *Contracting a Cure*, 25–55; cf. Wallis, *Medieval Medicine*, 384.

76 Bačić, *Stazama*, 92.

77 *Chilloresa* was Obercho's nickname, which means herniotomist. Obercho is a Slavic name. He was probably from the hinterland.

78 Jeremić and Tadić, *Prilozi*, 2:16, 3:134.

79 Grmek, "Izvještaji," 221, 231–2; Giorgio (Đuro) Baglivi (1668–1707) is certainly the most famous physician born in Dubrovnik. His parents, Anna de Lupis from Dubrovnik and his father Blasius Armeno, probably of Armenian origin, died when he was two years old. He was educated at the Jesuit College of Dubrovnik but at the age of fifteen, together with his brother, he was adopted by Pietro Angelo Baglivi, a prominent physician from Lecce, Italy and took Baglivi's name. He studied medicine in Naples, worked in hospitals in Padua, Venice, and Florence but settled in Bologna as an assistant of Marcello Malpighi at the university. Later Baglivi became a professor of anatomy in Rome, published his work *De praxi medica* (1696) and was appointed physician to two popes. His interest in physiological research and microscopic observation led him to perform experiments on animals. In his best known work, *De fibra motrice et morbosa* (1700), he describes the histology and the microscopic structure of muscle fibres. Baglivi was first to differentiate smooth from striated muscles. His contributions to the study of the nervous system remain invaluable (Grmek, "Giorgio Baglivi," 390–2; Ćosić, "Giorgio Baglivi," 128–30; Roje-Bedeković, "Gjuro Armeno Baglivi," 166–7; Mihalić, "Re-evaluation," 34–9). Appendini mentions Giorgio Baglivi among illustrious Ragusan physicians (Appendini, *Notizie*, 34–9).

80 Jeremić and Tadić, *Prilozi*, 2:17–18.

81 Bazala, *Pregled*, 79–83.

82 Jeremić and Tadić, *Prilozi*, 2:16.

83 Jeremić and Tadić, *Prilozi*, 2:23.

84 Jeremić and Tadić, *Prilozi*, 2:25.
85 Belicza and Blažina Tomić, "Dubrovački liječnici," 205–13.
86 Jeremić and Tadić, *Prilozi*, 2:33, 36, 37, 3:140–1.
87 Jeremić and Tadić, *Prilozi*, 2:37.
88 *Acta Consilii Rogatorum*, v. 3, f. 54, f. 166v.
89 Jeremić and Tadić, *Prilozi*, 2:43; Kordić, "Nekoliko zapisa," 89–94.
90 The *emin* was a customs officer who had to collect customs duty and supervise the salt trade. He also acted as an Ottoman representative who helped settle disputes between the Ottoman subjects and the Ragusan citizens. Miović, "Emin (Customs Officer) as Representative of the Ottoman Empire," 84.
91 Since 1541, the Ragusans were under increasing pressure from the Ottomans to get rid of Marin Stjepanov Zamagna. Ever since he had arrived in Spain as Ragusan ambassador in 1533, he had provided the Spanish with the strategic intelligence about the Ottoman military and political intentions. Zamagna's death in 1548 may not have been accidental. He may have become too much of a burden for Dubrovnik and the Senate may have ordered his murder at a time when Dubrovnik played a major role in the secret diplomacy between the Ottomans and the Europeans. Polić Bobić, "Activities," 188–90; Polić Bobić, *Među križom i polumjesecom*, 13, 59–62, 121–32.
92 Jeremić and Tadić, *Prilozi*, 2:25, 52–3; 3:151; Bazala, *Pregled*, 83. Appendini mentions Lujo Đurašević among illustrious Ragusan physicians (Appendini, *Notizie*, 33).
93 Jeremić and Tadić, *Prilozi*, 2:56–7, 3:153; Lučić, "Dubrovčani," 97–8; Tadić, *Dubrovački portreti*, 349–68.
94 Jeremić and Tadić, *Prilozi*, 2:56–7; Grmek, "Izvještaji," 109–10; Rešetar, "Toma," 136–41.
95 Jeremić and Tadić, *Prilozi*, 2:55–6; Stulli, *Povijest*, 56–7; Stulli, *Židovi u Dubrovniku*, 25–6; Miović, *The Jewish Ghetto*, 26; Belicza and Blažina Tomić, "Dubrovački liječnici," 207.
96 Lučić, "Dubrovčani," 95–7; Bačić, "Liječnici," 18–19. Mirko Dražen Grmek describes the cases of three physicians employed in Dubrovnik who took part in the medico-diplomatic missions to Bosnia in the eighteenth century: Matija Bratis in 1742, Marco Flori in 1747, and Giovanni Battista Pagani in 1754. Their tasks were to take care of the Ottoman dignitaries in Bosnia but they were also instructed to find out as much as possible about the political, economic, and health conditions (i.e., plague) in the area. During their audience with their politically powerful patients, they would try to influence the Ottoman dignitaries in their decisions concerning trade with Dubrovnik (Grmek, "Izvještaji," 97–114). Appendini mentions Marco Flori among illustrious Ragusan physicians (Appendini, *Notizie*, 39).
97 Miović, "Beylerbey of Bosnia," 59.
98 *Acta Consilii Maioris*, v. 20, 7v. Grmek studied the works and the career of Donato Muzi. Unless otherwise stated, the information about Muzi was cited from Grmek's article. Jeremić and Tadić cite the date of Muzi's contract as 28 March and the salary of 300 ducats. However, it is easy to confuse the words *madii* (May) and *martii* (March), especially if they are difficult to decipher. Grmek, "Renesansni učenjak Donato Muzi," 51; Jeremić and Tadić, *Prilozi*, 2:49.
99 After he left Dubrovnik, Muzi returned to Venice where he is mentioned from

1538 to 1554 as a *promotor* of the College of Physicians of Venice that granted medical degrees. The role of the *promotor* was to assist the graduating student during his exam and during the ceremony of graduation. Palmer, *The Studio*, 36, 101–42.

100 Palmer, *The Studio*, 31–4.

101 *Donati a Mutiis medici, in interpretationem Galeni super Quatordecim Aphorismos Hippocratis, Dialogus* qtd. in Grmek, "Renesansni učenjak Donato Muzi," 54.

102 Grmek, "Renesansni učenjak Donato Muzi," 65.

103 Glesinger, "Iz dubrovačkih dana," 121–52.

104 Doumerc, "Georges d'Armagnac," 123–5.

105 Spanish and Venetian archival sources demonstrate that throughout the sixteenth century, in times of crisis and war, Dubrovnik was an important source of strategic intelligence for both the Europeans and the Ottomans. Since Venice was involved in four wars with the Ottomans between 1463 and 1573, its usual role of transmitting strategic information was interrupted. Diplomats, secret agents, and travellers exchanged valuable intelligence in Dubrovnik. Owing to their pivotal role in providing information to all sides, the political, commercial, and diplomatic position of the Ragusans was enhanced during this period. See Polić Bobić, *Tajna diplomacija u Dubrovniku*. Compare note 91 above; Polić Bobić, *Među križom i polumjesecom*, 59.

106 Kumrular, "Ragusa," 144–5.

107 It is interesting to note that while the Senate accepted this leave of absence for political reasons, it had refused Santo's one-month unpaid leave of absence to go to Venice on 7 March 1532. *Acta Consilii Rogatorum*, v. 41, f. 40v, as cited by Glesinger, "Iz dubrovačkih dana," 121–52.

108 Suleiman continued with his army of 120,000 soldiers to the fort of Köszeg in Hungary where he was stopped by the Croatian baron Nikola Jurišić and his army of eight hundred soldiers.

109 For more about these momentous events in the sixteenth century, see Chapter 5.

110 Mariano Santo's biographers did not know about Antonio Rincón, Philippo Trivulzi, and the Dubrovnik connection. Therefore, they wrote that Santo took part in the war as a surgeon, but there is nothing to support that claim.

111 Jeremić and Tadić, *Prilozi*, 2:89–124, 3:5, 151; Glesinger, *Amatus Lusitanus*, 38–93.

CHAPTER FOUR

1 There has been an intimate connection between trade and disease throughout modern history. Commerce has been a major factor in the redistribution of diseases. Pathogens and their vectors circulated more widely than before, sometimes with catastrophic results. Harrison, *Contagion*, 276.

2 Conrad, "Epidemic," 77.

3 In the fourteenth century, the health officials were called Officials Against the Plague. In the fifteenth century, their title was *Officiales cazamortuorum*, *Signori Cazamorti*, or simply *Cazamorti*. And the term *health officials* has been used since the sixteenth century "Per dominos officiales cazzamortuorum personaliter impositum fuit preceptum" (*Diversa Cancellariae*, v. 39, f. 321). *Cazamortae* (pl.) is a term of Venetian origin consisting of the words *cazzar* = *(de)pellere* and

mortae, meaning to expel the dead. The Cazamorti are the Ragusan officials whose duty it was to make sure that plague would not spread ("officiales Ragusini qui vigilabant ne pestis contagio diffunderetur") (Kostrenčić, Gortan, and Herkov, *Lexicon Latinitatis Medii Aevi*, 1:200). "Quoddam offitium, cui nomen cazamortae, in quo ex potioribus et mortis timidioribus quinque elliguntur nobiles" (Diversis, *Opis*, 83; 168). The *Cazamorti* were the persons in the Ragusan Republic whom the government would send to the place of plague infection to make sure that the disease would not spread and they were given total control over life and death. The word is undoubtedly of Romance origin; if there were such a word in Italian (*cacciamorto*, Venetian: *cazzamorto*), it would mean the person who expels the dead (*Rječnik hrvatskoga ili srpskoga jezika*, 4:710). The health officials were very highly regarded and were always addressed most respectfully, being called *li magnifici Signori officiali sopra la sanità* (the magnificent gentlemen health officials) or *li spectabili signori officiali sopra la Sanità* (the distinguished gentlemen health officials) in the Ragusan *Libro deli Signori Chazamorbi* from the sixteenth century (*Libro deli Signori Chazamorbi, A tergo*, f. 91, 126).

4 *Liber viridis, caput* 49.

5 Razzi, *La storia*, 155. On the islet of Mrkan, less than two kilometres long, the ruins of the Benedictine monastery of St Michael and the vestiges of an ancient port were found. Vojnović, "Crkva," I:40, 168, 224.

6 Gelcich, *Delle istituzioni*, 37.

7 Crawshaw, *Plague Hospitals*, 15.

8 Grmek, "Le concept d'infection," 9–54. Campbell states that Dubrovnik promulgated the first quarantine regulation but that it was in fact a *trentina* (Campbell, *The Black Death*, 139). The following authors have also published the text of the Ragusan quarantine regulation: Lechner, *Das grosse Sterben*, 67; Jeremić and Tadić, *Prilozi*, 3:55; Bazala, "Delle peste," 723–56; Grmek, "Quarantaine à Dubrovnik," 30–3; Grmek, "Karantena," 3:591–7; Premuda, "Storia della quarantena," 45–64; Palmer, "L'azione della Repubblica," 103; Blažina Tomić, *Historical Development*, 73–6; Carmichael, "History," 198; Stuard, *A State*, 239–40.

9 Crawshaw, *Plague Hospitals*, 27.

10 They recognized these goods as potential carriers of plague infection but the connection with the rats and fleas was not made.

11 Carmichael, "The Last Plague," 133, 157–60.

12 Dubrovnik had three officials, known collectively as the *Massarii bladorum* or *Massari de le biave*, who were responsible for the state's grain supply. Their duty was to procure the grain, ensure the safe and legitimate unloading of grain cargo, and grant sale franchises. Rats, as plague hosts, have a particular predilection for grain. Diversis, *Opis*, 82; 168; Carter, *Dubrovnik*, 567, 581–2; Krekić, *Dubrovnik in the Fourteenth*, 107–8.

13 Contrary to medical opinion of the time, in the period between 1450 and 1470, city fathers in northern Italian cities also came to the conclusion that plague was contagious. Carmichael, "Plague Legislation," 513.

14 Regarding the habitual abandonment of plague-infected cities by the authorities, see Braudel, *The Mediterranean*, 1:81.

15 In later centuries, the plague regulations specified how many officials of each office had to stay in the city during the epidemic.

16 Lonza and Šundrica, *Odluke dubrovačkih vijeća*, 113.

17 "Ser marinus de Crosi, ser Pasqualis de Rasti, ser Symon de Goçe, in minori conscilio ad sonum campane more sollito congregato facti fuerunt officiales ad providendum super venientibus de locis pestiferis. Qui pro executione dicti officii habeant a presenti conscilio, ex auctoritate maioris conscilii ipsi minori conscilio attributa, illam auctoritatem quam antea habuerunt alii officiales super hoc deputati." Lonza and Šundrica, *Odluke dubrovačkih vijeća*, 76.

18 Lonza and Šundrica, *Odluke dubrovačkih vijeća*, 76.

19 Lonza and Šundrica, *Odluke dubrovačkih vijeća*, 80.

20 Lonza and Šundrica, *Odluke dubrovačkih vijeća*,130.

21 Lonza and Šundrica, *Odluke dubrovačkih vijeća*, 153–4.

22 Lonza and Šundrica, *Odluke dubrovačkih vijeća*, 331–2.

23 Jeremić and Tadić, *Prilozi*, 3:60; Lonza and Šundrica, *Odluke dubrovačkih vijeća*, 347.

24 "Fustigare aut brustulare … usque ad incisionem unius aurium" (*Odluke dubrovačkih vijeća*, 183). Corporal punishment was common in Europe until the eighteenth century (Lonza, *Pod plaštem pravde*, 151).

25 Lonza and Šundrica, *Odluke dubrovačkih vijeća*, 183.

26 *Reformationes*, v. 30, f. 7v.

27 "In Minori conscilio more solito congregato additi fuerunt pro officialibus invicem cum aliis officialibus prius deputatis contra venientes de locis pestiferis, cum modis et libertatibus prius datis." *Reformationes*, v. 30, f. 19v.

28 "Ellecti fuerunt officiales supra peste contra venientes a locis pestiferis cum modis et balya consuetis, salvo ubi dicitur ipsi ordines de pecunia, que pena arbitraria sit limitata ad ducatos centum, qui ordines sunt in libro minoris consilii die XXIII octobris 1394." *Reformationes*, v. 30, f. 29.

29 (In margine: contra venientes de locis pestiferis) "Prima pars est de dando arbitrium et liberam auctoritatem domino Rectori et eius minori conscilio providendi et regullandi contra quoscumque venientes de locis pestiferis et contra illos receptantes et se commiscentes cum illis modis, ordinibus et penis quibus videbitur dicto minori conscilio et faciendi propterea officialles pro premissis prout videbitur providendum." *Reformationes*, v. 30, f. 123v.

30 *Reformationes*, v. 30, f. 32.

31 *Liber viridis, caput* 91.

32 *Reformationes*, v. 30, f. 49v.

33 According to Grmek, the monastery of St Mary on the island of Mljet was probably the first lazaretto in the world. Grmek, "Concept," 52.

34 "Prima pars est quod de locis nostri districtus in quibus est vel erit pestis, non possint portari ad nostra loca sana aliqua blada nec frumenta, nec vestes vel alique alias res cuiuscumque generis sint, donec non erit bene et clare cessata ipsa pestis in ipsis locis sub pena ordinata." *Reformationes*, v. 30, f. 143v; *Liber viridis, caput* 91.

35 *Reformationes*, v. 30, f. 142v.

36 "In minori conscilio more solito congregato, captum fuit de faciendo fieri custodiam pro providendo contra pestilentiam ad Punctum et de mittendo duas barchas in illis partibus que custodiant quod nostri non acostant ad illa loca de Vigen et ad alia loca ubi est pestis, et de mittendo duos ex hominibus de Stagno qui ponant et custodiant, prout eisdem dabitur in comissione." *Reformationes*, v. 30, f. 67.

37 Jeremić and Tadić, *Prilozi*, 1:70.
38 "Item captum fuit de dicendo officialibus, quod illud quod dictum est et ordina-
tum per nos eis super facto Benedicti Contareno, quod debeant executioni man-
dare et debeant videre si sunt aliqui infirmi in ipsis duabus suis marcilianis, et
debeant expectare dies III quibus ipse statit in Spaleto, et possint ipsi officiales
imponere penas ex eorum officio ipsi Benedicto et ipsis marcilianis, quod non debeant intrare cathenam infra terminum unius mensis, secundum ordines compu-
tandi a die qua intravit Spaletum." *Reformationes*, v. 31, f. 6.
39 *Reformationes*, v. 31, f. 16v.
40 *Reformationes*, v. 31, f. 43v.
41 "In ipso minori Consilio data fuit libertas officialibus super peste, occasione que
dicitur presentialiter vigere in contrata de Obot, quod possint facere illam vetatio-
nem que sibi videbitur pro conservatione nostra et facere expensam pro custo-
dienda prout eisdem videbitur." *Reformationes*, v. 31, f. 70; Jeremić and Tadić,
Prilozi, 1:70.
42 *Reformationes*, v. 32, f. 22v, 190v; v. 33, f. 75v, 41, 56, 131v, 172v; v. 34, f. 47,
234; *Acta Minoris Consilii*, v.1, f. 82, 105v, 175v, v. 2, f. 34, 101, 162, 234; v. 3,
f. 39, 59, 109, 188, 275.
43 Jeremić and Tadić, *Prilozi*, 3:60; *Diversa Cancellariae*, v. 39, f. 321.
44 "Captum fuit de dando libertatem officialibus cazamortuorum tenendi unam
barkam armatam cum remis nove pro diebus quindecim ad expensas comunis que
debeat ire ad Insulas pro custodia venientium de locis infectis morbo." *Acta Minoris Consilii*, v. 1, f. 32v.
45 "Anno nativitatis eiusdem millesimo CCCCXXVI, indicione quarta, die XV mensis ianuarii, in maiori et generali consilio civitatis Ragusii, in quo interfuerunt
consiliarii LXXX, captum fuit et firmatum per LVII ex ipsis consiliariis de eli-
gendo in consilio maiori per angariam officiales cazamortuorum, ita tamen quod
ad ipsum officium elligi non debeant aliqui de consilio minori nec ex iudicibus
curie civilium." Ordo pro electione officialium cazamortuorum, *Liber viridis*,
caput 205; *Acta Consilii Maioris*, v. 3, f. 101v.
46 Čremošnik, "Činovnički stalež," 31–7; Stuard, "A Communal Program," 134–7.
About the salaries of the state officials, see Janeković-Römer, *Okvir*, 161–3;
Rheubottom, *Age, Marriage*, 39.
47 On 20 October 1417 "Facere expensas opportunas prout eis videbitur fora utile,
de denariis nostri communis" (*Acta Minoris Consilii*, v. 1, f. 160); 19 October
1420 "Quod expensis communis possint tenere barcham unam apud Insulas"
(*Acta Minoris Consilii*, v. 2, f. 148); On 13 November 1427 "Omnes expensas ex
inde necessarias et opportunas" (*Acta Minoris Consilii*, v. 4, f. 118).
48 On 30 May 1348, the Major Council decided that from that date on, due to the
great number of people who had died in Dubrovnik during the deadly plague outbreak, the age of entry into the Major Council would be lowered from twenty to
eighteen. In 1455, due to a demographic boom, the age of entry was again raised
to twenty. Foretić, *Povijest*, 1:336n42; *Monumenta ragusina*, 2:25; Jeremić and
Tadić, *Prilozi*, 1:67; Rešetar, "Dubrovačko," 10, as cited by Rheubottom, *Age,
Marriage*, 32.
49 About the temporary or permanent loss of the aristocratic title, see Lonza, *Pod
plaštem*, 158.

50 About refusing to serve and the penalties for it, see Janeković-Römer, *Okvir*, 154, 163–9, 241.

51 Janeković-Römer, *Okvir*, 153.

52 In Venice at the beginning of the sixteenth century, the *Provveditori alla Sanità* also served without salary. It seems that the main attraction of the post was the possibility of further advancement to higher positions, especially towards being elected to the Senate. The *Provveditori* could even seek election to a higher post before completing the anticipated term of office of one year. Palmer, *The Control of Plague*, 80–1.

53 *Ad Catenam* means "at the chain." In 1346, the city harbour was protected with a chain running from the pier to the St Luke Fortress on the northern side. In 1484, when the new breakwater Kaše was constructed, the chain ran from the breakwater to the foot of St John's Fortress on the southern side of the harbour. Diversis, *Opis*, 47; 145; Ničetić, *Povijest*, 162.

54 "Die. 28. februarii 1417. Officiales cazamortuorum: Voichna Vlach ad Pillas, Pribislavus Cuzanaz ad Sanctum Lucam, Nixa Gvosdarich ad Catenam." *Acta Minoris Consilii*, v. 1, f. 119v.

55 Lonza, "Election Procedure," 7–41. Lonza describes the election procedure of most public officials of the Ragusan Republic elected in the Major Council, but the article does not mention the election of the Cazamorti. See also the election procedures described in Chapter 1.

56 The authors gratefully acknowledge the contribution of Dr Nella Lonza, researcher at the Institute of the Croatian Academy of Arts and Sciences for the Historical Sciences in Dubrovnik, to our knowledge of the election procedure of the Minor Council.

57 Elections on 24 June 1390: "Ex auctoritate maioris conscilii ipsi minori conscilio attributa" (Lonza and Šundrica, *Odluke dubrovačkih vijeća, 1390–1392*, 76); Elections on 8 January 1392: "Facti fuerunt officiales in dicto minori conscilio ex auctoritate mayoris conscilii" (Lonza and Šundrica, *Odluke dubrovačkih vijeća, 1390–1392*, 183); Elections on 5 January 1397: "De dando arbitrium et liberam autoritatem domino rectori et eius minori conscilio eligendi" (*Liber viridis, caput* 91); Elections on 1 January 1418: "Electi sunt in minori consilio ex auctoritate maioiris consilii sibi data" (*Acta Minoris Consilii*, v. 1, f. 175v); Elections on 2 January 1419: "Electi fuerunt officiales cazamortuorum vigore libertatis habite a maiori consilio hac eadem die cum modis et auctoritatibus consuetis" (*Acta Minoris Consilii*, v. 2, f. 34); Elections on 8 January 1420: "Electi fuerunt officiales cazamortuorum vigore libertatis ista die habite a maiori consilio cum modis et auctoritate consueta" (*Acta Minoris Consilii*, v. 2, f. 101v).

58 "Officiales cazamortuorum. Non fuerunt electi ista die quia non fuerit data libertas in Maiori consilio, scilicet infra reperies die 2 presentis." *Acta Minoris Consilii*, v. 2, f. 32v.

59 *Liber viridis, caput* 205.

60 Elections on 6 June 1427, *Acta Minoris Consilii*, v. 4, f. 61; Elections in January 1428, *Acta Minoris Consilii*, v. 4, f. 130.

61 Andrija Bobaljević (Bobalio) (1399–1473) was elected to serve as Cazamorto at the age of forty-four, Junije Lukin Bunić (Bona) (ca 1440–1518) at the age of forty-seven, Ivan Stjepanov Gučetić (Goze) (ca 1451–1502) at the age of fifty,

Nikola Martinov Gučetić (Goze) (1473–1554) at the age of forty-nine, and Stjepan Junijev Gradić (Gradi) (ca 1443–1523) at the age of thirty-eight. The Ragusan Republic, while venerating the wisdom of age, avoided obsession with it. This changed in the eighteenth century. Janeković-Römer, *Okvir*, 116–27.

62 Gučetić (Goze), Bunić (Bona), Sorkočević (Sorgo), Gundulić (Gondola), Crijević (Cerva or Zrieva) Đurđević (Giorgi or Georgi) were the families who had the greatest number of members in the Major and Minor Council from 1440 to 1640. These families of common lineage were sometimes so big and had so many branches that, some of them, were no longer closely related (Janeković-Römer, *Okvir*, 178–9; Rheubottom, *Age, Marriage*, 102–22; Zlatar, "Huius ... est omnis," 54–5). For information about the origin, genealogy and development of these patrician families, see Vekarić, *Vlastela* 2:91–132, 180–98, 243–65, 292–326 and *Vlastela* 3:97–142, 259–94.

63 *Speculum Maioris Consilii*, series 21.1, v. 1 (1440–1499), v. 2 (1500–1599). Data concerning the election of the Cazamorti in earlier periods are available in the *Reformationes* and the deliberations of the Major and Minor Councils. Instructions for specific occasions can be found in the books of the Minor Council.

64 For example, on 27 October 1528, Mate Franov Bobaljević (Babalio) could no longer serve as a health official because he had been become a judge of the Criminal Court. *Libro deli Signori Chazamorbi, A tergo*, f. 117v.

65 Rheubottom, *Age, Marriage*, 43–6, 145–7.

66 "Captum fuit quod mandetur officialibus cazamortuorum, quod deinceps eveniente casu aliquo pestilentie in aliqua domo seu familia aliqua Ragusii, quod deus in sua misericordia dignetur avertere, pro quo casu, ipsi officiales discernerent et vellent aliquem dicturum familiarum Ragusii expellere et confinare, quod neminem possint expellere nec confinare, nisi prius notum fecerint domino Rectori et suo parvo consilio." *Acta Minoris Consilii*, v. 5, f. 91.

67 Janeković-Römer, *Okvir*, 230–1.

68 Diversis, *Opis*, 41, 141; 116–18, 168–9.

69 Diversis, *Opis*, 83; 168.

70 Providimentum et ordines regiminis et custodie civitatis Ragusii firmati in consilio Rogatorum heri et hodie ob dubium pestis, *Acta Consilii Rogatorum*, v. 6, f. 122–28, 131, 134, 136v. Similar special regulations were also adopted in 1430 and during previous plague outbreaks. *Acta Consilii Rogatorum*, v. 4, f. 249–254v.

71 The fact that only the oldest patrician survived could be the confirmation of the observation that the plague struck the young and healthy more than older people.

72 "Marinus Simonis de Restis ... existens solus in gubernando et custodiando urbem nostram ob mortem aliorum suorum sociorum salariatorum, de dando eidem ser Marino de Resti ex denariis nostri comunis yp. quingentos." *Acta Consilii Maioris*, v. 5, 148. Marin Šimunov Rastić (Resti) was a highly respected patrician who excelled in construction projects and was elected rector of the Republic on twelve occasions.

73 Diversis, *Opis*, 41–2, 79, 82–4, 97, 116–8; 141–2, 166, 168–9, 178–9,190–1; *Annales Ragusini Anonymi item Nicolai de Ragnina*, 55, 252; Janeković-Römer, *Okvir*, 154.

74 Jeremić and Tadić, *Prilozi*, 2:32.

75 "Se per lo avegnir occorresse morbo de epidimia in la citade nostra de Ragusa

morendo da doy in tre persone de essa epidimia, li officiali cazamorti siano tegnuti de denuntiarli al pizol conseglio, sotto pena de yperperi cinquanta per cadauno." *Liber viridis, caput* 319.

76 "Et dello angario, zoe cazamorti al mancho uno." *Liber viridis, caput* 351. The importance of wine in the Ragusan diet cannot be overstated. Most patricians owned a vineyard and needed to be present for the harvesting of their grapes and winemaking. This became the time of year when the Councils and the whole state apparatus suffered the most from absenteeism.

77 *Kopac* (masculine), *kopica* (feminine) means digger in the Croatian language, from the verb *kopati*, to dig.

78 "Prout habent officiales cazamorti salariati in civitate, remanentibus tamen ipsis officialibus cazamortuorum in eorum officio et in libertate ipsis attributa." *Acta Consilii Rogatorum*, v. 15, f. 97; Jeremić and Tadić, *Prilozi*, 3:90.

79 During the Venetian protection period (1205–1358), the rector, for example, received, over and above his salary of four hundred hyperperi, various taxes and fees from trials, customs duty, and fishing. After 1358, he received only a modest sum covering his expenses. A family with a very modest lifestyle needed fifty hyperperi per year to survive. Čremošnik, "Činovnički stalež," 31–7.

80 Blažina Tomić, "Uloga," 89–110.

81 The first building on St Peter was erected in 1431. Jeremić and Tadić, *Prilozi*, 1:112.

82 Jeremić and Tadić, *Prilozi*, 3:89–90; *Acta Consilii Rogatorum*, v. 15, f. 95v–96.

83 *Acta Consili Rogatorum*, v. 15, f. 143.

84 *Acta Consili Rogatorum*, v. 15, f. 149–150v.

85 "Et hoc ut pauperes qui tempore pestis moriuntur ibi ad Danzas, non veniant mori uti pecora, sed cicut Christicole sepeliantur in loco sacro." *Acta Consili Rogatorum*, v. 15, f. 182.

86 1466. A La Croma non mittendo Infecti. 26.III. MCCCCLXVI. Prima pars est de dando libertatem cazamortis quod possint facere ardere res infectas quae eis videbuntur et si haec pars copietur limitabitur a quanta infra debent dari dicta libertas et cuius expensis debeant facere conburere dictas res. Captum et firmatum fuit … 28 X 6.

Prima pars est quod dicti Cazamorti habeant libertatem faciendi ardere de quaqunque familia infecta res infectas quae eis videbuntur ab yperperis decem infra et vestum faceant lavare et hoc fiat expensis communis.

Captum et firmatum non fuit. [This paragraph was not adopted.]

Secunda pars est quod habeant dictam libertatem faciendi ardere infectas res ab yperperis quinque infra et vestum faciendi lavare, et hoc totum fiat ad expensis communis. Captum et firmatum fuit … 19 X 15.

Prima pars est (Cazamorti), quod Cazamorti debeant mittere infectos et infectandos ad Sanctum Petrum et non ad La Cromam aliquo modo et qui sunt in presentiarum ad La Cromam … debeant mitti ad Sanctum Petrum. Captum et firmatum fuit… omnes contra unum. (*Acta Consilii Rogatorum*, v. 19, f. 27)

87 Blažina Tomić, *Historical Development*, 86; Blažina Tomić, "Interakcija dubrovačkih vijeća," 1–16.

88 Čremošnik, "Činovnički stalež," 35–7.

89 In the sixteenth century, the Ragusans continued thinking about a lazaretto on Lokrum. On the 14 January 1534, the idea was discussed in the Senate. On 19

November, the Senate had decided to go ahead with this project. The walls of the building were built but the construction was stopped. More deliberations on this subject took place in 1553 and 1555 but the lazaretto remained unfinished. Its walls looked like those of a big theatre. The reasons were still the same: Lokrum was too close to the city and in case of war it could easily fall into the hands of the enemy. The lazaretto was eventually built at Ploče between 1590 and 1624, close to the port of Dubrovnik and the road that led to Bosnia and Istanbul. It is a monumental structure that consists of nine buildings (for people) and five courts (for merchandise). Razzi, *La storia*, 170; Jeremić and Tadić, *Prilozi*, 1:98, 113–15; *Acta Consilii Rogatorum*, v. 41, f. 261v–262; Janeković- Römer, "I lazzarettti di Dubrovnik," 246–7; Šundrica, *Tajna kutija*, 2:11–116.

90 Ordo super peste, *Liber croceus, caput 47*.

91 *Liber croceus, caput 60.*

92 Rheubottom, *Age, Marriage*, 133–4, 142.

93 *Acta Consilii Rogatorum* v. 24, f. 66v–67; Jeremić and Tadić, *Prilozi*, 1:86–90; 3:95–6.

94 On 13 March 1483, the Minor Council decided to no longer send the infected to Mrkan so that the bishop of Trebinje and Mrkan, who owned the island, could enjoy it without any impediment. *Acta Minoris Consilii*, v. 22, f. 79v.

95 Jeremić and Tadić, *Prilozi*, 1:119–21.

96 *Acta Consilii Rogatorum*, v. 24, f. 89v–90v; Jeremić and Tadić, *Prilozi*, 3:96–8.

97 *Acta Consilii Rogatorum*, v. 24, f. 66v–67; Jeremić and Tadić, *Prilozi*, 1:86–90; 3:95–6.

98 "Item, sel se trovasse alcuna cossa de tela a de panno in la via quando li copci portano ad sepellire alcuno over retornano, in tale caso li dicti copci debiano esser impicadi per la gola, et questo perche piu volte se ha trovato tanto ad Ragusa, quanto altrove che essi copci notrigano el male gittando cosse infecte in la via et in altri loghi dove tal cosse infecte se habiano a tochare." *Acta Consilii Rogatorum*, v. 24, f. 106–7; Jeremić and Tadić, *Prilozi*, 3:98–9.

99 "De privando ipsos vita, videlicet de faciendo ipsos suspendi per gulam, ita quod anima a corpore separetur; per XXI contra XVIII." *Acta Consilii Rogatorum*, v. 24, f. 125v–126; "Testamentum Givani Pupach qui suspensus fuit per gulam ad Danzas," *Testamenta de Notaria*, v. 24, f. 133v–134; Jeremić and Tadić, *Prilozi*, 3:99.

100 Since the 1610s, increasing rivalries between noble families led to the development of a fissure between the two main factions of the patriciate. This split continued to plague the political life of Dubrovnik until the end of the Republic. For centuries, the allegiance to nobility as a social rank had always taken precedence. However, the most recent research by Nenad Vekarić shows that the clan structure of the Ragusan patriciate – affiliation of patrician families into factions – was an ancient polarization between two sharply opposed groups. Between 1205 and the fall of the Republic in 1808, Dubrovnik saw three major political changeovers: in 1205, with the support of Venice, Damjan Juda's clan was overthrown in a coup and was succeeded by the Bobaljević (Bobali) clan, which, in 1358, was overthrown by the Gundulić-Gučetić (Gondola-Gozze) clan, with the support of the Hungarian king; in the 1620s, the Bobaljević clan, supported by Spain, took power and held on to it until 1808. The result over time, through an almost complete end to intermarriage between the two factions, was

the reduction of the demographic pool and the emergence of a group of families that monopolized power. Out of 232 marriages between 1667 and 1808, 93.5 percent were contracted within the same group. Ćosić and Vekarić, "The Factions," 45; Vekarić, *Vlastela*, 1:159–204; Janeković-Römer, *Okvir*, 178–9; Rheubottom, *Age, Marriage*, 102–22; Vekarić, *Nevidljive pukotine*, 31–84.

101 In 1978, Richard Palmer wrote, "It is possible that the appointment of [health] officials in Ragusa in 1397 marked the beginnings of Europe's first permanent Health Office." Palmer, *The Control of Plague*, 33.

102 Carmichael, *Plague and the Poor*, 122.

103 Bottero, "La peste in Milano," 17–28; Palmer, *The Control of Plague*, 33–5; Carmichael, "Plague Legislation," 512.

104 Carmichael, "Plague Legislation," 520–5.

105 Palmer, *The Control of Plague*, 36–7; Vanzan Marchini, "Venezia e l'invenzione del Lazzaretto," 18.

106 Palmer, *The Control of Plague*, 183–200. According to Frari, during the epidemic outbreak of 1403, Venice installed an ad hoc lazaretto in the convent of St Mary of Nazareth, situated on a small island in the lagoon. The word *lazaretto* is almost certainly derived from this name. Only the plague sufferers from Venice were treated there, not those who arrived from outside. Frari, *Della peste*, xliii; Grmek, "Le concept," 44.

107 Vanzan Marchini, "Venezia e l'invenzione del Lazzaretto," 24–7.

108 Stevens, "The Lazaretti," 45–7; Crawshaw, *Plague Hospitals*, 3–4, 35, 38, 234. See also Rodenwaldt, *Die Gesundheitsgesetzgebung*, 16–26, 79–91, 101–7.

109 In 1348, Venice and Florence had implemented the usual sanitary laws concerning the burial of the dead, cleaning of the streets and sewers, tanning of hides, selling of meat and fruit. All these measures reflect the concern with the quality of the air. The sick were forbidden from entering the city. Palmer, *The Control of Plague*, 18–22.

110 Palmer, *The Control of Plague*, 51–86, 230.

111 Palmer, "L'azione della Repubblica di Venezia," 104–6.

112 Northern European countries seemed to believe that they were far removed from the source of plague infection in the Levant that usually first struck the Mediterranean countries. Harrison, *Contagion*, 12.

113 Cipolla, *Public Health*, 18–9.

114 Cohn, *Cultures*, 80n8; Henderson, "Epidemics in Renaissance Florence," 165–86.

CHAPTER FIVE

1 In 1507, the Venetian Republic established the Board of Trade to protect the "prestige, profit and benefit which trade imparts" in the aftermath of the successful Portuguese voyage around the Cape of Good Hope. This demonstrates that the Venetians were truly worried about the impact of this event on their economy. Crawshaw, *Plague Hospitals*, 35–6.

2 Losses included Modon and Coron on the Peloponnese, the fortified ports of call used for all Venetian voyages to the Levant since 1204. The battle for Modon and Coron in 1499–1500 is described by a Ragusan chronicler (Crijević Tuberon, *Komentari*, 135–41, 165–71). The all-important Negroponte (Khalkis) in the Euboean Gulf had been lost in 1469. In the sixteenth century, Venice was involved in two more exhausting wars with the Ottomans that resulted in more territorial

losses: in 1537–40, the Aegean islands, Preveza; and in 1570–73, Cyprus, battle of Lepanto (Lane, *Venice*, 242–9; Madden, *Venice*, 280–301, 323–39; Crowley, *City of Fortune*, 328–75).

3 While Venice was at war, it begrudged Dubrovnik's neutrality and ability to continue trading with the Ottomans. During wars with Venice, the Ottomans not only lost a partner and acquired an enemy, but they also lost the strategic intelligence information that Venice usually provided about the Western powers, and they had to rely solely on Dubrovnik. For the role of Dubrovnik in sixteenth-century European diplomacy, see Polić Bobić, *Tajna diplomacija u Dubrovniku*.

4 As mentioned in Chapter 2, in spite of all the fear of overland infection, it seems that all major plague epidemics arrived in Dubrovnik by sea.

5 Diversis, *Opis*, 78–80; 165–7; Harris, *Dubrovnik*, 298–9.

6 Macan, "Dubrovački brabanti," 312–5; Mitić, "Organizacija kopnene i pomorske obrane," 104–5.

7 Diversis, *Opis*, 79; 166.

8 Mitić, *Konzulati*, 24–39.

9 Data from the *A recto* are enriched with information from other archival sources.

10 At that time, it was not known that the plague incubation period lasts only seven days. Thus, it was considered that a long quarantine period would ensure better protection of the Ragusan territory (see also Chapter 2).

11 *Libro deli Signori Chazamorbi, A tergo*, f. 1.

12 *Libro deli Signori Chazamorbi, A tergo*, f. 2.

13 *Libro deli Signori Chazamorbi, A recto*, f. 2.

14 *Acta Consilii Rogatorum*, v. 28, f. 228v.

15 *Libro deli Signori Chazamorbi, A recto*, f. 4v.

16 *Libro deli Signori Chazamorbi, A recto*, f. 5.

17 *Libro deli Signori Chazamorbi, A recto*, f. 6v.

18 Krekić, "Dubrovnik's Participation," 1–8.

19 Luka Nikolin Bunić (Bona) was elected to the Health Office in 1527. See Chapters 6 and 7.

20 *Libro deli Signori Chazamorbi, A recto*, f. 8–10.

21 *Diversa Notariae*, v. 67, f. 39.

22 *Liber viridis, caput* 91.

23 Razzi, *La Storia*, 71.

24 *Annales Ragusini Anonymi item Nicolai de Ragnina*, 91. Marin Sanudo maintains that the epidemic in 1503 was a continuation of the one in 1497. According to him, it was pervasive in Zadar in 1500 and also among the Turks in Dalmatia. It had been brought by the Venetians. Sanudo, "Odnošaji," 5:6.

25 "Captum fuit de dando libertatem officialibus Cazamortuorum quod possint conburi facere omnes res que sunt in domo in qua unus est mortuus in Zuliana, faciendo prius descriptionem dicturam rerum et extimando illarum valorem." *Acta Minoris Consilii*, v. 27. f. 229v.

26 "De dando libertatem officialibus cazamorbum quod infectis in Canali et alibi, si non obedient possint conburi facere domum et ipsos inobedientes in ipsis domibus possint conburi facere." *Acta Consilii Rogatorum*, v. 29, f. 131–131v.

27 "De dando libertatem officialibus Cazamorbum quod per totum mensem septembris proxime futuri, possint providere quod de terra firma non conducantur Ragusium lane, schlavine et alie res que ipsis videbuntur suspecte. Et possint ponere

contrafacientes et conburi facere res vestiarum que portarentur contra ordinem. Per omnes c. IV." *Acta Consilii Rogatorum*, v. 29, f. 156.

28 *Libro deli Signori Chazamorbi, A tergo*, f. 6.

29 *Schiavina* is a rough blanket, a clothing item, or rough fabric used by Slavs. *Lexicon Latinitatis Medii Aevi*, 2:1051; *Libro deli Signori Chazamorbi, A recto*, f. 19.

30 *Libro deli Signori Chazamorbi, A recto*, f. 13.

31 *Libro deli Signori Chazamorbi, A recto*, f. 13v.

32 *Libro deli Signori Chazamorbi, A recto*, f. 13v.

33 *Libro deli Signori Chazamorbi, A recto*, f. 14.

34 *Libro deli Signori Chazamorbi, A recto*, f. 14.

35 "Captum fuit de dando confine Petro Antonio de Castiglione qui venit Venetiis, … in domo Ser Nicolo de Zamagno ad Plocias, tamen cum custodia ponenda per officiales Cazamortum, expensis ipsius Petri Antonii." *Acta Minoris Consilii*, v. 27, f. 261.

36 *Acta Minoris Consilii*, v. 27, f. 261.

37 *Libro deli Signori Chazamorbi, A recto*, f. 15.

38 *Acta Minoris Consilii*, v. 27, f. 271.

39 *Libro deli Signori Chazamorbi, A recto*, f. 16v.

40 *Libro deli Signori Chazamorbi, A recto*, f. 17–17v.

41 *Libro deli Signori Chazamorbi, A recto*, f. 18.

42 "Captum fuit de dando libertatem officialibus Cazamortis, quod ad Insulam Zupane illis qui sunt infecti in loco deputato pro lazareto, necessitatis possint distribuere in elemosina de rebus cibariis usque ad amontantiam yperperorum triginta, quibus et prout dictis officialibus videbitur et placuerit in dicto loco." *Acta Minoris Consilii*, v. 28, f. 33.

43 *Acta Minoris Consilii*, v. 28, f. 41.

44 *Libro deli Signori Chazamorbi, A recto*, f. 22.

45 *Libro deli Signori Chazamorbi, A recto*, f. 23.

46 *Libro deli Signori Chazamorbi, A recto*, f. 25.

47 "Clarissimo viro ser Laurentio Ni. de Ragnina, dignissimo ambassiator della Signoria nostra fu al Sumo Pontifize, tornato da Roma, si obliga ut supra" (*Libro deli Signori Chazamorbi, A recto*, f. 26). Licences issued to enter Italian cities show that exceptions were always made for ambassadors and wealthy travellers even if they came from plague stricken areas (Carmichael, "Plague Legislation," 523).

48 *Libro deli Signori Chazamorbi, A recto*, f. 36v.

49 Popović, *Turska i Dubrovnik*, 92–4 ; Foretić, *Povijest*, 1:241; Miović, "Emin," 81–8; Miović, "Beylerbey," 37–69; Božić, *Dubrovnik i Turska*, 340–4.

50 Popović, *Turska i Dubrovnik*, 95. During the later Ottoman conflict with Venice, Sultan Selim II continued to send such letters to the Ragusans because he wanted to make sure that goods were not sold to Venetian merchants. Kumrular, "Ragusa", 48. About the role of the *emin*, see Chapter 7, note 5.

51 *Libro deli Signori Chazamorbi, A tergo*, f. 9.

52 *Libro deli Signori Chazamorbi, A tergo*, f. 9v.

53 *Acta Minoris Consilii*, v. 31, f. 195.

54 *Annales Ragusini Anonymi item Nicolai de Ragnina*, 98.

55 *Acta Minoris Consilii*, v. 32, f. 169v.

56 *Libro deli Signori Chazamorbi, A tergo*, f. 10.

57 *Libro deli Signori Chazamorbi, A tergo*, f. 10v.
58 Razzi, *La Storia*, 74; *Annales Ragusini Anonymi item Nicolai de Ragnina*, 276.
59 For the year 1520, there are no records of arrivals in the *A recto*; and in the *A tergo*, there are no records from 1517 to 1521 and then again from 1525 to 1526.
60 *Libro deli Signori Chazamorbi, A tergo*, f. 11.
61 *Libro deli Signori Chazamorbi, A tergo*, f. 11.
62 *Libro deli Signori Chazamorbi, A tergo*, f. 11v.
63 Foretić, *Povijest*, 1:271–2.
64 From 1514 to 1530, the Ottomans occupied the Croatian lands in the Dalmatian hinterland, eliminating this buffer zone between the Ottoman and Venetian territories. The Christian population of this area suffered total despair and abandonment. The economy of the Dalmatian coastal cities under Venetian protection was severely affected by these events. Doumerc, "Georges d'Armagnac," 123.
65 Dubrovnik made itself useful by providing strategic intelligence about the military movements of all participants in the war. Kumrular, "Ragusa," 143–54; Polić Bobić, "Activities," 86–93, 181–9; Polić Bobić, *Među križom i polumjesecom*, 49–85.
66 For the coronation of Suleiman in 1520 the Ragusans had already sent gifts worth 8,200 ducats, and in 1521, another 7,000 ducats. Razzi, *La storia*, 75.
67 Popović, *Turska i Dubrovnik*, 117–43.
68 *Libro deli Signori Chazamorbi, A recto*, f. 62v.
69 *Libro deli Signori Chazamorbi, A recto*, f. 63.
70 *Libro deli Signori Chazamorbi, A recto*, f. 64v.
71 *Libro deli Signori Chazamorbi, A recto*, f. 65.
72 *Libro deli Signori Chazamorbi, A recto*, f. 65v.
73 *Libro deli Signori Chazamorbi, A recto*, f. 65v.
74 *Libro deli Signori Chazamorbi, A recto*, f. 66v.
75 There is a locality called Borac in Herzegovina east of Livno and south of Šuica, and another one in central Serbia south of Rudnik and north of Gruža. *Libro deli Signori Chazamorbi, A recto*, f. 66v.
76 There are at least two localities in Bosnia called Vraneši, one near Sokolac, east of Sarajevo, one near Goražde. The one referred to is probably the first one because it is situated on the main road. *Libro deli Signori Chazamorbi, A recto*, f. 66v.
77 In the eighteenth century, the Criminal Court gradually stopped using this type of torture but it was still practised by the administrative institutions, including the health officials. Lonza, *Pod plaštem pravde*, 148–9, 198–9; Mitić, "Prilog upoznavanju kažnjavanja," 165–7.
78 Guerrini, *Empoli*, 20, 28, 30, 34.
79 Lonza, *Pod plaštem pravde*, 150–1; Mitić, *Dubrovačka država*, 66–75; 162; Diversis, *Opis*, 70; 160.
80 *Acta Consilii Rogatorum*, v. 37, f. 245v.
81 *Libro deli Signori Chazamorbi, A tergo*, f. 12.
82 *Libro deli Signori Chazamorbi, A recto*, f. 77v–90v.
83 *Libro deli Signori Chazamorbi, A recto*, f. 77v.
84 *Libro deli Signori Chazamorbi, A recto*, f. 78.
85 *Libro deli Signori Chazamorbi, A recto*, f. 89.
86 *Libro deli Signori Chazamorbi, A recto*, f. 84.

87 *Libro deli Signori Chazamorbi, A recto*, f. 85.
88 *Libro deli Signori Chazamorbi, A recto*, f. 86.
89 *Libro deli Signori Chazamorbi, A recto*, f. 90.
90 *Libro deli Signori Chazamorbi, A recto*, f. 87.
91 The names of the patricians whose houses had to be closed appear in *Libro deli Signori Chazamorbi, A recto*, f. 86v.
92 *Libro deli Signori Chazamorbi, A recto*, f. 88–88v.
93 *Libro deli Signori Chazamorbi, A recto*, f. 86v.
94 *Libro deli Signori Chazamorbi, A recto*, f. 86.
95 *Libro deli Signori Chazamorbi, A recto*, f. 88.
96 *Libro deli Signori Chazamorbi, A recto*, f. 88v.
97 *Libro deli Signori Chazamorbi, A recto*, f. 90v–101.
98 *Libro deli Signori Chazamorbi, A recto*, f. 94v.
99 *Libro deli Signori Chazamorbi, A recto*, f. 100.
100 For easier consultation, in Figure 5.1, we have used the names of present-day countries.
101 Albania refers only to the departure point named Albania in the manuscript and does not include all the places in that country such as Argento, Durrës, Lezhë, Pi(e)rgo, Scutari, Valona, or Vrego, which appear under their own names. The place names that we have not been able to identify are followed by a question mark in Table 5.1.
102 Carter, *Dubrovnik*, 587.
103 *Libro deli Signori Chazamorbi, A recto*, f. 30v, 91, 93, 94, 95, 99; *A tergo*, f. 14v, 21v, 27, 34v, 37, 45v, 48, 64, 66, 67–68v, 80v, 91, 93v, 104v, 110v, 111, 112v, 131, 131v.

CHAPTER SIX

1 Phlebotomy was one of the most frequently used forms of therapy. The principle behind this procedure was that bloodletting drew off corrupt matter from the body. Each of the four humours, all of which were contained in blood, was capable of being transformed by disordered complexion into a harmful secondary humour that had to be removed if the patient was to recover health. Siraisi, *Medieval and Early*, 139–40.
2 Grmek, "Renesansni učenjak Donato Muzi," 61–2. By its epidemiological characteristics, the Dubrovnik 1526–27 plague outbreak is very similar to the 1575–77 Venetian epidemic, which Rodenwaldt argued was due to the human flea vector (Rodenwaldt, *Pest in Venedig*, 224).
3 Razzi, *La storia*, 75–6; *Annales Ragusini Anonymi item Nicolai de Ragnina*, 280; Grmek, "Renesansni učenjak Donato Muzi," 61.
4 *Acta Consilii Rogatorum*, v. 38, f. 206. During every plague outbreak in every city, it was customary to identify and prosecute the first plague carrier, usually a foreigner. During the 1576 and 1630 plague epidemics in Milan, the authorities prosecuted, persecuted, and executed the *untori*, the plague spreaders. Adhering to the contagion theory, the physicians believed that plague could be carried in the form of unguents and salves, spread on doorways, walls of the city, benches of the churches, and elsewhere, which, of course, facilitated the spread of plague (Carmichael, "Contagion Theory," 254; Carmichael, "The Last Plague," 147–9). In Florence in November 1522, a German or a Flemish man was accused of

bringing plague into the city (Henderson, "Epidemics," 177; Naphy, *Plagues*, 28–34, 68–71, 138–41). See also Chapter 7, p. 195.

5 Henderson, "Epidemics," 176–86.
6 Sanudo, "Odnošaji skupnovlade mletačke," 8:256, 264.
7 Sanudo, "Odnošaji skupnovlade mletačke," 12:311. It appears that Sanudo's estimate of the number of people who succumbed to plague is exaggerated. According to the calculation of the Croatian historian Tomislav Raukar, Split had about five thousand inhabitants at that time. Due to the plague epidemic, that number declined to two thousand (Rafaelić, "Prilog poznavanju kužne epidemije," 194; Raukar, "Komunalna društva u Dalmaciji u XV stoljeću," 63–6; Raukar, *Hrvatsko srednjovjekovlje*, 174.
8 Jutronić, "Prilog proučavanju zdravstva," 277.
9 Carmichael, "The Last Plague," 133, 157–60.
10 Since 1416, during every plague outbreak, the Senate adopted ever more sophisticated regulations for the protection of the population during the epidemic. Jeremić and Tadić, *Prilozi*, 1:71–100. See also Chapter 4.
11 *Acta Consilii Rogatorum*, v. 38, f. 188v.
12 Finding the financial resources to implement plague control measures often seemed to be a problem in northern Italian cities. Plague control measures decided during an epidemic were regularly shelved later because of financial difficulties. Sources document, for example, events in seventeenth-century Florence and some smaller towns in its vicinity such as Monte Lupo, Pistoia, and Prato. Calvi, *Histories of a Plague Year*, 155–96; Cipolla, *Cristofano*, 32, 82–3, 91–5, 109–17, 127–39, 148–51; Cipolla, *Faith, Reason*, 19–20, 81; Cipolla, *Fighting the Plague*, 61, 66–75; Palmer, *The Control of Plague*, 66, 73–5, 80.
13 In the sixteenth century, the terms *officiali dela sanita* and *officiali sopra la sanita* – health officials (closer to the term that we use today) – replaced the term *Cazamorti*. In the manuscript *Libro deli Signori Chazamorbi, A tergo*, the health officials are called *Signori Cazamorbi* from 1500 to 1516. This term is used for the first time on 2 January 1500 (f. 1r) and last time on 17 October 1516. (f. 10v). The term *Signori Cazamorti* is used only once, on 13 July 1500 (f. 1v). The term *Signori Chazamorbi* was used for the first time on 4 January 1502 (f. 3), and last time on 11 February 1504 (f. 7). After 15 April 1522, they are called *Signori offiziali dela Sanità* (f. 11), and after 27 November 1527 (f. 91), *Signori officiali sopra la Sanità*. On 20 June 1528 (f. 111), they are called *Officiales sanitatis civitatis Ragusii*, and after 22 June 1528 (f. 113), only *Officiales sanitatis*. In the same book, *A recto*, they are called *Signori Chazamorbi, Ofiziali chazamorbi*, and *spetabili viri domini offiziali chazamorbo* on 23 June 1502 (f. 9). After 26 May 1524 (f. 63), they are called *Signori offiziali dela Sanità*.
14 *Acta Consilii Rogatorum*, v. 38, f. 206. Most of the relevant health regulations adopted in 1526–27 were transcribed from the State Archives of Dubrovnik collections by Lučić, "Arhivska građa o kugi," 22–54 and Jeremić and Tadić, *Prilozi*, 3:101–5.
15 *Acta Consilii Rogatorum*, v. 38, f. 192.
16 *Acta Consilii Rogatorum*, v. 38, f. 189.
17 *Acta Consilii Rogatorum*, v. 38, f. 188v–189v.
18 *Acta Consilii Rogatorum*, v. 38, f. 191. For more on the cult of St Roch, see also Chapter 2, p. 61–2.

19 *Acta Consilii Rogatorum*, v. 38, f. 192.
20 Jeremić and Tadić, *Prilozi*, 3:147–9; *Acta Consilii Rogatorum*, v. 38, f. 194v–195v.
21 Janeković-Römer, *Okvir*, 94–5.
22 *Acta Minoris Consilii*, v. 35, f. 216v.
23 *Acta Consilii Rogatorum*, v. 38, f. 197.
24 In Venice in 1557, however, set prices were determined by the Health Office as compensation for burned goods. The Health Office was given 5,304 ducats to compensate the owners of burned beds, bolsters, pillows, mattresses, blankets, and furs, items difficult to clean and disinfect. Stevens, "The Lazaretti," 213.
25 In the plague historiography, there is a lot of debate about whether plague affected people of a certain age or sex more than others. In Dubrovnik, it was reported that plague affected children and young people more than the old, men more often than women. The situation in Dubrovnik could be the result of increased exposure of certain groups to plague, such as the health officials, notaries, and priests. Stephen Ell claims that men had higher levels of iron and that such persons were more susceptible to plague. Ell, "Immunity as a Factor," 874.
26 *Acta Minoris Consilii*, v. 35, f. 218v, 219; *Acta Consilii Rogatorum*, v. 38, f. 200, 201v.
27 *Acta Consilii Rogatorum*, v. 38, f. 197.
28 *Acta Minoris Consilii*, v. 35, f. 217v–218v.
29 Even during the third plague pandemic, the burning of homes and whole sections of affected cities continued in Hong Kong (1894), Bombay (1896), and Vietnam (1898), among others places. In Honolulu (1900), three physicians ran the city for five months of the plague epidemic. They were empowered to incarcerate quarantined individuals in public detention camps and ultimately to destroy private property. In order to install modern water systems and sanitary sewers, and to improve the garbage disposal, they drew huge amounts of money from the Hawaiian treasury. On 20 January 1900, after twenty days of targeted burning, all of Chinatown burned down due to sudden high winds. Seven thousand people lost their homes on that day. The area was later rebuilt in brick and stone. In San Francisco (1900–05, 1907), to avoid burning the infected districts, preventive measures were taken, including a massive rat eradication campaign. Nevertheless, in 1906, after the earthquake, all of Chinatown went up in flames. Mollaret and Brossollet, *Yersin*, 158, 188, 197; Mohr, *Plague and Fire*, 88–141; Chase, *Barbary Plague*, 66, 144–7.
30 *Acta Minoris Consilii*, v. 35, f. 220.
31 Cipolla, *Cristofano*, 59.
32 *Acta Minoris Consilii*, v. 35, f. 219.
33 *Annales Ragusini Anonymi item Nicolai de Ragnina*, 282.
34 *Acta Consilii Rogatorum*, v. 38, f. 203.
35 *Acta Consilii Rogatorum*, v. 38, f. 203v.
36 *Acta Consilii Rogatorum*, v. 38, f. 207v.
37 *Acta Consilii Rogatorum*, v. 38, f. 209v.
38 *Acta Consilii Rogatorum*, v. 38, f. 208–209.
39 Health officials elected in 1527. On 8 December 1526 for January "1527: Prima pars est de dando supplementum per totum mensem januarii proxime secuturi D. Officialibus sanitatis cum eadem authoritate quam habent dicti officiales, attento

quod ipsimet hoc requirunt causa quorundam ipsorum, qui propter infirmitatem non possunt attendere et interesse dicto officio. Prima pars est de dando et faciendo dictum supplementum cum quatuor Nobilibus eligendis in presenti consilio. Electio dictorum quatuor pro supplemento D. Officialium sanitatis: Ser Stephanus Mar. de Bonda, Ser Dymiter Math. de Ragnina, ser Paschalis Tro. De Zrieva, ser Nicolaus Zor. De Palmota" (*Acta Consilii Rogatorum*, v. 38, f. 192). Elections on 14 January 1527, *Acta Consilii Maioris*, v. 8, f. 134v; Elections on 30 January 1527, *Acta Consilii Maioris*, v. 8, f. 135v; Elections on 21 February 1527, *Acta Minoris Consilii*, v. 35, f. 224v; Elections on 8 March 1527, *Acta Minoris Consilii*, v. 35, f 227v; Elections on 18 June and 25 November 1527, *Speculum Maioris Consilii*, weries 21.1, v. 2, f. 162; Elections on 27 September 1527, *Acta Consilii Maioris*, v. 8, f. 139.

40 *Speculum Maioris Consilii*, series 21.1, v. 2, f. 161v; *Acta Consilii Maioris*, v. 8, f. 114; *Libro deli Signori Chazamorbi, A tergo*, f. 25 v, 66, 70.

41 For the mortality of the Cazamorti in the fifteenth-century plague upsurges, see Chapter 4, p. 127.

42 Janeković-Römer, *Okvir*, 93; Ćosić and Vekarić, *Dubrovačka vlastela*, 100.

43 *Libro deli Signori Chazamorbi, A recto*, f. 77.

44 *Libro deli Signori Chazamorbi, A tergo*, f. 12.

45 The authors gratefully acknowledge the contribution of Nenad Vekarić, director of the Institute for the Historical Sciences of the Croatian Academy of Arts and Sciences in Dubrovnik.

46 *Acta Consilii Rogatorum*, v. 38, f. 211.

47 *Acta Consilii Rogatorum*, v. 38, f. 212v.

48 *Acta Consilii Rogatorum*, v. 38, f. 212v–216.

49 "Prima pars est de concedendo licentiam magistro Bartholomeo Barisono medico phisico et magistro Hieronymo Pavanello medico chirurgico, quod possint pro tribus mensibus se absentare a civitate nostra et ire quocunque eis videbitur, non livrando salarium et cum pacto quod pecunias quas habuerint a comuni nostro ante terminum, si eas fuerint lucrati in suo discessu, debeant restituere. Et hoc attento quod causa pestis non possunt neque audent exercere artem medendi propter manifesta pericula." Per XXVII contra XVI. *Acta Consilii Rogatorum*, v. 38, f. 212.

50 Jeremić and Tadić, *Prilozi*, 2:36, 40–1, 3:141, 143.

51 Grmek, "Renesansni učenjak Donato Muzi," 51; Jeremić and Tadić, *Prilozi*, 2:49. See also Chapter 3, p. 99–100.

52 Jeremić and Tadić, *Prilozi*, 2:147–70.

53 Seventy-four pharmacists are mentioned as having served in Dubrovnik in the sixteenth century, most of them in the latter part of the century. Kesterčanek mentions three pharmacies, all of them in the heart of the city: next to the St Blaise Church, across from the Rector's Palace, and south of the Rector's Palace. In the sixteenth century, there were eight more public pharmacies in Dubrovnik and another one in Ston. Kesterčanek, "Iz povijesti dubrovačke farmacije," 260–1; Kesterčanek, "Iz povijesti farmacije," 250.

54 *Acta Consilii Rogatorum*, v. 38, f. 216v.

55 *Liber croceus, caput* 239.

56 Jeremić and Tadić, *Prilozi*, 1:94–6.

57 Razzi, *La storia*, 75–6, 150.

58 *Acta Consilii Rogatorum*, v. 38, f. 194v–195v; Jeremić and Tadić, *Prilozi*, 2:49–50, 3:147–8.

59 Let us mention in passing that Mednić also had a wife, Ruža, and a daughter, whom he did not mention at all.

60 Doctors who wanted to serve in the Venetian lazarettos in the sixteenth century emphasized their pious motivation, loyalty, and self-sacrifice to justify their demands. This is how they marketed themselves. Stevens, "The Lazaretti," 115–16.

61 Jeremić and Tadić, *Prilozi*, 2:159–61.

62 In Venice in 1576, there were thirteen individuals who tried to sell "secret treatments" for plague to the state. Of those, six were used in the lazaretti. The individuals, often charlatans, stressed the originality of their recipe but they also stressed that it did not go against accepted rules. They confirmed that the medicine was to be applied externally and not to be ingested orally and finally expressed pious and charitable intentions to gain acceptance for their recipe. Stevens, "The Lazaretti," 127–43; Gentilcore, *Medical*, 118; Preto, *Peste*, 90–7, 189–215.

63 Cipolla, "A Plague Doctor," 68.

64 Jeremić and Tadić, *Prilozi*, 2:42, 3:144; *Acta Consilii Rogatorum*, v. 24, f. 227. See also Table 3.1.

65 *Acta Consilii Rogatorum*, v. 38, f. 231; *Diversa Notariae*, v. 99, f. 151–151v.

66 "1527. Prima pars est de accomitendo Dominus sanitatis processum faciendum contra Jacobum Rizum medicum pestis Venetiis missum, qui Gravosii habitat pro excessibus et robariis per eum, ut dicitur, factis et cum libertate intromittendi ipsum et famulum et omnimodo providendi. Per omnes" (*Acta Consilii Rogatorum*, v. 38, f. 262v; Sept. 1527). "Prima pars est de dando libertatem Domino Rectori et suo minori consilio quod cum interventu D. Sanitatis et illorum de vicenda, possint videre, decidere et terminare, absolvere et condemnare magistrum Jacobum Rizium medicum pestis, viso eius processu et si quid extremi criminis esset, consulendi presens consilium. Per omnes" (*Acta Consilii Rogatorum*, v. 38, f. 276).

67 *Libro deli Signori Chazamorbi, A tergo*, f. 82v.

68 *Acta Consilii Rogatorum*, v. 38, f. 232v.

69 *Acta Consilii Rogatorum*, v. 38, f. 234v.

70 *Acta Consilii Rogatorum*, v. 38, f. 233.

71 *Acta Consilii Rogatorum*, v. 38, f. 235–235v.

72 *Acta Consilii Rogatorum*, v. 38, f. 242.

73 *Acta Consilii Rogatorum*, v. 38, f. 247v.

74 *Annales Ragusini Anonymi item Nicolai de Ragnin*a, 102, 280–2; Razzi, *La Storia*, 75–6.

75 Vekarić, "The Population of the Dubrovnik Republic," 26–8; Vekarić, *Vlastela*, 1: table 39, p. 145, 248. For more data on the population see also Chapter 1, p. 11, 13.

76 *Acta Consilii Rogatorum*, v. 39, f. 18–18v.

77 *Acta Consilii Rogatorum*, v. 39, f. 17–17v; Jeremić and Tadić, *Prilozi*, 2:148–9.

78 *Diversa Notariae*, v. 101, f. 34.

79 *Annales Ragusini Anonymi item Nicolai de Ragnina*, 102, 283–4.

80 *Acta Consilii Rogatorum*, v. 41, f. 188v–190, f. 207, f. 208, f. 212, 215v, 217.

81 *Acta Consilii Rogatorum*, v. 41, f. 189v, 256v.

82 "Et Deus omnipotens mediante intercessione dictae gloriose virginis liberet

civitatem nostram a presenti pestilentia." *Acta Consilii Rogatorum*, v. 41, f. 208; Razzi, *La storia*, 80.

83 *Acta Consilii Rogatorum*, v. 41, f. 211.
84 *Acta Consilii Rogatorum*, v. 41, f. 232.
85 Jeremić and Tadić, *Prilozi*, 1:108.
86 Miović-Perić, *Na razmeđu*, 117–32.
87 Stevens, "The Lazaretti," 191, 237–8; Crawshaw, *Plague Hospitals*, 10, 186–91.
88 In 1576, the Venetian Senate forced the Health Office to rescind the order of se-
    questration and quarantine, causing the number of deaths to soar. The official his-
    torian of Venice, Andrea Morosini wrote, "If noised abroad that the city was in
    the grip of a pestilential disease, terror would arise in every estate, customs rev-
    enue would be diminished, traders of Europe and Asia would recoil from the city
    and the enemies of the Republic would be incited to revolt" (qtd. in Cohn, *Cul-
    tures*, 126). It was decided to stop sending the survivors of plague to the
    Lazaretto Nuovo, mostly for financial reasons. Tragically, Venice lost another
    46,000 lives in the 1630 epidemic (Stevens, "The Lazaretti," 119; Cohn, *Cultures
    of Plague*, 180–1).
89 Cohn, *Cultures*, 98.
90 Cohn, *Cultures*, 213–37, 294–300.
91 Cohn, *Cultures*, 80–93.
92 Christensen, "Appearance," 21.

CHAPTER·SEVEN

1 *Acta Consilii Rogatorum*, v. 38, f. 253v–254. About the quorum problems see
   Raukar, "Consilium generale," 87–103; Lonza, *Pod plaštem pravde*, 44–5;
   Janeković-Römer, *Okvir*, 103.
2 *Acta Consilii Rogatorum*, v. 38, f. 192; *Acta Minoris Consilii*, v. 35, f. 227v.
3 Whereas, in Venice after 1563, the criminal archive of the Health Office is no
   longer extant. Cases are sometimes referred to briefly in the records of the notary.
   Palmer, *The Control of Plague*, 227–9.
4 *Libro deli Signori Chazamorbi, A tergo*, f. 31v. The Primo family, which belonged to the much-respected confraternity of St Anthony, had formed a genuine
   dynasty of chancellors in Dubrovnik. Trojan Primo, son of Pasko, was a second-
   generation chancellor. His sons Ivan-Petar Lukin and Jeronim Trojanov, as well
   as the sons of Ivan-Petar, Luka and Pasko, were all chancellors, spanning almost
   the whole sixteenth century. Pešorda Vardić, *U predvorju vlasti*, 167.
5 In later centuries, the *emin*, the Ottoman customs official, had to make sure that
   the Ottoman subjects arriving in Dubrovnik respected the quarantine regulations.
   The office of the emin was situated in the lazaretto complex at Ploče, the western
   suburb of Dubrovnik where the road from Bosnia ended. As soon as the Ottoman
   subjects arrived, the emin made them sign a statement declaring that they would
   respect the plague control measures of the Republic. Since the Ottoman subjects
   often refused to obey plague control regulations, escaped, or did as they pleased,
   the emin had a hard time enforcing these rules. He then had no choice but to report them to the Bosnian *beylerbey*, the highest Ottoman official in Bosnia. If an
   Ottoman subject died of the plague in the lazaretto, the Ragusans often asked the
   emin to be their witness and confirm it in writing for the Ottoman authorities to
   avoid trouble. In such cases, the Ragusans were afraid of being accused of having

killed the Ottoman subject. The extant statements date from the eighteenth century. They often refer to the Bosnian *haj*, pilgrims and merchants arriving from Alexandria. The emin was an Ottoman customs officer who had to collect customs duty and supervise the salt trade. He was also an unofficial consular representative who acted as a witness, investigator, and even judge, but, above all, he helped settle disputes between the Ottoman subjects and the Ragusan citizens. Miović, "Emin," 87.

6 In the eighteenth century, the Health Office participated in a highly appreciated international network and remained in constant touch with their counterparts in Croatian and Italian ports, especially Rijeka, Venice, and Ancona. These ports used to send reports concerning the presence of epidemic diseases in their area while Dubrovnik offered information about the health situation, not only in the Ragusan Republic, but also in Bosnia-Herzegovina, Albania, other regions of the Balkans, the Levant, and even North Africa. Miović-Perić, *Na razmeđu*, 119.

7 *Libro deli Signori Chazamorbi, A recto*, f. 90v.

8 For methods of disinfection used in sixteenth-century Venice, see Stevens, "The Lazaretti," 169; Crawshaw, *Plague Hospitals*, 209–22.

9 According to Rocco Benedetti, during the 1576 plague epidemic in Venice, men and women who had returned from the lazaretto in good health were put to work within the city. They were asked to treat the sick and disinfect goods. It is not clear whether they were paid or had to perform these services in return for the care they had received by the state. Benedetti, *Relatione*, 25, as cited by Crawshaw, *Plague Hospitals*, 207.

10 The authorities realized only later, in the seventeenth and eighteenth centuries, that the gravediggers should get better remuneration and their wages were increased. It seems that in fifteenth-century Venice the salaries of gravediggers, also called *pizzigamorti* (body clearers), were higher than those of other men and women hired to do various jobs in the lazaretti. In the sixteenth century, their salaries leveled out but in 1576, during a major plague outbreak in Venice, additional quantities of wine were sent for the sustenance of the body clearers; also special monetary rewards of one hundred ducats, one and a half times what a body clearer would make in a year, were promised to those who survived until the end of the outbreak. There is no mention of plague survivors among the body clearers in Venice. Miović-Perić, *Na razmeđu*, 135; Stevens, "The Lazaretti," 165; Crawshaw, *Plague Hospitals*, 196–7.

11 Out of 135 folios, the trials in 1527 filled eighty; in 1528, twenty-six folios; in 1529, only twelve; and in 1530, just four folios.

12 Diversis, *Opis*, 68–72; 159–61; Razzi, *La storia*, 127; Lonza, *Pod plaštem*, 79–90; Janeković-Römer, *Okvir*, 131–5.

13 Harris, *Dubrovnik*, 133.

14 See also Chapter 8, p. 211–12.

15 The judges of the Criminal Court received symbolic salaries: twelve to fifteen hyperperi per year plus 10 percent of the monetary fines assessed. In 1624, these salaries were lowered to ten hyperperi. Lonza, *Pod plaštem*, 53–5; Ordo sex iudicum de Criminali, *Liber viridis, caput* 492.

16 A chancellor dedicated to the Criminal Court – *cancelliero de criminale* – is mentioned in a 1473 regulation concerning the fees of chancellors and notaries. *Liber croceus, caput* 67, 75; Foretić, "Dubrovački arhiv," 335.

17 Diversis devotes several pages of his book to their profession. Diversis, *Opis*, 76–8; 164–5.
18 *Libro deli Signori Chazamorbi, A recto*, f. 16v, 23 (Pasqual), f. 93,100 (Marino); a tergo, f. 10v, 11v, 12 (Pasqual), 31v (Troyano Pasqual de Primi), f. 135 (Marino).
19 When, for example, in the eighteenth century, there was a conflict between the chancellors and the head of the confraternity of St Anthony over who would go first in the official processions, the Senate sided with the chancellors. Their high social standing as elite citizens was thus confirmed. Lonza, *Pod plaštem*, 83.
20 Lonza, *Pod plaštem*, 79–90; Gulin, "Srednjovjekovni," 186–93.
21 *Speculum Maioris Consilii*, v. 2, f. 161v; Lonza, *Pod plaštem*, 43; Janeković–Römer, *Okvir*, 176–82.
22 *Speculum Maioris Consilii*, v. 2, f. 162.
23 Carmichael, *Plague and the Poor*, 77.
24 Cohn, *Cultures*, 88.
25 *Libro deli Signori Chazamorbi, A tergo*, f. 13v. For more on the 14 October 1482 regulation, refer to Chapter 4.
26 Lentić, *Dubrovački zlatari*, 7. Regarding the luxurious clothes of the Ragusan nobility, see Janeković-Römer, *Okvir*, 349–52.
27 Stevens, "The Lazaretti," 161–9; Crawshaw, "The Beasts of Burial," 577–82; Crawshaw, *Plague Hospitals*, 113.
28 Benedetti, *Relatione*, 29, as cited by Stevens, "The Lazaretti," 166–7. Theatrical executions were also practised in Palermo during the 1576 plague outbreak in order to deter theft of infected goods. Cohn, *Cultures*, 81.
29 Canobbio, *Successo*, 19, as cited by Stevens, "The Lazaretti," 167.
30 Calvi, *Histories of a Plague Year*, 155–96.
31 Regarding immunity to plague, see Chapter 2, p. 45–6.
32 *Libro deli Signori Chazamorbi, A tergo*, f. 19v.
33 Konavle is the agricultural region southeast of Dubrovnik. Pile is the western suburb of Dubrovnik, right at the city entrance gate of the same name.
34 *Libro deli Signori Chazamorbi, A tergo*, f. 53.
35 *Libro deli Signori Chazamorbi, A tergo*, f. 64.
36 *Libro deli Signori Chazamorbi, A tergo*, f. 66. The beginning of the execution ritual was announced by a special bell two hours after dawn. This was the signal for the procession to leave the city. The sentenced was accompanied by guards and soldiers while Franciscan friars prayed for his soul. It was the duty of the members of the confraternity of St Roch to prepare the sentenced, reconciled to his fate, to confront death in a calm manner. The executions were usually performed at Dance, on the summit of a steep hill by the sea, situated just outside the city walls, nowadays a lovely city park called Gradac. This location was chosen because it was visible to all travellers arriving in the city, by land and by sea. The gallows at Gradac can be seen in the pictures of the city from that period. The sight of the body left hanging for several days played an important role in the state ritual the purpose of which was to elicit public scorn and to terrify. With a high mass celebrated for his soul in the nearby church, the executed was buried at Dance. At the beginning of the eighteenth century, death sentences represented 5 percent of the sentences pronounced. By the end of the century, that proportion had dropped to 1 percent but few of them were actually carried out. Lonza, *Pod plaštem pravde*, 141–7; Lonza, *Kazalište vlasti*, 123–30.

37 *Libro deli Signori Chazamorbi, A tergo,* f. 67v–68.

38 During the plague outbreak in Bombay in 1894, the Indian Plague Commission reported cases where no rats – dead, sick or healthy – could be found but plague was transmitted by merchandise, mostly grain and rice, and by means of clothes. Walløe, "Medieval and Modern Bubonic Plague," 69–70.

39 *Libro deli Signori Chazamorbi, A tergo,* f. 79–79v.

40 The 1484 rules for the lazaretti in Venice required all workers returning from the lazaretti to the city to wear a white sign on their clothes. In Siena in 1485, physicians, priests, and "contacts" of plague cases were all required to wear a sign, usually a white stole, when they moved around the city. In Florence in 1522–23, the "contacts" had to wear a white sign on their arms as a warning to others. Stevens, "The Lazaretti," 163; Crawshaw, *Plague Hospitals,* 131; Carmichael, "Plague Legislation," 523; Henderson, "Epidemics," 182.

41 Being exposed at the column of shame had truly grave consequences not only for the individual but also for the reputation of his whole family. From the recorded appeals and requests for the change of sentence, it becomes evident that the sentence of riding a donkey through the streets of the city or standing for one hour at the column of shame were considered terrifying to such a degree that the sentenced were willing to exchange them for a year in prison or a ten-year banishment. Orlando's (Roland's) column, erected in 1419, served as a column of shame until 1808. Flying the flag of the Ragusan Republic, Orlando's column came to be recognized as a powerful symbol of justice at a time when the Republic was de facto functioning as an independent state under the protection of the Croatian-Hungarian king. Also, related to the legend of Orlando defending Dubrovnik from the Saracens, the column became the place where the town criers usually read important announcements and new regulations. As well, the forearm of Orlando came to be known as a measure of length – namely, the Ragusan *ell,* which was about fifty-one to fify-five centimetres long (Lonza, *Pod plaštem pravde,* 160–2; Lonza, *Kazalište vlasti,* 118–23; Kunčević, "On Ragusan," 31–6). Diversis mentions that various criminals are tied to this column, and whipped, and sometimes their beard is also burned: "Nam ad illam ligantur, et fistigantur aliquando scelesti homines, quibus etiam interdum barba comburitur" (Diversis, *Opis,* 95; 177).

42 *Libro deli Signori Chazamorbi, A tergo,* f. 22.

43 *Libro deli Signori Chazamorbi, A tergo,* f. 45–7.

44 *Libro deli Signori Chazamorbi, A tergo,* f. 22, 89, 91, 92–92v, 93, 94, 119v, 126v, 127v, 129, 133v.

45 For example, in the Geneva plague outbreaks of the sixteenth and seventeenth centuries, the same type of torture (*la corde*) was used during the trials of plague spreaders, some of whom were laundresses. Naphy, *Plagues,* 24–8, 58, 68, 138–41.

46 The Appeals Court was created in 1445. In Dubrovnik it was possible to appeal the sentence but not in the cases of plague control measures. In Venice, the criminal sentences of the Health Office were without appeal until 1563 when the Senate decided to allow them. Diversis, *Opis,* 71; 163–4; Lonza, *Pod plaštem,* 246–50; Palmer, *The Control of Plague,* 227.

47 *Libro deli Signori Chazamorbi, A tergo,* f. 85v.

48 *Libro deli Signori Chazamorbi, A tergo,* f. 92–92v, f. 93, f. 116.

49 Punishment by the ritual rounds on a donkey does not ever appear in isolation. It

usually precedes the exposure on the column of shame, branding with the mark of disgrace, and the banishment from the Republic. It regularly precedes the death penalty. Its basic purpose is to humiliate and shame the sentenced in front of the multitude, demonstrating to all his guilt and his crime. Accompanied by drummers, guards, and soldiers, the ritual rounds on a donkey and the major religious processions shared the same route through the heart of the city. Both left the Rector's Palace and continued through Ulica od Puča, turning right on Široka Ulica and returning to the Rector's Palace through the largest street in the city, the Placa. Mitić, *Dubrovačka država*, 71–3; Lonza, *Pod plaštem pravde*, 159–60; Lonza, *Kazalište vlasti*, 120.

50 The suspicion that animals were responsible for the transmission plague was always present. We now know that plague can be transmitted by many species of animals, including domestic animals, carnivores, and many varieties of rodents. Ell, "Immunity as a Factor," 869.

51 *Libro deli Signori Chazamorbi, A tergo*, f. 114v.

52 *Libro deli Signori Chazamorbi, A tergo*, f. 115, at the margin.

53 *Libro deli Signori Chazamorbi, A tergo*, f. 105–105v, 106–106v.

54 In Venice, between 1541 and 1558, more than twenty employees of the Health Office were tried for theft of infected clothing, theft from the lazaretto, taking bribes, and giving licence to infected goods, among other offences. Palmer, *Control of Plague*, 235–6. For denunciations of crimes committed in the lazaretto by the Health Office employees, see Crawshaw, *Plague Hospitals*, 226–8.

55 *Libro deli Signori Chazamorbi, A tergo*, f. 106v. *Raša* in Croatian or *raxo* in the language of the manuscript was a sort of rough woven fabric that was produced in Dubrovnik and on the islands. The cattle rearing Vlachs in Bosnia-Herzegovina and Serbia produced the greatest amount of raša (Roller, *Dubrovački zanati*, 22–32; Lučić, *Obrti i usluge*, 72–84; Dinić-Knežević, *Tkanine u privredi*, 11–15).

56 "Dizemo et criminalmente ad morte sententiamo prefato Giorgi de Marchetto, sia conduto fora della zitta alle Pille et li sia, infra le porte, inpicato per le canne della gola, ad eo che l anima si parta dal corpo suspenso senza anima rimanga ad exemplo et castiga deli altri simil exzessi cometer volesseno." *Libro deli Signori Chazamorbi, A tergo*, f. 109v.

57 Naphy, *Plagues*, 28–34, 68–71, 138–41.

58 Calvi, *Histories of a Plague Year*, 155–96.

59 Cipolla, *Faith, Reason*, 13–14.

60 Calvi, *Histories of a Plague Year*, 179–80.

61 *Libro deli Signori Chazamorbi, A tergo*, f. 113v.

CHAPTER EIGHT

1 *Libro deli Signori Chazamorbi, A tergo*, f. 14v.

2 *Libro deli Signori Chazamorbi, A tergo*, f. 13–13v.

3 *Libro deli Signori Chazamorbi, A tergo*, f. 60.

4 *Libro deli Signori Chazamorbi, A tergo*, f. 41.

5 *Libro deli Signori Chazamorbi, A tergo*, f. 91. *Latino vulgare* denotes the Italian language, mostly the Venetian dialect of the sixteenth century, used by the scribes keeping records of the meetings of the three Ragusan ruling Councils, the courts and the administration, in general. *Materno linguagio* was the Croatian mother tongue spoken by all social classes.

6 *Libro deli Signori Chazamorbi, A tergo*, f. 91.

7 In Venice, the Health Office depended on the denunciations of the offenders by the citizens who were paid if their information led to a successful prosecution. Palmer, *The Control of Plague*, 227.

8 *Libro deli Signori Chazamorbi, A tergo*, f. 93v.

9 *Kaznac* was the local authority of a *kaznačina*, a territorial unit, approximately the size of a village. Lonza, *Pod plaštem pravde*, 99.

10 *Libro deli Signori Chazamorbi, A tergo*, f. 94.

11 *Libro deli Signori Chazamorbi, A tergo*, f. 98–103.

12 Gabela, also called *portum Narenti* in Latin or Narente by Ragusans and Drijeva by its Slavic name, was a major trading place between Ragusans and Bosnians on the geographically and economically pivotal Neretva Delta. Sea salt was brought to Gabela from the Adriatic salt pans, and especially from Ston. The Ragusan merchants held a quasi-monopoly on sea salt trade. Gabela was built around a marketplace, with its own customs office, warehouses, shops, and churches, and it was home to a permanent Ragusan colony. Harris, *Dubrovnik*, 153–4.

13 Janeković-Römer, "Dubrovačko 15. stoljeće," 18–30.

14 *Aspra*, from Byzantine Greek, means money, but here it refers to Turkish silver coins.

15 Ston, on the Pelješac Peninsula, was and still is an important sea salt-producing centre. Peričić, "Prilog poznavanju," 139–44.

16 *Libro deli Signori Chazamorbi, A tergo*, f. 99.

17 To quickly isolate the plague-stricken and those suspected of infection from the healthy population, the authorities would send persons coming from the islands and from the coastal areas of Župa and Primorje to the nearby rocky islets. Living conditions on those islets were exceptionally difficult.

18 *Gipon* was a tunic worn under armor in the fourteenth century and later adapted for civilian use.

19 *Libro deli Signori Chazamorbi, A tergo*, f. 102.

20 *Libro deli Signori Chazamorbi, A tergo*, f. 98, 103v.

21 "Prete Vizenzo disse haver diligentemente domandato et interrogato ala confession la ditta moglier de quondam Boxo." *Libro deli Signori Chazamorbi, A tergo*, f. 100.

22 There was an exchange place for goods from the Ottoman-controlled territory at Ploče, called Tabor. Miović-Perić, *Na razmeđu*, 119, 122–4.

23 Diversis reports that sailors from infected ships would sometimes leave infected persons somewhere along the coast of the Ragusan Republic. If that were the case, one or two armed boats would leave right away to investigate. Their commander would not let anyone arriving from infected areas enter the Ragusan territory. If the local counts heard of a case of plague, they had to report it to the *Cazamorti*. Fabric from infected areas was not allowed to be imported without being quarantined for at least a month on the bottom of some tower. Similar treatment was reserved for other types of goods. Diversis, *Opis*, 83–4; 169.

24 *Libro deli Signori Chazamorbi, A recto*, f. 93v.

25 "Et per lo simel sia bruxata la caxa de Giurag Matilovich in Mochoxiza che venne de Tarstino per terra in Ombla senza lizenzia. E anche sia bruxata la caxa de Antonio Zvitchovich de Gionchetto sotto Comolaz ... De comandamento deli Signori officiali sopra la Sanita, fo commesso a ser Polo Ni. de Luchari che andasse in perzona in Mochoxiza e in Gionchetto a far brusar le ditte caxe talmente

che non si trovino la vestigia de quelle." *Libro deli Signori Chazamorbi, A tergo*, f. 103v.

26 *Libro deli Signori Chazamorbi, A recto*, f. 92.

27 "Questo ad perpetuam rei memoriam et exemplo deli altri." *Libro deli Signori Chazamorbi, A tergo*, f. 117–117v.

28 Trsteno, twenty-four kilometres northwest of Dubrovnik, was the summer residence of the famous patrician family Gučetić (Goze) who, in 1494, founded an arboretum with classical fountains, villas, and a profusion of horticultural species. The Renaissance buildings were renovated after the 1667 earthquake. The Arboretum of Trsteno, home to more than three hundred species of trees from the Mediterranean area, can still be visited to this day. Grujić, "Dubrovačka," 141–67; Lučić, "Gozze/Gučetići," 14–16; Harris, *Dubrovnik*, 314–15.

29 *Libro deli Signori Chazamorbi, A tergo*, f. 124.

30 Putting a miter on the head of the sentenced, painted with the scenes of hell, was sometimes part of the ritual rounds through the city. The miter, a symbol of high religious dignitaries, was transformed into a shaming punishment and subjected to ridicule. Lonza, *Pod plaštem pravde*, 160.

31 "Et le caxe de ambi duo, zoe del ditto Michan in Bersecine e de Petar in Tersteno, siano bruxate." *Libro deli Signori Chazamorbi, A tergo*, f. 123–126v.

32 *Libro deli Signori Chazamorbi, A tergo*, f. 120.

33 On 22 June 1528, five health officials were present as trial judges and two were absent. *Libro deli Signori Chazamorbi, A tergo*, f. 112.

34 New trial judges in 1528: Mato Franov Bobaljević (Babalio) and Nikola Franov Sorkočević (Sorgo); in 1529: Dominik Martinov Ragnina, Dimitar Martinov Ragnina, Andro Mihov Rastić (Resti), and Andro Lukin Sorkočević (Sorgo). Names of trial judges for 1530 are not mentioned. *Libro deli Signori Chazamorbi, A tergo*, f. 93v–131.

35 *Libro deli Signori Chazamorbi, A tergo*, f. 80, 110.

36 Pavao Marinov Gradić (Gradi), 1478–1558; Marin Stjepanov Džamonjić (Giamagno), 1479–1548; Mato Franov Bobaljević (Babalio), 1480–1549. We do not have the year of birth or death of Nikola Franov Sorkočević (Sorgo). *Libro deli Signori Chazamorbi, A tergo*, f. 93v, f. 108v, f. 110. The information about the patricians was kindly provided by Nenad Vekarić, director of the Institute for the Historical Sciences of the Croatian Academy of Arts and Sciences in Dubrovnik.

37 For example, Frano Pandolfov Benešić (Benessa), Miho Marinov Bučinčić (Bocignolo), Stjepan Marinov Bunčić (Bonda), Paskoje Trojanov Crijević (Zrieva), and Dimitar Matov Ragnina, who were elected as health officials in 1527, are not mentioned as trial judges in *Libro deli Signori Chazamorbi, A tergo*.

CHAPTER NINE

1 Cipolla, *Fighting the Plague*, 89–110.

2 Many taverns in Dubrovnik were owned by patricians. Commoners were employed as tavern keepers. Wine served in taverns was considered indispensable to people's health. Therefore, the government put as much effort into supplying the city with wine as it did with grain. The wine commerce was strictly regulated and supervised by special government employees – *officiales supra vino*. They controlled the quality and the price of wine served in taverns. It was forbidden to serve wine that was mixed with honey or spices. The opening hours of taverns,

which had to be housed in stone buildings, were also specified. To avoid criminal actions by inebriated citizens at night, the taverns had to close after the third bell (*post tertiam campanam*), probably around 22:00 hours in winter and around 23:00 hours in the summer months. The taverns were usually located in wider streets, squares, and close to churches and monasteries where people gathered. In the fourteenth and the fifteenth centuries, there were 132 tavern owners in Dubrovnik. Women, who are most often cited as pouring wine in taverns, sometimes had trouble with their patrons. Every year, five *Officiales contrabanoris vini* – officers against trade in contraband wine – were elected. Four armed vessels were prepared to intercept this illicit trade. Ravančić, *Život u krčmama*, 20–35, 43, 55–6, 67, 75–84; Ravančić, "Javni prostor," 57–61; Janeković-Römer, "Post tertiam campanam," 10–11; Rheubottom, *Age, Marriage*, 20.

3 *Libro deli Signori Chazamorbi, A recto*, f. 92v.
4 *Libro deli Signori Chazamorbi, A recto*, f. 94.
5 *Libro deli Signori Chazamorbi, A tergo*, f. 23v – 24.
6 *Libro deli Signori Chazamorbi, A tergo*, f. 37.
7 *Libro deli Signori Chazamorbi, A tergo*, f. 74–75.
8 *Libro deli Signori Chazamorbi, A tergo*, f. 82v.
9 *Libro deli Signori Chazamorbi, A tergo*, f. 90–90v.
10 Ledenice is a community in the hinterland of the Bay of Kotor, in present-day Montenegro.
11 *Libro deli Signori Chazamorbi, A tergo*, f. 11v.
12 *Libro deli Signori Chazamorbi, A recto*, f. 90.
13 *Libro deli Signori Chazamorbi, A tergo*, f. 96v.
14 Ragnina mentions Pietro Pantella in 1432, while the Anonymous chronicler and Razzi report his activities in 1433. *Annales Ragusini Anonymi item Nicolai de Ragnina*, 55, 251; Razzi, *La storia*, 55.
15 Hrabak, *Vuna*, 63–93; Spremić, *Dubrovnik*, 147–52; Fejić, *Španci*, 78–89; Hrabak, "Učešće Katalonaca," 42, 66–8.
16 Roller, *Dubrovački zanati*, 5–84; Krekić, *Dubrovnik in the 14th and 15th Centuries*, 56; Lučić, *Obrti i usluge*, 73–84; Dinić-Knežević, *Tkanine u privredi*, 87–92, 245–9. There were two standards for fabrics, the small one of 36 Ragusan ells and the big one of 60 ells in length. Since Diversis does not specify the size, it could mean between 73,400 or 122,400 metres of fabric. Diversis also mentions that at that time the Ragusans started thinking about building an aqueduct for the city because a good water supply was crucial for textile manufacturing. Seferović and Stojan report that several additional workshops for rolling and washing cloth, as well as more than ten mills were planned in 1440s, but were never built because the water output of the new aqueduct was not sufficient to support this activity during the dry season. Diversis reports that an addition to the aqueduct was contemplated but it was reconstructed only in 1550. Seferović and Stojan, "The Miracle," 72–82; Diversis, *Opis*, 61, 109–11; 154, 186–7.
17 The craftsmen involved in the textile manufacturing all belonged to their own professional confraternities. Roller, *Dubrovački zanati*, 173–260.
18 *Libro deli Signori Chazamorbi, A tergo*, f. 96v; *Liber viridis, caput* 152, 107. Textile production in Dubrovnik was highly regulated. *Camera artis lanae*, the Chamber of wool craft, was founded on 30 January 1416 by the Major Council. Every year, three officials were elected to supervise all aspects of textile

production. Another three officials and two assistants were added later. The scribe of the Chamber had to mark all the pieces of fabric produced with a stamp of St Blaise. Otherwise, the fabric was considered contraband and could not be sold. Illegal bales of fabric were cut into small pieces to prevent their sale and the producers were fined. Roller, *Dubrovački zanati*, 13–22; Harris, *Dubrovnik*, 182.

19 Foretić, "Dubrovnik," 265–75; Lučić, *Prošlost dubrovačke Astareje*, 33–6; Krekić, *Dubrovnik in the 14th and 15th Centuries*, 23–62; Carter, *Dubrovnik*, 70–4; Foretić, *Povijest Dubrovnika do 1808*, 1:32–6; Blažina Tomić, *Historical Development*, 16; Prelog, "Dubrovnik: prostor i vrijeme," 30; Mitić, *Dubrovačka država*, 33–7; Stulli, *Židovi u Dubrovniku*, 17–19; Dinić-Knežević, *Migracije stanovništva*, 233–52. ·

20 *Libro deli Signori Chazamorbi, A tergo*, f. 110.

21 Concealing of plague cases, both by individuals and officials, continued in the third plague pandemic in Hong Kong (1894), Bombay (1896), Vietnam (1898), Honolulu (1900), San Francisco (1900–05, 1907), and many other cities. The consequences of a plague epidemic were so disastrous for every community that each affected city tried to deny the presence of plague even when it was obvious that plague was rampant. Families would hide their plague-stricken relatives and city officials would ask physicians not to disclose or to change the fateful diagnosis. In San Francisco (1900–05), federal health officials sent from Washington worked diligently to eradicate plague from Chinatown while the California state officials, afraid that the city or the state would be quarantined, systematically denied its presence for five years. The physicians who risked their lives daily for the common good were attacked and ridiculed. They were even accused by the media of deliberately introducing plague to the city. Mollaret and Brossollet, *Yersin*, 154, 187–8, 197–8; Mohr, *Plague and Fire*, 79–80; Chase, *Barbary Plague*, 46–55, 64–74, 86, 115.

22 *Libro deli Signori Chazamorbi, A tergo*, f. 110v.

23 Compare the situation in Venice during the plague outbreak of 1555–58; Health Office employees – boatmen, disinfectors, chaplains, body clearers, and doctors – were often accused of wrongdoing by denunciation. Fines were issued and a proportion of the money was given to the accuser. Stevens, "The Lazaretti," 174–6.

24 *Libro deli Signori Chazamorbi, A tergo*, f. 111v–112v.

25 The Church of St Mary the Great is the cathedral of Dubrovnik.

26 In Venice during the 1575–77 plague epidemic, the state spent large amounts of money to disinfect goods. Crawshaw, *Plague Hospitals*, 209–22.

27 *Libro deli Signori Chazamorbi, A tergo*, f. 111.

28 It is the church of the Sts Peter, Lawrence, and Andrew, the three martyrs from Kotor, but in the manuscript it is called the church of St Peter and St Lawrence. *Libro deli Signori Chazamorbi, A tergo*, f. 113.

29 *Libro deli Signori Chazamorbi, A tergo*, f. 113.

30 *Libro deli Signori Chazamorbi, A tergo*, f. 12v.

31 *Libro deli Signori Chazamorbi, A tergo*, f. 15.

32 *Libro deli Signori Chazamorbi, A tergo*, f. 42.

33 *Libro deli Signori Chazamorbi, A tergo*, f. 77.

34 The fish market is situated close to the Dominican monastery.

35 *Libro deli Signori Chazamorbi, A tergo*, f. 95v–96.

36 *Libro deli Signori Chazamorbi, A tergo,* f. 86, 87.
37 *Libro deli Signori Chazamorbi, A tergo,* f. 99v, 113.
38 Lonza, *Kazalište,* 267–95.
39 Cohn, *Cultures,* 283–93.
40 Palmer, *The Control of Plague,* 319–21.
41 Bowers, *Plague, Politics,* 106–28; Bowers, "Balancing Individual," 335–58.
42 Cook and Cook, *The Plague Files,* 12, 141–67, 210.
43 Cavallo, *Charity,* 44–57.

APPENDIX A

1 Šundrica, "Kako je nastala," 28–35; Tadić, "Dubrovački arhiv," 111–15.
2 The oldest document in the archives is the bull of Pope Benedict VIII dated 21 September 1022. It refers to the authority of the Ragusan archbishop over subordinate bishoprics. The second oldest document is dated 1023 and refers to the foundation of the Benedictine monastery on the island of Lokrum. For the period 1022 to 1208, there are twenty-four documents preserved in the State Archives. Foretić, "Dubrovački arhiv," 315.
3 The archives probably existed before that time but as part of church archives and were considered private property of the notaries. Local priests served as notaries at that time. Čremošnik, "Kada," 57–60.
4 Since the seventeenth century and until the end of the Republic, these duties were performed by Ragusan commoners. This profession usually remained within families and was often passed on from one generation to the next, from father to son. It was the highest social rank that the commoners could attain. Lonza, *Pod plaštem,* 81.
5 Diversis, *Opis,* 76–8, 164–5.
6 In the Middle Ages, the work of chancellors and notaries was regulated by laws adopted by the Ragusan Councils in 1313, 1345, 1366, 1385, 1428, and 1473. Foretić, "Dubrovački arhiv," 336.
7 Čremošnik, "Dubrovačka kancelarija," 232–41; Marinović, "Postanak," 12–16; Foretić, *Povijest,* 1 6–10; Ćosić, "Prinos," 123–45; Harris, *Dubrovnik,* 125.
8 Gelčić, "Dubrovački arhiv," 537–44.
9 Foretić, "Dubrovački arhiv," 209–15; Foretić, "O Dubrovačkom arhivu," 52–64; Foretić, "Dosadašnji rezultati," 445–61; Blažina Tomić, *Historical Development,* 1–5; Stulli, "Dva pokušaja," 203–60; Carter, *Dubrovnik,* 587–91.
10 Voje, *Poslovna uspešnost,* 65.
11 Lonza, "Pred gosparom knezom," 25–54; Lonza and Janeković-Römer, "Dubrovački *Liber de maleficiis,*" 173–228; Lonza, "Tužba, osveta, nagodba," 57–104; Lonza, "Srednjovjekovni zapisnici," 45–74.
12 Janeković-Römer, "*Post tertiam campanam,*" 7–14; Ravančić, "*In taberna quando erant,*" 33–44.
13 The oldest Ottoman document dates from 1458. It is a receipt (*firman*) issued by Sultan Mehmed II concerning the payment of the tribute (*harač*) by Dubrovnik. Miović and Selmani, "Turska kancelarija," 279–82. See also Miović, *Dubrovačka Republika u spisima osmanskih sultana.*
14 Foretić, "Pregled stanja," 68–75.
15 Miović and Selmani, "Turska kancelarija," 252–78.

APPENDIX B
1 Diversis, *Opis*, 39–40; 140–1.

APPENDIX C
1 Mount Krstac (Cresta) is actually Mount Srđ (Sergius), 412 metres, which dominates the city of Dubrovnik from the north side and is part of the Dinaric chain of Alps extending along the entire length of the Dalmatian coastline. The church, which is still standing, was built on a steep hill just above the port of Gruž. It was the first votive church against plague built in Dubrovnik.
2 Placa is the main street in Dubrovnik.
3 St Mary the Great is the cathedral of Dubrovnik.
4 St Andrew and St Mary in Kaštel (de Castello) were situated in the oldest part of the city.
5 Višnjica is a small coastal village east of Dubrovnik. Saint James in Višnjica was a Benedictine monastery established in 1222 by the patrician Ivan Gundulić (Gondola) and his wife Dobroslava.
6 Angelo de Leticia did not want the priest to be a foreigner.
7 Monte Sant'Angelo is situated on the Gargano promontory, north of Manfredonia in Italy. There is a sacred cave in which Saint Michael the Archangel is said to have appeared. It is a well-known shrine and a place of pilgrimage.
8 *Primitia* was a legacy for those who wanted to become nuns or priests and for the celebration of the first Mass of a new priest.
9 Pakljena is situated on the island of Šipan, near Suđurađ.
10 *Testamenta de Notaria*, v. 5, f. 2v–4v.
11 *Testamenta de Notaria*, v. 5, f. 2v–4v. Transcription by Ravančić, *Vrijeme umiranja*, 164–5.

References

MANUSCRIPT SOURCES IN THE STATE ARCHIVES OF DUBROVNIK
(DRŽAVNI ARHIV U DUBROVNIKU OR DAD), CROATIA

Acta Consilii Maioris
Acta Consilii Rogatorum
Acta Minoris Consilii
Diversa Cancellariae
Diversa Notariae
Lettere di Levante (Lettere e Commissioni)
Libro deli Signori Cazamorbi, Sanitas, Series 55, v. 1, 1500–1530
Monumenta Ragusina
Reformationes
Speculum Maioris Consilii
Testamenta de Notaria

PUBLISHED SOURCES

Note: In the Croatian language, C, Č, and Ć are separate letters as are S and Š, and Z and Ž. They are arranged in separate alphabetical order after the letters C, S, or Z. All Croatian, Bosnian, Serbian, and Slovenian titles have been translated into English.

Aboudharam, Gérard, Michel Signoli, E. Crubezy, G. Larrouy, B. Ludes, Olivier Dutour, Didier Raoult, and Michel Drancourt. "La mémoire des dents: Le cas de la peste." In *Peste: Entre épidémies et sociétés. Fourth International Congress on the Evolution and Palaeoepidemiology of the Infectious Diseases, 2001, Marseilles, France*. Édité par Michel Signoli, Dominique Chevé, Pascal Adalian, Gilles Boëtsch, and Olivier Dutour, 207–16. Florence: Firenze University Press, 2007.
Amundsen, Darrel W. "Medieval Canon Law on Medicine and Surgical Practice by the Clergy." *Bulletin of the History of Medicine* 52 (1978): 22–44.
Annales Ragusini Anonymi item Nicolai de Ragnina. Zagabriae: JAZU, Monumenta spectantia historiam Slavorum meridionalium 14, digessit Speratus Nodilo, 1883.

Appendini, Francesco Maria. *Notizie istorico-critiche sulla antichità, storia, e letteratura de'Ragusei: Divise in due tomi e dedicate all'eccelso Senato della Rupublica Ragusa.* Vol. 2. Dubrovnik: Martecchini, 1803.

Bacalexi, Dina. "Trois traducteurs de Galien au XVIe siècle et leur regard sur la tradition arabe." In *Pratique et pensée médicales à la Renaissance: Actes du Colloque international d'études humanistes, Tours, 2–6 juillet 2007.* Edited by Jacqueline Vons, 201–21. Paris: De Boccard, 2009.

Bačić, Jurica. "Liječnici Dubrovačke Republike na službi u Banjaluci krajem XVI stoljeća" [Physicians of the Ragusan Republic serving in Banja Luka at the end of the sixteenth century]. *Acta historiae medicinae stomatologiae pharmaciae medicinae veterinae* (Belgrade) 24 (1984): 17–21.

– "Magister Kristofor-fizik (prva liječnička mirovina u starom Dubrovniku, 1399. g.)" [Magister Christophorus, physicus, the first physician to receive a pension in Dubrovnik in 1399]. *Liječnički vjesnik* (Zagreb) (1968):108.

– *Stazama medicine starog Dubrovnika* [Medicine in old-time Dubrovnik]. Rijeka: Izdavački centar Rijeka, 1988.

Badurina, Anđelko. "Likovnost Dubrovnika u vizitaciji biskupa Sormana 1573.–4. godine" [Fine arts of Dubrovnik in the bishop Sormano 1573–74 report]. In *Likovna kultura Dubrovnika 15. i 16. stoljeća* [Fine arts in Dubrovnik in the fifteenth and sixteenth centuries]. Edited by Igor Fisković, 280–1. Scientific conference accompanying the exhibition "The Golden Age of Dubrovnik." Zagreb: Znanstvena djela Muzejsko-Galerijskog Centra 2, 1991.

– "Sakralna arhitektura" [Religious architecture]. In *Zlatno doba Dubrovnika XV. i XVI. stoljeće: Urbanizam, arhitektura, skulptura, slikarstvo, iluminirani rukopisi, zlatarstvo* [The Golden Age of Dubrovnik in the fifteenth and sixteenth centuries: Urban planning, architecture, sculpture, painting, illuminated manuscripts and goldsmithing]. Exhibition catalogue, 324–31. Edited by Milan Prelog, Marija Planić-Lončarić, Anđelko Badurina, Nada Grujić, Igor Fisković, Vladimir Marković, Ivo Lentić, Ivica Prlender, and Tonko Maroević. Zagreb: Muzej Topić Mimara, 1987.

Barker, Sheila. "The Making of a Plague Saint: Saint Sebastian's Imagery and Cult before the Counter-Reformation." In *Piety and Plague: From Byzantium to the Baroque.* Edited by Franco Mormando and Thomas Worcester, 90–131. Kirksville, MO: Truman State University Press, 2007.

Battelli, Giulio. *Lezioni di paleografia.* Città del Vaticano: Pont. Scuola vaticana di paleografia e diplomatica, 1949.

Bazala, Vladimir. "Calendarium Pestis." *Acta Historica Medicinae Pharmaciae Veterinae* 1 (1962): 55–65.

– "Delle peste e dei modi di preservarsene nella Repubblica di Ragusa-Dubrovnik." In *Atti XIX Congresso Internazionale della Storia di Medicina.* Roma, 1954: 723–56.

– *Pregled povijesti zdravstvene kulture Dubrovačke Republike* [Review of the history of health culture in the Ragusan Republic]. Zagreb: Dubrovački horizonti, 1972.

Belamarić, Joško. "Sveti Vlaho i dubrovačka obitelj svetaca zaštitnika" [Saint Blaise and the Ragusan protection saints]. In *Tisuću godina uspostave dubrovačke (nad)biskupije: Zbornik radova znanstvenoga skupa u povodu tisuću godina uspostave dubrovačke (nad)biskupije /metropolije (998–1998)* [One thousand years of the Ragusan (Arch)bishopric]. Edited by Želimir Puljić and Nediljko Ante Ančić, 703–31. Dubrovnik: Biskupski ordinarijat; Split: Crkva u svijetu, 2001.

Belicza, Biserka, and Zlata Blažina Tomić. "Dubrovački liječnici u službi dubrovačke diplomacije u srednjem vijeku i renesansi" [Ragusan physicians as diplomats in the Middle Ages and the Renaissance]. In *Hrvatska Srednjovjekovna diplomacija* [Croatian mediaeval diplomacy]. Edited by Mladen Andrlić and Mirko Valentić. *Zbornik Diplomatske akademije* [Proceedings of the Diplomatic Academy] 2 (1999): 205–13.

Benedetti, Rocco. *Relatione d'alcuni casi occorsi in Venetia al tempo della peste l'anno 1576 et 1577 con le provisioni, rimedii et orationi fatte à Dio benedetto per la sua liberatione.* Bologna, 1630.

Benedictow, Ole Jørgen. *The Black Death, 1346–1353: The Complete History.* Woodbridge, UK: Boydell Press, 2004.

Beritić, Lukša. "Dubrovački vodovod" [The Ragusan aqueduct]. *Anali Historijskog instituta JAZU u Dubrovniku* 8–9 (1962): 99–116.

– "Stonske utvrde" [The fortifications of Ston]. *Anali Historijskog instituta JAZU u Dubrovniku* 3 (1954): 297–354.

– "Stonske utvrde 2" [The fortifications of Ston 2]. *Anali Historijskog instituta JAZU u Dubrovniku* 4–5 (1956):71–152.

Biegman, Nicolaas H. *The Turco-Ragusan Relationship: According to the Firmans of Murad III (1575–1595) Extant in the State Archives of Dubrovnik.* The Hague and Paris: Mouton, 1967.

Biraben, Jean Noël. *Les hommes et la peste en France et dans les pays européens et mediterranéens.* Vol. 1, *La peste dans l'histoire*; Paris-La Haye: Mouton, 1975.

– *Les hommes et la peste en France et dans les pays européens et mediterranéens.* Vol. 2, *Les hommes face à la peste.* Paris-La Haye: Mouton, 1976.

Bischoff, Bernhard. *Latin Palaeography: Antiquity and the Middle Ages.* Cambridge: Cambridge University Press, 1990.

Blažina Tomić, Zlata. "Historical Development of the Laws and Regulations Concerning Public Health in Dubrovnik (Ragusa) from the 13th to the 15th Century." MA thesis, McGill University, Montreal, 1981.

– "Interakcija dubrovačkih vijeća i javnih zdravstvenih službenika (*officiales cazzamortuorum*) za vrijeme epidemija u četrnaestom i petnaestom stoljeću" [Interaction of the Ragusan Councils and the *Cazamorti* during the epidemics in the fourteenth and the fifteenth centuries]. *Rasprave i Građa za povijest znanosti HAZU* 7 (1992): 1–16.

– *Kacamorti i kuga: utemeljenje i razvoj zdravstvene službe u Dubrovniku* [The Cazamorti and the plague: Founding and development of the Health Office in Dubrovnik]. Zagreb, Dubrovnik: HAZU, Zavod za povijesne znanosti u Dubrovniku, 2007.

– "The Status of the Medical Profession in Dubrovnik (Ragusa) from the 13th to the 15th Century." In *It Is Good to Know: Essays and Appreciations in Honour of the 90th Birthday of Dr. Harold Nathan Segall.* Edited by Faith Wallis, 18–50. Montreal: Osler Library, McGill University, 1989.

– "Uloga javnih zdravstvenih službenika – kacamorata, vijeća i medicinske profesije u sprečavanju kuge u Dubrovniku u prvoj polovici 16. stoljeća" [The role of the Health Officials, the Councils, and the medical profession in preventing plague in Dubrovnik in the first half of the sixteenth century]. PhD diss., University of Zagreb, 2001.

Boeckl, Christine M. *Images of Plague and Pestilence: Iconography and Iconology.* Kirksville, MO: Truman State University Press, 2000.

Bottero, Aldo. "La peste in Milano nel 1399–1400 e l'opera di Gian Galeazzo Visconti." *Atti e Memorie del'Accademia di Storia dell"Arte. Sanitaria La Rassegna di Clinica, Terapia e Scienze Affini* 41, fasc. 6 (1942): 17–28.

Bos, Kirsten, V. Schuenemann, G.B. Golding, H. Burbano, N. Waglechner, B. Coombes, J. McPhee, et al. "A Draft Genome of *Yersinia pestis* from Victims of the Black Death." *Nature*, 478 (27 October 2011): 506–10. doi:10.1038/nature10549. http://www.nature.com/nature/journal/vaop/ncurrent/pdf/nature10549.pdf.

Bowers, Kristy Wilson. "Balancing Individual Needs and Communal Needs: Plague and Public Health in Early Modern Seville." *Bulletin of the History of Medicine* 81 (2007): 335–58.

– "Plague, Politics and Municipal Relations in Sixteenth-Century Seville." PhD diss., Indiana University, Bloomington, 2001.

Božić, Ivan. *Dubrovnik i Turska u XIV i XV veku* [Dubrovnik and Turkey in the 14th and 15th centuries]. Belgrade: Istorijski institut SAN, knjiga 3, 1952.

Braudel, Fernand. *The Mediterranean and the Mediterranean World in the Age of Philip II*. Translated by Sian Reynolds. 2 vols. [Translation from French, *Méditerranée et le monde méditerranéen à l'époque de Philippe II*]. New York: Harper and Row, 1972.

Brown, Michelle. *A Guide to Western Historical Scripts from Antiquity to 1600*. Toronto: University of Toronto Press, 1990.

Buconić Gović, Tereza. *Dubrovačke crkvice* [Small churches in Dubrovnik]. Dubrovnik: [published by the author], 2002.

Buklijaš, Tatjana. *"Per relationem medicorum* – povijesnomedicinska građa u dubrovačkim kaznenim spisima iz 15. stoljeća (1421–1431)" [*Per relationem medicorum*: Fifteenth-century Ragusan criminal records as medical history sources]. *Anali Zavoda za povijesne znanosti HAZU u Dubrovniku* 39 (2001): 49–120.

Buklijaš, Tatjana, and Irena Benyovsky. "Domus Christi in Late Medieval Dubrovnik: A Therapy for the Body and Soul." *Dubrovnik Annals* 8 (2004): 81–107.

Bullough, Vernon. "Population and the Study and Practice of Medieval Medicine." *Bulletin of the History of Medicine* 36 (1962): 62–9.

Butler, Thomas C. *Plague and Other Yersinia Infections*. New York: Plenum Medical Book Company, 1983.

Bylebyl, Jerome J. "The School of Padua: Humanistic Medicine in the Sixteenth Century." In *Health, Medicine and Mortality in the Sixteenth Century*. Edited by Charles Webster, 335–70. Cambridge: Cambridge University Press, 1979.

Calvi, Giulia. *Histories of a Plague Year*. Translated by Dario Biocca and Briant Ragan, Jr. Berkeley: University of California Press, 1989.

Campbell, Anna Montgomery. *The Black Death and Men of Learning*. New York: Columbia University Press, 1931.

Canobbio, Alessandro. *Il successo della peste occorsa in Padoua l'anno MDLXXVI*. Venice: Paolo Megietti libraro in Padova, 1577.

Carmichael, Ann G. "Bubonic Plague." In *The Cambridge World History of Human Disease*. Edited by Kenneth F. Kiple, 628–31. Cambridge: Cambridge University Press 1993.

– "Contagion Theory and Contagion Practice in Fifteenth-Century Milan." *Renaissance Quarterly* 44 (1991): 213–56.

– *Epidemic Diseases in Early Renaissance Florence*. Ann Arbor: University Microfilms, 1980.

- "History of Public Health and Sanitation in the West before 1700." In *The Cambridge World History of Human Disease*. Edited by Kenneth F. Kiple, 192–200. Cambridge: Cambridge University Press, 1993.
- "The Last Plague: The Uses of Memory in Renaissance Epidemics." *Journal of the History of Medicine* 53 (1998): 132–60.
- *Plague and the Poor in Renaissance Florence*. Cambridge: Cambridge University Press, 1986.
- "Plague Legislation in the Italian Renaissance." *Bulletin of the History of Medicine* 57 (1983): 508–25.
Carniel, Elisabeth. "Plague Today." In *Pestilential Complexities: Understanding Medieval Plague*. Edited by Vivian Nutton, 115–22. London: Wellcome Trust for the History of Medicine at UCL, 2008.
Carter, Francis W. *Dubrovnik (Ragusa), a Classic City-State*. London: Seminar Press, 1972.
Cavallo, Sandra. *Charity and Power in Early Modern Italy: Benefactors and Their Motives in Turin 1541–1789*. Cambridge: Cambridge University Press, 1995.
Chambers, David, and Brian Pullan, eds. *Venice: A Documentary History, 1450–1630*. Toronto: Toronto University Press in association with the Renaissance Society of America, 2001.
Chase, Marilyn. *The Barbary Plague: The Black Death in Victorian San Francisco*. New York: Random House, 2003.
Christakos, George, Ricardo A. Olea, Marc L. Serre, Hwa-Lung Yu, and Lin-Lin Wang, eds. *Interdisciplinary Public Health Reasoning and Epidemic Modelling: The Case of Black Death*. New York: Springer, 2005.
Christensen, Peter. "Appearance and Disappearance of Plague: Still a Puzzle?" In *Living with Black Death*. Edited by Lars Bisgaard and Leif Søndergaard, 11–21. Odense: University Press of Southern Denmark, 2009.
Cipolla, Carlo M. *Cristofano and the Plague: A Study in the History of Public Health in the Age of Galileo*. Berkeley: University of California Press, 1973.
   Faith, Reason, and the Plague in the Seventeenth-Century Tuscany. Ithaca, NY: Cornell University Press, 1979.
- *Fighting the Plague in the Seventeenth-Century Italy*. Madison: University of Winsconsin Press, 1981.
- *Miasmas and Diseases*. New Haven: Yale University Press, 1992.
- "A Plague Doctor." In *The Medieval City*. Edited by Harry A. Miskimin, 65–72. New Haven: Yale University Press, 1977.
- *Public Health and the Medical Profession in the Renaissance*. Cambridge: Cambridge University Press, 1976.
Clifford, Timothy. "Dubrovnik: Italian Art, c. 1400–1800." In *Croatia: Aspects of Art, Architecture and Cultural Heritage*. Introduction by John Julius Norwich, 148–73. London: Frances Lincoln, 2009.
Cohn, Samuel Kline. *Cultures of Plague: Medical Thought at the End of the Renaissance*. Oxford: Oxford University Press, 2010.
Constantine VII Porphyrogenitus. *De administrando imperio*. English and Greek text. Greek text edited by Gy. Moravcsik. English translation by R.J.H. Jenkins. Washington: Dumbarton Oaks Center for Byzantine Studies, 1967.
Conrad, Lawrence I. "Epidemic Disease in Formal and Popular Thought in Early Islamic Society." In *Epidemics and Ideas: Essays on the Historical Perception of*

Pestilence, edited by Terence Ranger and Paul Slack, 77–99. Cambridge: Cambridge University Press, 1992.

Cook, Alexandra Parma, and Noble David Cook. *The Plague Files: Crisis Management in the Sixteenth-Century Seville*. Baton Rouge: Louisiana State University Press, 2009.

Corradi, Alfonso. *Annali delle epidemie occorse in Italia, dale prime memorie fino al 1850*. 5 vols. Bologna: Arnaldo Forni, 1865–1894.

Crawshaw, Jane L. Stevens. "The Beasts of Burial: Pizzigamorti and Public Health for the Plague in Early Modern Venice." *Social History of Medicine* 24 (2011): 570–87.

– *Plague Hospitals: Public Health for the City in Early Modern Venice*. Farnham, UK: Ashgate, 2012.

Crijević Tuberon, Ludovik. *Komentari o mojem vremenu* [Comments about my time]. Zagreb: Hrvatski institut za povijest, 2001.

Crowley, Roger. *City of Fortune: How Venice Won and Lost a Naval Empire*. London: Faber and Faber, 2011.

Čizmić, Frane. *Državni grb Dubrovačke Republike / The State Coat of Arms of the Dubrovnik Republic*. Catalogue of an Exhibition Held in the Rector's Palace, February–April 2010. Dubrovnik: Dubrovački muzeji, Kulturno-povijesni muzej, 2010.

Čoralić, Lovorka. "The Ragusans in Venice from the Thirteenth to the Eighteenth Century." *Dubrovnik Annals* 3 (1999): 13–40. A longer version of this article was previously published in Croatian under the title: "Dubrovčani u Veneciji od XII. do XVIII. stoljeća." *Anali Zavoda za povijesne znanosti HAZU u Dubrovniku* 32 (1994): 15–57.

Čremošnik, Gregor. "Činovnički stalež u srednjem vijeku u Dubrovniku" [Salaried state employees in mediaeval Dubrovnik]. *Dubrovački horizonti* 30 (1990): 31–7.

– "Dubrovačka kancelarija do godine 1300. i najstarije knjige dubrovačke arhive" [The Dubrovnik chancery until the year 1300 and the oldest books of the Archives of Dubrovnik]. *Glasnik Zemaljskog muzeja* (Sarajevo) 39 (1927): 231–53.

– "Dubrovački pečati srednjega vijeka" [Ragusan mediaeval seals]. *Anali Historijskog instituta JAZU u Dubrovniku* 4–5 (1956): 31–47.

– "Kada je postao dubrovački arhiv?" [When were the Archives of Dubrovnik founded?] *Glasnik Zemaljskog muzeja BiH* (Sarajevo) 44 (1932): 57–61.

– "Nekoliko ljekarskih ugovora iz Dubrovnika" [Several contracts of Ragusan physicians]. In *Zbornik iz dubrovačke prošlosti Milanu Rešetaru o 70-oj godišnjici života prijatelji i učenici*. [Papers about the history of Dubrovnik collected in honour of Milan Rešetar for his 70th birthday], 43–5. Dubrovnik: Knjižara Jadran, 1931.

– "Postanak i razvoj srpske ili hrvatske kancelarije u Dubrovniku" [Origin and development of the Serbian or Croatian chancery in Dubrovnik]. *Anali Historijskog instituta JAZU u Dubrovniku* 1 (1952): 73–84.

Ćosić, Stjepan. "Giorgio Baglivi. *De fibra motrice et morbosa*. Book Review" [Giorgio Baglivi. The nature of the motor fibre and its disorders]. *Dubrovnik Annals* 5 (2001): 128–30. This article was previously published in Croatian under the title: "Gjuro Baglivi, De fibra motrice et morbosa / O zdravom i bolesnom motoričkom vlaknu. Zagreb: Prometej i Medicinski fakultet Sveučilišta u Zagrebu, 1997." *Anali Zavoda za povijesne znanosti HAZU u Dubrovniku* 38 (2000): 400–2.

– "Prinos poznavanju tajništva i arhiva Dubrovačke Republike" [The chancery and the Archives of the Ragusan Republic]. *Arhivski vjesnik* 37 (1994): 123–45.

Ćosić, Stjepan, and Nenad Vekarić. *Dubrovačka vlastela između roda i države:*

pathologische Untersuchungen. Vol. 7. Edited by August Hirsch. Reprint of the Berlin Edition, 1865. Hildesheim: Olms, 1964.

Henderson, John. "Epidemics in Renaissance Florence: Medical Theory and Government Response." In *Maladies et sociétés (XIIe – XVIIIe siècles): Actes du Colloque de Bielefeld, novembre 1986*. Edited by Neithard Bulst and Robert Delort, 165–86. Paris: CNRS, 1989.

– "Healing the Body and Saving the Soul: Hospitals in Renaissance Florence." *Journal of the Society for Renaissance Studies* 15 (2001): 188–216.

– *The Renaissance Hospital: Healing the Body and Healing the Soul*. New Haven: Yale University Press, 2006.

Herlihy, David. *The Black Death and the Transformation of the West*. Cambridge, MA: Harvard University Press, 1997.

Hippocrates. *Hippocratic Writings*. Edited by G.E.R. Lloyd. Harmondworth: Penguin 1978.

Hirst, Leonard Fabian. *The Conquest of Plague: A Study of the Evolution of Epidemiology*. Oxford: Clarendon Press, 1953.

Hopkins, Andrew. "Combating Plague: Devotional Paintings, Architectural Programs, and Votive Processions in Early Modern Venice." In *Hope and Healing: Painting in Italy in a Time of Plague, 1500–1800*. Edited by Gauvin Alexander Bailey, Pamela M. Jones, Franco Mormando, and Thomas W. Worcester, 137–52. Worcester: Clark University, College of the Holy Cross, Worcester Art Museum; Chicago: University of Chicago Press, 2005.

Howard-Jones, Norman. "Kitasato, Yersin and the Plague Bacillus." *Clio Medica* 10 (1975): 23–7.

Hrabak, Bogumil. *Izvoz žitarica iz Osmanlijskog carstva u XIV, XV i XVI stoljeću* [Export of grain from the Ottoman Empire in the fourteenth, fifteenth and sixteenth centuries]. Priština: (s.n.) 1971.

– "Kuga u balkanskim zemljama pod Turcima od 1450–1600" [Plague in the Balkan lands under Turkish rule, 1450–1600]. *Istoriski glasnik* (Belgrade) 1–2 (1957): 19–37.

– "Učešće Katalonaca u dubrovačkom prometu zrnastom hranom, solju, metalima, koraljima i kreditima (do 1520. godine)" [Participation of the Catalonians in the grain, salt, metals, corals and credit trade in Dubrovnik until 1520]. *Anali Zavoda za povijesne znanosti JAZU u Dubrovniku* 22–23 (1985): 41–78.

– *Vuna s Pirinejskog poluostrva u Dubrovniku u XV veku* [Wool from the Pyrenean Peninsula in fifteenth-century Dubrovnik]. Belgrade: Istorijski institut, Prosveta, 1980.

Ivančević, Radovan. *Art Treasures of Croatia*. Zagreb: Motovun, 1993.

– "Sorkočevićev ljetnikovac na Lapadu i problem klasične renesanse" [The Sorkočević family villa in Lapad and the issue of classical Renaissance]. In *Likovna kultura Dubrovnika 15. i 16. stoljeća* [Fine arts in Dubrovnik in the fifteenth and sixteenth centuries]. Scientific conference accompanying the exhibition "The Golden Age of Dubrovnik." Edited by Igor Fisković, 75–81. Zagreb: Znanstvena djela Muzejsko-Galerijskog Centra 2, 1991.

Janeković-Römer, Zdenka. "Dubrovačko 15. stoljeće: vrijeme rada i bogaćenja" [The fifteenth century in Dubrovnik: working hard and accumulating wealth]. In *Opis slavnoga grada Dubrovnika* by Filip de Diversis, 18–30. Zagreb: Dom i svijet, 2004.

– "Gradation of Differences: Ethnic and Religious Minorities in Medieval Dubrovnik."

In *Segregation, Integration, Assimilation: Religious and Ethnic Groups in the Medieval Towns of Central and Eastern Europe*. Edited by Derek Keene, Balázs Nagy, and Katalin Szende, 115–34. Surrey, UK: Ashgate, 2009.

– "I lazzaretti di Dubrovnik (Ragusa)." In *Rotte mediterranee e baluardi di sanita: Venezia e i lazzaretti mediterranei*. Edited by Nelli-Elena Vanzan Marchini, 246–7. Milano: Skira, 2004.

– "Na razmeđi ovog i onog svijeta. Prožimanje pojavnog i transcedentalnog u dubrovačkim oporukama kasnoga srednjeg vijeka" [On the crossroads between this world and the next: The permeation of the real and transcendental elements in Ragusan testaments of the late Middle Ages]. *Otium* (Zagreb) 2 (1994): 3–16.

– "Nasilje zakona: gradska vlast i privatni život u kasnosrednjovjekovnom i ranonovovjekovnom Dubrovniku" [The violence of the law: Government and privacy in late mediaeval and early modern Dubrovnik]. *Anali Zavoda za povijesne znanosti HAZU u Dubrovniku* 41 (2003): 9–44.

– "Noble Women in Fifteenth-Century Ragusa." In *Women and Power in East Central Europe – Medieval and Modern*. Edited by Marianne Sághy. Special issue of *East Central Europe* 20–23 (1996): 141–70.

– *Okvir slobode: dubrovačka vlastela između srednjovjekovlja i humanizma* [Framework of freedom: The Ragusan patriciate between the Middle Ages and humanism]. Dubrovnik: Zavod za povijesne znanosti HAZU u Dubrovniku, 1999.

– "O poslaničkoj službi i diplomatskom protokolu Dubrovačke Republike u XV. stoljeću" [The consular office and diplomatic protocol of the Ragusan Republic in the fifteenth century]. In *Hrvatska Srednjovjekovna diplomacija* [Croatian mediaeval diplomacy]. Edited by Mladen Andrlić and Mirko Valentić. *Zbornik Diplomatske akademije* [Proceedings of the Diplomatic Academy] 2 (1999): 193–204.

– "*Post tertiam campanam* – noćni život Dubrovnika u srednjem vijeku" [After the third bell: Night life in Dubrovnik in the Middle Ages]. *Anali Zavoda za povijesne znanosti HAZU u Dubrovniku* 32 (1994): 7–14.

– "*Pro anima mea et predecessorum meorum*: Death and the Family in 15th-Century Dubrovnik." *Otium* (Zagreb) 3 (1995): 25–34.

– "Public Rituals in the Political Discourse of Humanist Dubrovnik." Translated by Alexander D. Hoyt. *Dubrovnik Annals* 6 (2002): 7–43. This article was previously published in Croatian under the title: "Javni rituali u poličkom diskursu humanističkog Dubrovnika." *Radovi Zavoda za hrvatsku povijest* 29 (1996): 68–86.

– *Rod i grad: dubrovačka obitelj od 13. do 15. stoljeća*. [Kinship and the city: The Ragusan family from the thirteenth to the fifteenth centuries]. Dubrovnik: Zavod za povijesne znanosti HAZU u Dubrovniku; Zagreb: Zavod za hrvatsku povijest Filozofskog fakulteta u Zagrebu, 1994.

– *Višegradski ugovor: Temelj Dubrovačke Republike* [The Treaty of Višegrad: The basis of the Ragusan Republic]. Zagreb: Golden Marketing, 2003.

Jeremić, Risto, and Jorjo Tadić. *Prilozi za istoriju zdravstvene kulture starog Dubrovnika* [Contributions to the history of health culture of old-time Dubrovnik]. 3 vols. Belgrade: Centralni higijenski zavod, 1938–40.

Jutronić, Andre. "Prilog proučavanju zdravstva na Braču" [Contribution to the study of health culture on the island of Brač]. *Anali Historijskog instituta JAZU u Dubrovniku* 2 (1953): 277–82.

Kaznačić-Hrdalo, Ana. "Dioba i ubikacija Slanskog primorja u doba pripojenja Dubrovniku godine 1399" [The distribution of land in Slano Primorje in 1399 when it became part of the Ragusan Republic]. *Anali Zavoda za povijesne znanosti Istraživačkog centra* JAZU *u Dubrovniku* 17 (1979): 17–48.

Kesterčanek, Zdenka. "Iz povijesti farmacije u Dubrovniku u XVI stoljeću" [Excerpts from the history of Ragusan pharmacy in the sixteenth century]. *Anali Historijskog instituta* JAZU *u Dubrovniku* 6–7 (1959): 249–66.

– "Iz povijesti dubrovačke farmacije u XVI stoljeću: biografski prinosi" [History of Ragusan pharmacy in the sixteenth century: biographical data]. *Anali Historijskog instituta* JAZU *u Dubrovniku* 8–9 (1962): 255–74.

– "Roko Fasano, dubrovački ljekarnik XVI stoljeća" [Roko Fasano, a pharmacist in sixteenth-century Dubrovnik]. *Anali Historijskog instituta* JAZU *u Dubrovniku* 2 (1953): 267–76.

Kisić, Anica. "Pomorska ikonografija u likovnoj kulturi Dubrovnika 15. i 16. stoljeća" [Maritime iconography in the art of Dubrovnik in the fifteenth and sixteenth centuries]. In *Likovna kultura Dubrovnika 15. i 16. stoljeća* [Fine arts in Dubrovnik in the fifteenth and sixteenth centuries]. Scientific conference accompanying the exhibition "The Golden Age of Dubrovnik." Edited by Igor Fisković, 242–9. Zagreb: Znanstvena djela Muzejsko-Galerijskog Centra 2, 1991.

– *Zavjetne slike hrvatskih pomoraca: ex voto Adriatico.* [Votive paintings of Croatian mariners]. Zagreb: Matica hrvatska, 2000.

Kisić, Anica, and Vinicije B. Lupis. *Miho Pracat: O 400. obljetnici smrti* [Miho Pracat: On the occasion of the 400th anniversary of his death]. Dubrovnik: Matica hrvatska, 2007.

Klaić, Nada. *Povijest Hrvata u ranom srednjem vijeku* [History of Croats in the early Middle Ages]. Zagreb: Školska knjiga, 1975.

– *Povijest Hrvata u razvijenom srednjem vijeku* [History of Croats in the late Middle Ages]. Zagreb: Školska knjiga, 1976.

Knjiga odredaba dubrovačke carinarnice 1277 / Liber statutorum doane Ragusii MCCLXXVII [The Ragusan Customs Statute of 1278]. Transcribed, prepared, and translated by Josip Lučić. Dubrovnik: Historijski arhiv Dubrovnik, 1989.

Kordić, Šime. "Nekoliko zapisa iz Dubrovačkog arhiva o zdravstvenim vezama Dubrovnika s Bosnom u XIV i XV stoljeću" [Records from the Archives of Dubrovnik about the health connections between Bosnia and Dubrovnik in the fourteenth and fifteenth centuries]. *Saopćenja* (Zagreb) 15 (1972): 89–94.

Kostrenčić, Marko, Veljko Gortan, and Zlatko Herkov, eds. *Lexicon Latinitatis Medii Aevi Iugoslaviae* [Lexicon of the Mediaeval Latin of Yugoslavia], vol. 1. Zagreb: JAZU, 1978.

Kotruljević, Beno. *Libro del arte dela mercatura. Knjiga o vještini trgovanja.* [On the Art of Trade]. Edited and translated by Zdenka Janeković-Römer. Zagreb and Dubrovnik: Zavod za povijesne znanosti HAZU u Dubrovniku; Hrvatski računovođa, 2009.

Krasić, Stjepan. *Zdravstvena kultura i nekadašnja ljekarna Dominikanskog samostana u Dubrovniku./Health Care and the Old Pharmacy in the Dominican Monastery in Dubrovnik.* Bilingual Croatian and English ed. Dubrovnik: Matica hrvatska, 2010.

Krasić, Stjepan, and Serafino Razzi. *Povijest dubrovačke metropolije i dubrovačkih nadbiskupa: (X. – XVI. stoljeća)* [History of the Ragusan Metropolitan Church and the Ragusan archbishops from the 10th to the 16th century]. Dubrovnik: Biskupski ordinarijat; Split: Crkva u svijetu, 1999.

Krekić, Bariša. "Contribution to the Study of the Ragusan Presence in Venice in the Fourteenth Century." *Dubrovnik Annals* 5 (2001): 7–45.

– *Dubrovnik in the 14th and 15th Centuries: A City Between East and West*. Norman: University of Oklahoma Press, 1972.
– *Dubrovnik, Italy and the Balkans in the Late Middle Ages*, vol. XVII. London: Variorum, 1980.
– *Dubrovnik (Raguse) et le Levant au Moyen Age*. Paris: Mouton, 1961.
– "Dubrovnik's Participation in the War against the Ottomans in 1443 and 1444." In *Dubrovnik, Italy and the Balkans in the Late Middle Ages*, vol. XVII: 1–17. London: Variorum, 1980.
– "Images of Urban Life: Contributions to the Study of Daily Life in Dubrovnik at the Time of Humanism and the Renaissance." In *Dubrovnik: A Mediterranean Urban Society, 1300–1600*, vol. V: 1–38. Aldershot, UK: Variorum, 1997.
– "Influence politique et pouvoir économique à Dubrovnik (Raguse) du XIIIe au XVIe siècle." In *Dubrovnik: A Mediterranean Urban Society, 1300–1600*, vol. I: 241–58. Aldershot, UK: Variorum, 1997.
– "La navigation ragusaine entre Venise et la Méditerranée orientale aux XIVe et XVe siècles." *Dubrovnik: A Mediterranean Urban Society, 1300–1600*, vol. XIII: 129–30. Aldershot, UK: Variorum, 1997.
– "Le port de Dubrovnik (Raguse), entreprise d'état, plaque tournante du commerce de la ville (XIIe–XVIe siècle)." In *Dubrovnik: A Mediterranean Urban Society, 1300–1600*, vol. XIV: 653–73. Aldershot, UK: Variorum, 1997.
– *Unequal Rivals*. Dubrovnik: Zavod za povijesne znanosti HAZU u Dubrovniku, 2007.
– "Venetians in Dubrovnik (Ragusa) and Ragusans in Venice as Real Estate Owners in the Fourteenth Century" In *Dubrovnik: A Mediterranean Urban Society, 1300–1600*, vol. XI: 1–48. Aldershot, UK: Variorum, 1997.
Krivošić, Stjepan. *Stanovništvo Dubrovnika i demografske promjene u prošlosti* [The population of Dubrovnik and the demographic changes in the past]. Dubrovnik: Zavod za povijesne znanosti HAZU u Dubrovniku, 1990.
Krizman, Bogdan. *O dubrovačkoj diplomaciji* [About Ragusan diplomacy]. Zagreb: Školska knjiga, 1951.
Kumrular, Özlem. "Ragusa: Una fuente de información entre el Occidente y Oriente – Ragusa, Venecia y la Sublime Puerta." In *Tajna diplomacija u Dubrovniku u XVI. stoljeću/Secret Diplomacy in the 16th Century Dubrovnik*. Edited by Mirjana Polić Bobić, 38–48, 143–54. Zagreb: Sveučilište u Zagrebu/University of Zagreb, 2011.
Kunčević, Lovro. "Dubrovačka slika Venecije i venecijanska slika Dubrovnika u ranom novom vijeku" [Ragusan image of Venice and Venetian image of Ragusa in the Early Modern Period]. *Anali Zavoda za povijesne znanosti HAZU u Dubrovniku* 50 (2012): 9–37.
– "Janus-faced Sovereignty: The International Status of the Ragusan Republic in the Early Modern Period." In *The European Tributary States of the Ottoman Empire in the Sixteenth and Seventeenth Centuries*. Edited by Gábor Kármán and Lovro Kunčević, 91–121. Leiden, Boston: Brill, 2013.
– "On Ragusan *Libertas* in the Late Middle Ages." *Dubrovnik Annals* 14 (2010): 25–69. This article was previously published in Croatian under the title: "O dubrovačkoj *Libertas* u kasnom srednjem vijeku." *Anali Zavoda za povijesne znanosti HAZU u Dubrovniku* 46 (2008): 9–64.
– "Retorika granice kršćanstva u diplomaciji renesansnog Dubrovnika" [The rhetoric of the frontier of Christendom in the diplomacy of Renaissance Dubrovnik]. *Anali Zavoda za povijesne znanosti HAZU u Dubrovniku* 48 (2010): 179–211.

Kurtović, Esad. "Motivi Sandaljeve prodaje Konavala Dubrovčanima" [The motives of Sandalj Hranić's sale of Konavle to the Ragusans]. *Anali Zavoda za povijesne znanosti HAZU u Dubrovniku* 38 (2000): 103–20.

Lane, Frederic Chapin. *Venice: A Maritime Republic*. Baltimore: Johns Hopkins University Press, 1973.

Lechner, Karl. *Das grosse Sterben in Deutschland 1348 bis 1351. und die folgenden Pestepidemien bis zum Schlusse des 14. Jahrhunderts.* Reprint of the edition Innsbruck: Wagnersche Universitätsbuchhandlung, 1884. Walluf bei Wiesbaden: Sandig, 1974.

Lentić, Ivo. *Dubrovački zlatari, 1600–1900* [The goldsmiths of Dubrovnik, 1600–1900]. Book 34. Zagreb: Društvo povjesničara umjetnosti SR Hrvatske, 1984.

– "Zlatarstvo" [Goldsmithing]. In *Zlatno doba Dubrovnika XV. i XVI. stoljeće: Urbanizam, arhitektura, skulptura, slikarstvo, iluminirani rukopisi, zlatarstvo* [The Golden Age of Dubrovnik in the fifteenth and sixteenth centuries: Urban planning, architecture, sculpture, painting, illuminated manuscripts and goldsmithing]. Exhibition catalogue, 384, 389. Edited by Milan Prelog, Marija Planić-Lončarić, Anđelko Badurina, Nada Grujić, Igor Fisković, Vladimir Marković, Ivo Lentić, Ivica Prlender, and Tonko Maroević. Zagreb: Muzej Topić Mimara, 1987.

Le Roy Ladurie, Emmanuel. *The Mind and Method of the Historian.* Translated by Sian Reynolds and Ben Reynolds. English translation of *Territoire de l'historien.* Chicago: University of Chicago Press, 1984.

Lexicon Latinitatis Medii Aevi Iugoslaviae [Lexicon of the Mediaeval Latin of Yugoslavia]. Vol. 1. Edited by Marko Kostrenčić, Veljko Gortan, and Zlatko Herkov. Zagreb: JAZU, 1978.

Liber croceus [The yellow book]. Edited by Branislav Nedeljković. Belgrade: SANU, Zbornik za istoriju, jezik i književnost srpskog naroda, odelenje III, knj. XXIV, 1997.

Liber viridis [The green book]. Edited by Branislav Nedeljković. Belgrade: SANU, Zbornik za istoriju, jezik i književnost srpskog naroda, odelenje III, knj. XXIII, 1984.

Libro deli Signori Chazamorbi. Sanitas, Series 55, v. 1, 1500–1530 [The book of the Health Officials. Health series 55, v. 1, 1500–30]. Edited by Zlata Blažina Tomić, Vesna Blažina, and Zdravko Šundrica. Zagreb, Dubrovnik: Zavod za povijesne znanosti HAZU, forthcoming.

Little, Lester K., ed. *Plague and the End of Antiquity: The Pandemic of 541–750.* Cambridge: Cambridge University Press, 2007.

Lisičar, Vicko. *Lopud: Historički i savremeni prikaz* [Lopud: A historical and contemporary description]. Dubrovnik: Dubrovačka hrvatska tiskara, 1931.

Lonza, Nella. "Election Procedure in the Republic of Dubrovnik." *Dubrovnik Annals* 8 (2004): 7–41. A longer version of this article was previously published in Croatian under the title: "Izborni postupak Dubrovačke Republike." *Anali Zavoda za povijesne znanosti HAZU u Dubrovniku* 38 (2000): 9–52.

– *Kazalište vlasti: Ceremonijal i državni blagdani Dubrovačke Republike u 17. i 18. stoljeću* [The theater of power: Ceremony and state holidays of the Ragusan Republic in the seventeenth and eighteenth centuries]. Zagreb and Dubrovnik: Zavod za povijesne znanosti HAZU u Dubrovniku, 2009.

– "Na marginama Lastovskog statuta iz XIV. stoljeća" [Notes on the fourteenth-century manuscript of the Statutes of Lastovo]. *Anali Zavoda za povijesne znanosti HAZU* 36 (1998): 7–32.

– "*Obliti privatorum publica curate*: A Ragusan Political Epigraph and Its Historical

Background." Translated by Vesna Baće. *Dubrovnik Annals* 11 (2007): 25–47. This article was previously published in Croatian under the title: "Obliti privatorum publica curate: preci i srodnjaci jedne političke maksime." *Anali Zavoda za povijesne znanosti HAZU u Dubrovniku* 44 (2006): 25–46.

– *Pod plaštem pravde: Kaznenopravni sustav Dubrovačke Republike u XVIII. stoljeću* [Under the cloak of justice: The criminal justice system of the Ragusan Republic in the eighteenth century]. Dubrovnik: Zavod za povijesne znanosti HAZU, 1997.

– "Pred gosparom knezom i njegovim sucima …: Dubrovački kazneni postupci s početka XIV stoljeća" [In front of the lord rector and his judges: Criminal procedure in Dubrovnik at the beginning of the fourteenth century]. *Anali Zavoda za povijesne znanosti HAZU u Dubrovniku* 30 (1992): 25–54.

– "Srednjovjekovni zapisnici dubrovačkog kaznenog suda: Izvorne cjeline i arhivsko stanje" [Criminal records of mediaeval Dubrovnik: A survey]. *Anali Zavoda za povijesne znanosti HAZU u Dubrovniku* 41 (2003): 45–74.

– "State Funerals in Dubrovnik in the Seventeenth and Eighteenth Centuries." *Dubrovnik Annals* 9 (2005): 71–89. Translated by Davies d.o.o. This article was previously published in Croatian under the title: "Državni pogrebi u Dubrovniku (17.–18. stoljeće)." *Anali Zavoda za povijesne znanosti HAZU u Dubrovniku* 42 (2004): 131–48.

– "Tužba, osveta, nagodba: Modeli reagiranja na zločin u srednjovjekovnom Dubrovniku" [Settling disputes in mediaeval Dubrovnik by court proceedings, revenge, or out-of-court settlement]. *Anali Zavoda za povijesne znanosti HAZU u Dubrovniku* 40 (2002): 57–104.

Lonza, Nella, and Zdenka Janeković-Römer. "Dubrovački *Liber de maleficiis* iz 1312.–1313" [The Ragusan criminal records of 1312–13]. *Radovi Zavoda za hrvatsku povijest* 25 (1992): 173–228.

Lonza, Nella, and Zdravko Šundrica, eds. *Odluke dubrovačkih vijeća, 1390–1392* [The decisions of the Ragusan Councils, 1390–92]. Zagreb-Dubrovnik: Zavod za povijesne znanosti HAZU u Dubrovniku, 2005.

Lučić, Josip. "Arhivska građa o kugi u Dubrovniku godine 1526.–1527. i obitelj Držić" [Archival material about plague in Dubrovnik in 1526–27 and about the family Držić]. *Rasprave i građa HAZU* (Zagreb) 7 (1992): 17–58.

– "Dubrovčani i Hasan paša Predojević" [The Ragusans and Hasan Pasha Predojević]. In *Dubrovačko povijesno iverje* [Sketches from the Ragusan history]. Dubrovnik: Matica Hrvatska, 1997: 91–108.

– "Gozze/Gučetići i Trsteno u XV. i XVI. Stoljeću" [The Gozze/Gučetić family in Trsteno in the fifteenth and sixteenth centuries]. *Anali Zavoda za povijesne znanosti HAZU u Dubrovniku* 33 (1995): 7–20.

– "Najstarija zemljišna knjiga u Hrvatskoj – Dubrovački zemljišnik diobe zemlje u Stonu i Pelješcu iz godine 1336" [The oldest cadastral book in Croatia: The Ragusan cadastral book of land allotment in Ston and Pelješac in 1336]. *Anali Zavoda za povijesne znanosti Istraživačkog centra JAZU u Dubrovniku* 18 (1980): 57–89.

– *Obrti i usluge u Dubrovniku do početka XIV stoljeća* [Crafts and services in Dubrovnik until the beginning of the fourteenth century]. Zagreb: Sveučilište u Zagrebu, Institut za hrvatsku povijest, Odjel za hrvatsku povijest, 1979.

– "Povijest Dubrovnika od VII stoljeća do godine 1205" [History of Dubrovnik from the seventh century until the year 1205]. Supplement. *Anali Historijskog instituta JAZU u Dubrovniku* 13–14 (1976): 6–139.

– *Prošlost dubrovačke Astareje, Župe, Šumeta, Zatona, Gruža i okolice grada do 1366* [The Past of the Ragusan Astareja, Župa, Šumet, Zaton, Gruž and the surroundings of the city until 1366]. Dubrovnik: Matica hrvatska, 1970.

Luetić, Josip. "Dubrovačka međunarodna pomorska djelatnost u XIV stoljeću" [The Ragusan international maritime activity in the fourteenth century]. *Rad JAZU* (Zagreb) 384 (1980): 57–83.

– "Dubrovački galijun druge polovine XVI stoljeća" [The Ragusan galleon in the second half of the sixteenth century]. *Anali Historijskog instituta JAZU u Dubrovniku* 6–7 (1959): 129–41.

– *Pomorci i jedrenjaci Republike Dubrovačke* [The sailors and the sailing ships of the Ragusan Republic]. Zagreb: Nakladni zavod Matice hrvatske, 1984.

Lupis, Vinicije B. "Benediktinci i njihova baština na dubrovačkom području" [The cultural heritage of the Benedictines in the Ragusan region]. In *Benediktinci na području Dubrovačke nadbiskupije. Zbornik radova* [The Benedictines in the Ragusan Archbishopric]. Edited by Želimir Puljić and Marijan Sivrić, 317–37. Dubrovnik: Dubrovačka biskupija, 2010.

– "Nove spoznaje o sakralnoj baštini Blata" [New insights about the religious heritage of Blato]. In *Blato do kraja 18. stoljeća* [Blato until the end of the 18th century]. Edited by Teo Šeparović, vol. 3, 90–164. Blato: Općina Blato, 2005.

– "Oltarna pala Navještenja Blažene Djevice Marije iz crkve Gospe Nuncijate u Dubrovniku" [The altar painting of Annunciation of the Blessed Virgin Mary from the church of the Annunciation in Dubrovnik]. *Dubrovnik* 19 (2008): 117–20.

– *Sakralna baština Stona i okolice* [The religious heritage of Ston and its surroundings]. Ston: Matica hrvatska, 2000.

– *Ston u srednjem vijeku* [Ston in the Middle Ages]. Split: Muzej hrvatskih arheoloških spomenika, 2010.

– *Trstenica u srednjem vijeku* [Trstenica in the Middle Ages]. Split: Muzej hrvatskih arheoloških spomenika, 2010.

– "Umjetnička baština Svetišta sv. Marije od milosti na Dančama" [The artistic heritage of the church of Saint Mary of Compassion at Dančе]. *Dubrovački horizonti* 37 (2008): 57–65.

– "Zavjetne slike peljeških pomoraca u Italiji" [Votive paintings of the Pelješac mariners in Italy]. *Naše more* (Dubrovnik) 47 (2000): 230–4.

Macan, Trpimir. "Dubrovački brabanti u XVI stoljeću" [The Ragusan barabanti in the sixteenth century]. *Anali Historijskog instituta JAZU u Dubrovniku* 8–9 (1962): 301–23.

Madden, Thomas F. *Venice: A New History.* New York: Penguin, 2012.

Mahnken, Irmgard. *Dubrovački patricijat u XIV veku* [The Ragusan patriciate in the fourteenth century]. Belgrade: SANU, Posebna izdanja, knjiga 340/1, 2, Odelenje društvenih nauka, knj. 36, 1960.

Marinković, Ana. "Territorial Expansion of the Ragusan Commune/Republic and the Churches Of Its Patron Saints." *Dubrovnik Annals* 13 (2009): 7–23. This article was previously published in Croatian under the title: "Teritorijalno širenje Dubrovačke Komune/Republike i crkve njezinih svetaca zaštitnika." *Anali Zavoda za povijesne znanosti HAZU u Dubrovniku* 45 (2007): 219–34.

Marinović, Ante. "Postanak i prvi spisi kancelarija srednjovjekovnih dalmatinskih gradova, posebno Dubrovnika i Kotora u 13. i 14. stoljeću" [The establishment of the first chanceries in Dalmatian mediaeval cities, especially in Dubrovnik and Kotor in the 13th and the 14th centuries]. *Anali Zavoda za povijesne znanosti Istraživačkog centra JAZU u Dubrovniku* 22–23 (1985): 7–24.

– "Pravni status benediktinske opatije Svete Marije na jezeru na Mljetu (prema sred-njovjekovnom statutu otoka Mljeta iz 1345. godine)" [The legal status of the Bene-dictine monastery of Saint Mary on the island of Mljet according to the 1345 mediaeval statute of the island of Mljet]. In *Benediktinci na području Dubrovačke nadbiskupije. Zbornik radova* [The Benedictines in the Ragusan Archbishopric]. Ed-ited by Želimir Puljić and Marijan Sivrić, 277–96. Dubrovnik: Dubrovačka biskupija, 2010.

– "Prilog poznavanju dubrovačkih bratovština" [About Ragusan confraternities]. *Anali Historijskog instituta JAZU u Dubrovniku* 1 (1952): 233–46.

Marković, Vladimir. "Slikarstvo" [Painting] in *Zlatno doba Dubrovnika XV. i XVI. stol-jeće: Urbanizam, arhitektura, skulptura, slikarstvo, iluminirani rukopisi, zlatarstvo* [The Golden Age of Dubrovnik in the fifteenth and sixteenth centuries: Urban plan-ning, architecture, sculpture, painting, illuminated manuscripts and goldsmithing]. Exhibition catalogue, 324–31, 357, 361–2. Edited by Milan Prelog, Marija Planić-Lončarić, Anđelko Badurina, Nada Grujić, Igor Fisković, Vladimir Marković, Ivo Lentić, Ivica Prlender, and Tonko Maroević. Zagreb: Muzej Topić Mimara, 1987.

Marshall, Louise. "Manipulating the Sacred: Image and Plague in Renaissance Italy." *Renaissance Quarterly* 45 (1994): 485–532.

McCormick, Michael. "Rats, Communications, and Plague: Toward an Ecological His-tory." *Journal of Interdisciplinary History and Allied Sciences* 34 (2003): 1–25.

– "Toward a Molecular History of Justinianic Pandemic." In *Plague and the End of An-tiquity: The Pandemic of 541–750*. Edited by Lester K. Little, 290–312. Cambridge: Cambridge University Press, 2007.

Meiss, Millard. *Painting in Florence and Siena after the Black Death*. Princeton: Princeton University Press, 1951.

Meyer, Karl Friedrich. "Pneumonic Plague." *Bacteriological Review* 25 (1961): 249–61.

Mihalić, Neva G. "Re-evaluation of the epistemic foundation of Baglivi's medical doc-trine and his anatomico-physiological theory." *Liječnički vjesnik* 131 (2009): 34–9.

Miličić, Dubravka. "Počeci dubrovačkog ljekarništva od XIII do XVI st" [Beginnings of the Ragusan pharmacy from the thirteenth until the sixteenth century]. In *Spomenica 650-godišnjice ljekarne Male braće u Dubrovniku* [The 650th anniversary of the Franciscan friars' pharmacy in Dubrovnik]. Edited by Hrvoje Tartalja, 69–76. Zagreb: Institut za povijest prirodnih, matematičkih i medicinskih nauka JAZU; Pliva, 1968.

Miović, Vesna. "Beylerbey of Bosnia and Sancakbey of Herzegovina in the Diplomacy of the Dubrovnik Republic." *Dubrovnik Annals* 9 (2005): 37–69. This article was previously published in the Croatian language under the title: "Bosanski beglergeg i hercegovački sandžakbeg i diplomacija Dubrovačke Republike." *Anali Zavoda za povijesne znanosti HAZU u Dubrovniku* 38 (2000): 121–64.

– "Diplomatic Relations between the Ottoman Empire and the Republic of Dubrovnik." In *The European Tributary States of the Ottoman Empire in the Six-teenth and Seventeenth Centuries*. Edited by Gábor Kármán and Lovro Kunčević, 187–208. Leiden: Brill, 2013.

– *Dubrovačka diplomacija u Istambulu* [Ragusan diplomacy in Istanbul]. Zagreb and Dubrovnik: Zavod za povijesne znanosti HAZU u Dubrovniku, 2003.

– *Dubrovačka Republika u spisima osmanskih sultana: S analitičkim inventarom sul-*

tanskih spisa serije Acta Turcarum Državnog arhiva u Dubrovniku [The Ragusan Republic in the papers of the Ottoman sultans: An analytical inventory of the sultans' papers in the series *Acta Turcarum* held in the State Archives of Dubrovnik]. Dubrovnik: Državni arhiv u Dubrovniku, 2005.

– "Emin (Customs Officer) as Representative of the Ottoman Empire in the Republic of Dubrovnik." *Dubrovnik Annals* 7 (2003): 81–8. This article was previously published in the Croatian language under the title: "Emin na Pločama kao predstavnik Osmnalija na području Dubrovačke Republike." *Anali Zavoda za povijesne znanosti HAZU u Dubrovniku* 37 (1999): 205–15.

– *The Jewish Ghetto in the Dubrovnik Republic (1546–1808)*. Zagreb, Dubrovnik: Zavod za povijesne znanosti HAZU u Dubrovniku, 2005.

– "Turske priznanice o uplaćenom dubrovačkom haraču" [Turkish receipts for the payment of Ragusan tribute]. *Anali Zavoda za povijesne znanosti HAZU u Dubrovniku* 42 (2004): 53–77.

Miović, Vesna, and Nikša Selmani. "Turska kancelarija i *Acta Turcarum* od vremena Dubrovačke Republike do danas" [Turkish chancery and *Acta Turcarum* from the era of the Ragusan Republic until the present]. *Anali Zavoda za povijesne znanosti HAZU u Dubrovniku* 45 (2007): 235–84.

Miović-Perić, Vesna. "Dragomans of the Dubrovnik Republic: Their Training and Careers." *Dubrovnik Annals* 5 (2001): 81–94.

– "Dnevnik dubrovačkog dragomana Miha Zarinija" [The diary of Miho Zarini, a Ragusan dragoman]. *Anali Zavoda za povijesne znanosti HAZU u Dubrovniku* 33 (1995): 93–135.

– *Na razmeđu: Osmansko-dubrovačka granica (1667–1806)*. [On the boundary: The Ottoman-Ragusan frontier, 1667–1806]. Dubrovnik: Zavod za povijesne znanosti HAZU u Dubrovniku, 1997.

Mitić, Ilija. *Dubrovačka država u međunarodnoj zajednici od 1358. do 1815.* [The international relations of the Ragusan state, 1358–1815]. Zagreb: Nakladni zavod Matice hrvatske, 1988.

– "Dubrovački konzularni predstavnici na Siciliji od kraja XIV do početka XIX stoljeća" [Ragusan consular representatives in Sicily from the end of the 14th until the beginning of the 19th century]. *Radovi Instituta za povijest Filozofskog fakulteta Sveučilišta u Zagrebu* 16 (1983): 97–108.

– "Dubrovački konzulati u Španiji i Portugalu" [Ragusan consulates in Spain and Portugal]. *Anali Historijskog instituta JAZU u Dubrovniku* 8–9 (1962): 597–620.

– "Imigracijska politika Dubrovačke Republike s posebnim obzirom na ustanovu svjetovnog azila" [The immigration policy of the Ragusan Republic and the right of asylum]. *Anali Zavoda za povijesne znanosti Istraživačkog centra JAZU u Dubrovniku* 17 (1979): 125–64.

– "Kada se Dubrovnik počeo nazivati Republikom" [The date when Dubrovnik started calling itself a Republic]. *Pomorski zbornik* (Rijeka) 25 (1987): 487–93.

– *Konzulati i konzularna služba starog Dubrovnika* [Consulates and consular service of old-time Dubrovnik]. Dubrovnik: Historijski institut JAZU, 1973.

– "Organizacija kopnene i pomorske obrane dubrovačke države – Republike od stjecanja nezavisnosti 1358. do dolaska Francuza 1806. godine" [The organization of defence of the Ragusan Republic from independence in 1358 until the arrival of the French in 1806]. *Anali Zavoda za povijesne znanosti IC JAZU u Dubrovniku* 24–25 (1987): 97–138.

– "Prilog proučavanju odnosa Dubrovnika i Sicilije od druge polovice XIV do početka XIX stoljeća" [Contribution to the study of the relations between Dubrovnik and Sicily from the second half of the fourteenth century until the beginning of the nineteenth century]. *Anali Zavoda za povijesne znanosti Istraživačkog centra JAZU u Dubrovniku* 18 (1980): 105–33.

– "Prilog upoznavanju načina kažnjavanja u Dubrovačkoj Republici" [Types of punishments in the Ragusan Republic]. *Anali Zavoda za povijesne znanosti IC JAZU u Dubrovniku* 22–23 (1985): 153–73.

– "Predstavnici stranih država u Dubrovniku za vrijeme Republike." [Representatives of foreign countries in the Ragusan Republic]. *Pomorski zbornik* (Zadar) 4 (1966): 381–401.

Mohr, James C. *Plague and Fire: Battling Black Death and the 1900 Burning of Honolulu's Chinatown.* New York: Oxford University Press, 2005.

Mollaret, Henri H., and Jacqueline Brossolet. *Yersin: Un pasteurien en Indochine.* Paris: Belin, 1993.

Molnár, Antal. *Le Saint-Siège, Raguse et les missions catholiques de la Hongrie ottomane 1572–1647.* Rome: Accademia d'Ungheria; Budapest: Bibliothèque Nationale de Hongrie, Société pour l'Encyclopédie de l'Histoire de l'Église en Hongrie, 2007.

Monumenta ragusina: Libri reformationum [Ragusan documents: Books of the reformations]. Zagreb: JAZU, Monumenta spectantia historiam Slavorum meridionalium. Vol. IX, tome I, 1879; Vol. XIII, tome II, 1882; Vol. XXVII, tome III, 1895.

Mormando, Franco. "Introduction: Response to the Plague in Early Modern Italy: What the Primary Sources, Printed and Painted, Reveal." In *Hope and Healing: Painting in Italy in a Time of Plague, 1500–1800.* Edited by Gauvin Alexander Bailey, Pamela M. Jones, Franco Mormando, and Thomas W. Worcester, 1–44. Worcester: Clark University, College of the Holy Cross, Worcester Art Museum; Chicago: University of Chicago Press, 2005.

Musis, Gabriele de. "Historia de morbo sive mortalitate quae fuit anno Domini 1348." In *Archiv für die gesammte Medizin.* Edited by Heinrich Häser. Vol. 2, *Dokumente zur Geschichte des schwarzen Todes.* Edited by August Wilhelm Eduard Theodor Henschel, 26–59. Berlin, 1842.

Mustać, Ivo. "Dubrovačko humanističko školstvo i ilirski zavodi u Italiji u 16. i 17. stoljeću" [Humanistic education in Dubrovnik and the Illyrian institutions in Italy in the sixteenth and seventeenth centuries]. *Dubrovački horizonti* 30 (1990): 43–9.

Naphy, William G. *Plagues, Poisons and Potions: Plague-Spreading Conspiracies in the Western Alps c. 1530–1640.* Manchester: Manchester University Press, 2002.

Naphy, William, and Andrew Spicer. *Plague: Black Death and Pestilence in Europe.* Stroud, UK: Tempus, 2004.

Nicoud, Marilyn. "Pratiquer la medicine dans l'Italie de la fin du Moyen Âge: Enquête sur les statuts communaux et les statuts de métier." In *Pratique et pensée médicales à la Renaissance: Actes du Colloque international d'études humanistes, Tours, 2–6 juillet 2007.* Edited by Jacqueline Vons, 9–23. Paris: De Boccard, 2009.

Ničetić, Antun. "Galije trireme i bireme bile su tijekom više stoljeća ratni brodovi Dubrovnika" [Trireme and bireme galleys, the war ships of the Ragusan Republic during several centuries]. *Anali Zavoda za povijesne znanosti HAZU u Dubrovniku* 40 (2002): 9–56.

– *Nove spoznaje o postanku Dubrovnika, o njegovom brodarstvu i plovidbi svetoga*

Pavla [New insights into the founding of Dubrovnik, its shipping and the navigation of Saint Paul]. Dubrovnik: Sveučilište u Dubrovniku, 2005.

- "O otoku Lokrumu sjedištu benediktinske opatije Svete Marije" [The island of Lokrum and the Benedictine monastery of Saint Mary]. In *Benediktinci na području Dubrovačke nadbiskupije. Zbornik radova* [The Benedictines in the Ragusan Archbishopric]. Edited by Želimir Puljić and Marijan Sivrić, 339–64. Dubrovnik: Dubrovačka biskupija, 2010.

- *Povijest dubrovačke luke* [History of the port of Dubrovnik]. Dubrovnik: Zavod za povijesne znanosti HAZU u Dubrovniku, Pomorski fakultet Dubrovnik, 1996.

Nockels Fabbri, Christiane. "Treating Medieval Plague: The Wonderful Virtues of Theriac." *Early Science and Medicine* 12 (2007): 247–83.

Nodilo, Marija. "Vrt u benediktinskom samostanu Svete Marije na Mljetu" [The garden of the Benedictine monastery of Saint Mary on the island of Mljet]. In *Benediktinci na području Dubrovačke nadbiskupije. Zbornik radova* [The Benedictines in the Ragusan Archbishopric]. Edited by Želimir Puljić and Marijan Sivrić, 383–95. Dubrovnik: Dubrovačka biskupija, 2010.

Novak, Grga. "Povijest Dubrovnika od najstarijih vremena do početka VII stoljeća (do propasti Epidaura)" [History of Dubrovnik from prehistoric times until the beginning of the seventh century]. *Anali Historijskog instituta JAZU u Dubrovniku* 10–11 (1962–1963). Supplement. 1–84.

Novak, Viktor, ed. *Supetarski kartular* [The chronicle of Saint Peter]. Zagreb: JAZU, 1952.

Nutton, Vivian. "Continuity and Rediscovery? The City Physician in Antiquity and Medieval Italy." In *The Town and State Physician in Europe from the Middle Ages to the Enlightenment.* Edited by Andrew W. Russell. Wolfenbüttel: Herzog Bibliothek, *Wolfenbütteler Forschungen* 17 (1981): 9–46.

- "Humoralism." In *Companion Encyclopedia of the History of Medicine.* 2 vols. Edited by W.F. Barnum and Roy Porter, 1:281–91. London: Routledge, 1993.

Obad, Stijepo, Serđo Dokoza, and Suzana Martinović. *Južne granice Dalmacije od XV. st. do danas* [The southern borders of Dalmatia from the fifteenth century until the present time]. Zadar: Državni arhiv u Zadru, 1999.

Odluke veća Dubrovačke Republike [The decisions of the Ragusan Councils]. Vol.1. Edited by Mihajlo Dinić. Belgrade: SKA, Zbornik za istoriju, jezik i književnost srpskog naroda, odelenje III, knj. XV, 1955.

Ostojić, Ivan. "Benediktinci i Benediktinski samostani na prostoru Dubrovačke nadbiskupije" [The Benedictines and Benedictine monasteries in the Ragusan Republic]. In *Benediktinci na području Dubrovačke nadbiskupije. Zbornik radova* [The Benedictines in the Ragusan Archbishopric]. Edited by Želimir Puljić and Marijan Sivrić, 113–92. Dubrovnik: Dubrovačka biskupija, 2010.

Palmer, Richard John. "L'azione della Repubblica di Venezia nel controllo della peste: Lo sviluppo della politica governativa." In *Venezia e la Peste, 1348–1797.* Venezia: Comune di Venezia, Assessorato alla cultura e belle arti, Marsilio, 1979: 103–10.

- "The Control of Plague in Venice and Northern Italy, 1348–1600." PhD diss., University of Kent at Canterbury, 1978.

- "Physicians and Surgeons in 16th Century Venice." *Medical History* 23 (1979): 451–60.

- "Physicians and the State in Post-Medieval Italy." In *The Town and State Physicians*

in Europe from the Middle Ages to the Enlightenment. Edited by Andrew W. Russell.
  Wolfenbüttel: Herzog Bibliothek, Wolfenbütteler Forschungen, 17 (1981): 47–61.
– The Studio of Venice and Its Graduates in the Sixteenth Century. Trieste: Edizioni
  Lint, 1983.
Park, Katharine. Doctors and Medicine in Early Renaissance Florence. Princeton:
  Princeton University Press, 1985.
– "Medicine and Society in Medieval Europe, 500–1500." In Medicine in Society.
  Edited by Andrew Wear, 59–90. Cambridge: Cambridge University Press, 1992.
Pejić, Pijo. "Zapadno redovništvo u povijesti Dubrovačke nabiskupije u srednjem
  vijeku" [Western religious orders in the history of the Ragusan Archbishopric in the
  Middle Ages]. In Tisuću godina uspostave dubrovačke (nad)biskupije: zbornik
  radova znanstvenoga skupa u povodu tisuću godina uspostave dubrovačke
  (nad)biskupije /metropolije (998–1998) [One thousand years of the Ragusan
  (Arch)bishopric]. Edited by Želimir Puljić and Nediljko Ante Ančić, 669–86.
  Dubrovnik: Biskupski ordinarijat; Split: Crkva u svijetu, 2001.
Peković, Željko. Crkva Sv. Petra Velikog: Dubrovačka predromanička katedrala (998–
  1022) i njezina skulptura [The church of Saint Peter the Great: The pre-Romanesque
  cathedral of Dubrovnik and its sculptures, 998–1022]. Dubrovnik: Omega Engineer-
  ing; Split: Centar Studia Mediterranea pri Filozofskom fakultetu u Splitu, 2010.
– Nastanak i razvoj katedralnog sklopa u Dubrovniku" [Origin and development of the
  cathedral complex in Dubrovnik]. In Tisuću godina uspostave dubrovačke
  (nad)biskupije: Zbornik radova znanstvenoga skupa u povodu tisuću godina
  uspostave dubrovačke (nad)biskupije /metropolije (998–1998) [One thousand years
  of the Ragusan (Arch)bishopric]. Edited by Želimir Puljić and Nediljko Ante Ančić,
  517–76. Dubrovnik: Biskupski ordinarijat; Split: Crkva u svijetu, 2001.
– "Prva katedrala izronila iz povijesti" [The first cathedral rediscovered]. Dubrovački
  list 7 October 2010, http://dulist.hr/content/view/10935/99/.
Peković, Željko, and Ivica Žile. Ranosrednjovjekovna crkva Sigurata na Prijekome u
  Dubrovniku [The early mediaeval church of Sigurata at Prijeko in Dubrovnik]. Kat-
  alozi i monografije, 6. Split: Muzej hrvatskih arheoloških spomenika, 1999.
Pelling, Margaret. "Contagion/Germ Theory/Specificity." In Companion Encyclopedia
  of the History of Medicine. 2 vols. Edited by W.F. Barnum and Roy Porter, 1:309–33.
  London: Routledge, 1993.
Peričić, Šime. "Prilog poznavanju stonske solane" [A contribution to the history of salt
  production in Ston]. Anali Zavoda za povijesne znanosti HAZU u Dubrovniku 43
  (2005): 139–63.
Pešorda-Vardić, Zrinka. "The Crown, the King and the City: Dubrovnik, Hungary and
  the Dynastic Controversy, 1382–1390." Translated by Vesna Baće. Dubrovnik Annals
  10 (2006): 7–29. This article was previously published in Croatian under the title:
  "Kruna, kralj i Grad: odnos Dubrovnika prema ugarskoj kruni na početku
  protudvorskog pokreta." Povijesni prilozi (Zagreb) 26 (2004): 19–37.
– U predvorju vlasti: Dubrovački antunini u kasnom srednjem vijeku [In the antecham-
  ber of power: members of the confraternity of St Anthony in late mediaeval
  Dubrovnik]. Zagreb: HAZU Zavod za povijesne znanosti, Hrvatski institut za povijest, 2012.
Planić-Lončarić, Marija. Planirana izgradnja na području Dubrovačke Republike
  [Planned construction on the territory of the Ragusan Republic]. Studije i
  monografije, vol. 1. Zagreb: Institut za povijest umjetnosti, 1980.

Šišić, Bruno. *Dubrovnik Renaissance Gardens: Genesis and Design Characteristics.* Zagreb and Dubrovnik: Zavod za povijesne znanosti HAZU, Agronomski fakultet Sveučilišta u Zagrebu, Centar za povijesne vrtove i razvoj krajobraza u Dubrovniku, 2008.

– "The Gardens of the Benedictine Abbey on the Island of Lokrum." *Dubrovnik Annals* 7 (2003): 99–122. This article was previously published in Croatian under the title: "Vrtovi benediktinske opatije na otoku Lokrumu." *Anali Zavoda za povijesne znanosti HAZU u Dubrovniku* 39 (2001): 397–426.

– "Tragom domaćeg iskustva u vrtno-arhitektonskom stvaralaštvu renesansnog Dubrovnika" [The Renaissance garden architecture in Dubrovnik]. In *Likovna kultura Dubrovnika 15. i 16. stoljeća* [Fine arts in Dubrovnik in the fifteenth and sixteenth centuries]. Scientific conference accompanying the exhibition "The Golden Age of Dubrovnik." Edited by Igor Fisković, 82–90. Zagreb: Znanstvena djela Muzejsko-Galerijskog Centra 2, 1991.

Šundrica, Zdravko. "Kako je nastala i kako je sačuvana bogata arhivska građa Dubrovačkog arhiva" [The founding and the conservation of the exquisite collections of the Archives of Dubrovnik]. *Arhivist* (Belgrade) 29 (1979): 23–36.

– "O darovima u dubrovačkoj diplomaciji" [About gifts in Ragusan diplomacy]. *Naše more* 6 (1959): 53–7.

– *Tajna kutija Dubrovačkog arhiva II.* [The secret box of the Archives of Dubrovnik 2]. Zagreb and Dubrovnik: HAZU, Zavod za povijesne znanosti u Dubrovniku, 2009.

Tadić, Jorjo. "Dubrovački arhiv kao izvor za istoriju zdravstvene službe" [The Archives of Dubrovnik as a source for the history of the Health Office]. In *Spomenica 650-godišnjice ljekarne Male braće u Dubrovniku* [The 650th anniversary of the Franciscan friars' pharmacy in Dubrovnik]. Edited by Hrvoje Tartalja, 111–15. Zagreb: Institut za povijest prirodnih, matematičkih i medicinskih nauka JAZU; Pliva, 1968.

– *Dubrovački portreti* [The Dubrovnik Portraits]. Belgrade: Srpska književna zadruga, kolo 44, knjiga 305, 1948: 349–68.

– "Dubrovnik od postanka do kraja XV stoljeća" [Dubrovnik from the foundation until the fifteenth century]. In *Historija naroda Jugoslavije* [History of the peoples of Yugoslavia]. Edited by Bogo Grafenauer, Dušan Perović, and Jaroslav Šidak. Zagreb: Školska knjiga, 1953: 629–67.

– "Organizacija dubrovačkog pomorstva u XVI veku" [Organization of the Ragusan shipping in the sixteenth century]. *Istorijski časopis* (Belgrade) 1 (1949): 1–53.

– *Pisma i uputstva Dubrovačke Republike* [Letters and instructions of the Ragusan Republic]. Belgrade: SKA, Zbornik za istoriju, jezik i književnost srpskog naroda, III, 4, 1935.

– "Le port de Raguse et sa flotte au XVIe siècle." In *Le navire et l'économie maritime du Moyen Age au XVIIIe siècle principalement en Méditerrannée: Travaux du Deuxième colloque international d'histoire maritime tenu, les 17 et 18 mai, 1957, à l'Académie de marine.* Edited by Michel Mollat, Commandant Denoix, and Olivier de Prat, 9–20. Paris: S.E.V.P.E.N., 1958.

– *Španija i Dubrovnik.* [Spain and Dubrovnik]. Belgrade: SKA, posebna izdanja, knjiga 93, 1932.

Tartalja, Hrvoje. "Dubrovačko ljekarništvo" [Ragusan pharmacy]. In *Veteris Ragusae medicina et pharmacia.* Edited by Lavoslav Glesinger, 23–34. Zagreb: Institut za povijest prirodnih, matematičkih i medicinskih nauka JAZU, Pliva, 1968.

– "Znameniti dubrovački ljekarnici" [Famous Ragusan pharmacists]. In *Spomenica 650-godišnjice ljekarne Male braće u Dubrovniku* [The 650th anniversary of the Franciscan friars' pharmacy in Dubrovnik. Edited by Hrvoje Tartalja, 77–88. Zagreb: Institut za povijest prirodnih, matematičkih i medicinskih nauka JAZU; Pliva, 1968.

Temkin, Owsei. *Galenism: Rise and Decline of Medical Philosophy*. Ithaca, NY: Cornell University Press, 1973.

Theilmann, John Meier, and Frances Cate. "A Plague of Plagues: The Problem of Plague Diagnosis in Medieval England." *Journal of Interdisciplinary History* 37 (2007): 371–93.

Vanzan Marchini, Nelli-Elena. "Venezia e l'invenzione del Lazzaretto." In *Rotte mediterranee e baluardi di sanità: Venezia e i lazzaretti mediterranei*. Edited by Nelli-Elena Vanzan Marchini, 17–47. Milano: Skira, 2004.

Vekarić, Nenad. *Nevidljive pukotine: dubrovački vlasteoski klanovi* [Invisible fissures: the Ragusan patrician clans]. Zagreb and Dubrovnik: Zavod za povijesne znanosti HAZU u Dubrovniku, 2009.

– "The Population of the Dubrovnik Republic in the Fifteenth, Sixteenth and Seventeenth Centuries." *Dubrovnik Annals* 2 (1998): 7–28. A longer version of this article was previously published in Croatian under the title: "Broj stanovnika Dubrovačke Republike u 15., 16. i 17. stoljeću." *Anali Zavoda za povijesne znanosti HAZU u Dubrovniku* 29 (1991): 7–22.

– "The Proportion of the Ragusan Nobility at the Closing of the Major Council in 1332." *Dubrovnik Annals* 16 (2012): 7–22. This article was previously published in Croatian under the title: "Udio plemstva u stanovništvu Dubrovnika u trenutku zatvaranja vijeća 1332. godine." *Rad HAZU* (Zagreb) 510 (2011): 31–46.

– *Vlastela grada Dubrovnika 1: korijeni, struktura i razvoj dubrovačkog plemstva* [The patricians of Dubrovnik. Volume 1: Roots, structure and development of the Ragusan patricians]. Zagreb and Dubrovnik: HAZU, Zavod za povijesne znanosti u Dubrovniku, 2011.

– *Vlastela grada Dubrovnika 2: Vlasteoski rodovi (A–L)* [The patricians of Dubrovnik. Volume 2: Patrician families A–L]. Zagreb and Dubrovnik: HAZU, Zavod za povijesne znanosti u Dubrovniku, 2012.

– *Vlastela grada Dubrovnika 3: Vlasteoski rodovi (M–Z)* [The patricians of Dubrovnik. Volume 3: Patrician families M–Z]. Zagreb and Dubrovnik: HAZU, Zavod za povijesne znanosti u Dubrovniku, 2012.

Vekarić, Stjepan. "Dubrovačka trgovačka flota 1599. godine" [The Ragusan merchant fleet in 1599]. *Anali Historijskog instituta JAZU u Dubrovniku* 3 (1954): 427–32.

– *Naši jedrenjaci* [Croatian sailing ships]. Split: Književni krug, 1977.

– "Vrste i tipovi dubrovačkih brodova XIV stoljeća" [Types of Ragusan ships in the fourteenth century]. *Anali Zavoda za povijesne znanosti u Dubrovniku* 11–12 (1962–1963): 19–42.

Velnić, Vinko. "Ljekarna Male braće u Dubrovniku: Historijat i njene kulturne tekovine" [The Franciscan friars' pharmacy in Dubrovnik: Its history and cultural heritage]. In *Spomenica 650-godišnjice ljekarne Male braće u Dubrovniku* [The 650th anniversary of the Franciscan friars' pharmacy in Dubrovnik]. Edited by Hrvoje Tartalja, 13–26. Zagreb: Institut za povijest prirodnih, matematičkih i medicinskih nauka JAZU; Pliva, 1968.

Viseltear, Arthur Jack. "The Pneumonic Plague Epidemic of 1924 in Los Angeles." *Journal of Biology and Medicine* 47 (1974): 40–1.

Voje, Ignacij. *Poslovna uspešnost trgovcev v srednjeveškem Dubrovniku* [The business success of merchants in mediaeval Dubrovnik]. Ljubljana: Znanstveni inštitut Filozofske fakultete, 2003.

Vojnović, Kosta. *Bratovštine i obrtne korporacije u Republici Dubrovačkoj od XIII do konca XVIII vijeka* [Confraternities and craft guilds in the Ragusan Republic from the thirteenth until the end of the eighteenth century]. Vol. 1. Zagreb: Monumenta historico-juridica Slavorum Meridionalium, JAZU, 1899.

– "Crkva i država u dubrovačkoj republici" [The Church and the state in the Ragusan Republic] Part I: *Rad JAZU* (Zagreb) 119 (1894): 32–142; Part II: *Rad JAZU* (Zagreb) 121 (1895): 1–91.

– "Državni rizničari Dubrovačke Republike" [State treasurers of the Ragusan Republic]. *Rad JA* (Zagreb) 127 (1896): 1–101.

– "O državnom ustrojstvu republike Dubrovačke" [The political system of the Ragusan Republic]. *Rad JAZU* (Zagreb) 103 (1891): 24–67.

Wallis, Faith, ed. *Medieval Medicine: A Reader*. Toronto: Toronto University Press, 2010.

Walløe, Lars. "Medieval and Modern Bubonic Plague: Some Clinical Continuities." In *Pestilential Complexities: Understanding Medieval Plague*. Edited by Vivian Nutton, 59–73. London: Wellcome Trust for the History of Medicine at UCL, 2008.

Wiechmann, Ingrid, and Gisela Grupe. "Detection of Yersinia Pestis DNA in Two Early Medieval Skeletal Finds from Ashheim (Upper Bavaria, 6th century A.D.)." *American Journal of Physical Anthropology* 126 (2005): 48–55.

Worcester, Thomas. "Saint Roch vs. Plague, Famine and Fear." In *Hope and Healing: Painting in Italy in a Time of Plague, 1500–1800*. Edited by Gauvin Alexander Bailey, Pamela M. Jones, Franco Mormando, and Thomas W. Worcester, 153–76. Worcester: Clark University, College of the Holy Cross, Worcester Art Museum; Chicago: University of Chicago Press, 2005.

World Health Organization. *Plague Manual: Epidemiology, Distribution, Surveillance and Control*. Edited by David T. Dennis, Kenneth L. Gage, Norman Gratz, Jack D. Poland, and Evgueni Tikhomirov. Geneva, 1999. http://www.who.int/csr/resources/publications/plague/whocdscsredc99.2a.pdf.

Wray, Shona Kelly. *Communities and Crisis: Bologna during the Black Death*. Leiden: Brill, 2009.

Ziegler, Philip. *The Black Death*. London: Collins, 1969.

Zlatar, Zdenko. *Between the Double Eagle and the Crescent: The Republic of Dubrovnik and the Origins of the Eastern Question*. Boulder, CO: East European Monographs; New York: Columbia University Press, 1992.

– "Huius ... est omnis reipublicae potestas: Dubrovnik's Patrician Houses and Their Participation in Power (1440–1640)." *Dubrovnik Annals* 6 (2002): 45–65. This article was previously published in Croatian under the title: "Huius ... est omnis reipublicae potestas: sudjelovanje vlasteoskih rodova u vlasti (1440–1640)." *Anali Zavoda za povijesne znanosti HAZU u Dubrovniku* 40 (2002): 185–99.

– "Udio vlastele u dubrovačkoj kreditnoj trgovini (1520–1623): Kvantitativna analiza vjerovnika" [Participation of the patriciate in the Ragusan credit trade: Quantitative analysis of the creditors]. *Anali Zavoda za povijesne znanosti HAZU u Dubrovniku* 45 (2007): 131–8.

Zovko, Valentina. "Metode i tehnike komunikacije između vlasti i poslanika u pregovorima oko proširenja dubrovačkih granica" [Communication methods and techniques of the Ragusan government and its envoys in the negotiations for the expansion of Dubrovnik's borders]. *Anali Zavoda za povijesne znanosti HAZU u Dubrovniku* 52 (2014): 21–49.

Žile, Ivica. "Archaeological Findings within the Historic Nucleus of the City of Dubrovnik." Translated by Vesna Baće. *Dubrovnik Annals* 12 (2008): 73–92. This article was previously published in Croatian under the following title: "Arheološki nalazi unutar perimetra povijesne jezgre grada Dubrovnika." *Opuscula Archaeolog-* *ica* (Zagreb) 23–4 (1999–2000): 336–46.

– "Kameni namještaj i arhitektonska plastika prve dubrovačke katedrale" [Stone furniture and architectural plastic art of the first Dubrovnik cathedral]. In *Tisuću godina uspostave dubrovačke (nad)biskupije: zbornik radova znanstvenoga skupa u povodu tisuću godina uspostave dubrovačke (nad)biskupije /metropolije (998–1998).* [One thousand years of the Ragusan (Arch)bishopric]. Edited by Želimir Puljić and Nediljko Ante Ančić, 445–515. Dubrovnik: Biskupski ordinarijat; Split: Crkva u svijetu, 2001.

– ed. *Novije znanstvene spoznaje o genezi grada Dubrovnika* [The latest scientific findings concerning the founding of the city of Dubrovnik]. *Dubrovnik* 4 (1997): 5–275.

Index

Catalan (Catellanus), Jacob the; Catalan (Catellanus), Johannes; Dolce Calderia, Johannes della; health care; Ivan from Trogir; Johannes; Johannes de Ancona; Johannes de Padua; Johannes de Recanato; Mednić, Ivan; Michael from Lecce; Obercho Chilloresa; Papia, Johannes de Aldoardis de; Pavanellus, Hieronymus; pharmacists; physicians; plague doctors; Reginis de Feltro, Johannes Mathias de; Reginus, Petrus; Salama, Joseph; Squadro, Mihajlo; Stilo, Johannes de; Stilo, Thomasius de; Teolo, Johannes de; Thoma
Susorina, Ivan, 149
Syracuse, 163, 247

Šibenik, 15; plague epidemic, 46, 163
Šimša, Mihoč Božov, 189
Šipan, 11; arrivals from, 154; plague in, 52, 143, 147, 177
Škorpion, isolation in, 204–5, 207, 214
Šumet, 30, 198
Šundrica, Zdravko, 58. See also State Archives of Dubrovnik

Tabak, Suliman, 204
Taverns, 29, 89, 213, 244, 312n2. See also Ravančić, Gordan
Teolo, Johannes de, 92. See also surgeons
Termoli, 15
theriac, 88–9, 124, 285n47
Thessaloniki, 56
Thoma (surgeon), 89. See also surgeons
Thomas (physician), 89. See also physicians
Tomado Mihov from Župa, 115
Tomašević, Bartulić, 142; Stjepan, 95
Tomašić, Đivo, 149
Tomić, Petar, 206
Torela, Peroto, 142
Tortus de Piceno, Cesar, 91. See also physicians
trade. See maritime trade; overland trade
Trani, 147, 247
Travnik, 95
Treaty of Višegrad. See Ragusan Republic

Trebinje, 11, 96–7; plague in, 146, 153
Trivulzi, Philippo, 100; as agent of the French king François I, 101; and Mariano Santo, 101
Trogir, 15, 72
Trstenica, 214. See also Pelješac Peninsula
Trstenik, 143. See also Pelješac Peninsula
Trsteno, 153, 207, 210, 214
Tudišić (Theodoysi, Tudisi), Đivo, 251; Nikola Franov, 174, 178. See also patricians
Turčinović, Julije Cvjetkov, 154
Turin, plague in, 228
Turkish Chancery, 244, 274n136. See also relations with the Ottomans; State Archives of Dubrovnik

Uguiccius from Padua, 87. See also physicians
Ulcinj, plague in, 110–11
Usrijenac, Stjepan Nikolin, 34. See also votive tablets, silver

Valencia, 247
Valona (Vlorë), 53, 56, 247
Vanzan Marchini, Nelli-Elena, 61
Vasto (Guasto), 247
Vegetiis, Bartholomeus de, 91. See also physicians
Vekarić, Nenad, 13, 17, 170, 178
Veneziano, Paolo, 50
Venice, 11, 16–18, 39, 87, 108, 134, 247; body clearers, 187; cult of St Roch, 61; founding of the Health Office, 136; lazarettos, 135–6, 181–2, 238; and the Ottomans, 138–9; trade, 172, 180; trade ban, 52
Ventura, Giovanni, 87. See also physicians
Vicko (guard), 214; son of Božo Radovanov, 205
Victoriis from Faenza, Antonius de, 95. See also physicians
Viganj, plague in, 114
Villani, Matteo, 91
Vlachs, 144, 149, 271n114
Vlahotić, Andrija, 207